Functional Connectivity

Editor

JAY J. PILLAI

NEUROIMAGING CLINICS OF NORTH AMERICA

www.neuroimaging.theclinics.com

Consulting Editor
SURESH K. MUKHERJI

November 2017 • Volume 27 • Number 4

ELSEVIER

1600 John F. Kennedy Boulevard • Suite 1800 • Philadelphia, Pennsylvania, 19103-2899

http://www.neuroimaging.theclinics.com

NEUROIMAGING CLINICS OF NORTH AMERICA Volume 27, Number 4
November 2017 ISSN 1052-5149, ISBN 13: 978-0-323-54891-5

Editor: John Vassallo (j.vassallo@elsevier.com)
Developmental Editor: Casey Potter

Neuroimaging Clinics of North America (ISSN 1052-5149) is published quarterly by Elsevier Inc., 360 Park Avenue South, New York, NY 10010-1710. Months of issue are February, May, August, and November. Business and editorial offices: 1600 John F. Kennedy Blvd., Suite 1800, Philadelphia, PA 19103-2899. Business and editorial offices: 6277 Sea Harbor Drive, Orlando, FL 32887-4800. Periodicals postage paid at New York, NY, and additional mailing offices. Subscription prices are USD 365 per year for US individuals, USD 581 per year for US institutions, USD 100 per year for US students and residents, USD 415 per year for Canadian individuals, USD 740 per year for Canadian institutions, USD 525 per year for international individuals, USD 740 per year for international institutions and USD 260 per year for Canadian and foreign students and residents. To receive student/resident rate, orders must be accompanied by name of affiliated institution, date of term, and the *signature* of program/residency coordinator on institution letterhead. Orders will be billed at individual rate until proof of status is received. Foreign air speed delivery is included in all *Clinics* subscription prices. All prices are subject to change without notice. POSTMASTER: Send address changes to *Neuroimaging Clinics of North America*, Elsevier Health Sciences Division, Subscription **Customer Service, 3251 Riverport Lane, Maryland Heights, MO 63043. Telephone: 1-800-654-2452 (U.S. and Canada); 314-447-8871 (outside U.S. and Canada). Fax: 314-447-8029. E-mail: journalscustomer service-usa@elsevier.com (for print support); journalsonlinesupport-usa@elsevier.com (for online support).**

Reprints. For copies of 100 or more of articles in this publication, please contact the Commercial Reprints Department, Elsevier Inc., 360 Park Avenue South, New York, NY 10010-1710. Tel.: 212-633-3874; Fax: 212-633-3820; E-mail: reprints@ elsevier.com.

Neuroimaging Clinics of North America is covered by *Excerpta Medica/EMBASE,* the RSNA Index of Imaging Literature, *MEDLINE/PubMed (Index Medicus),* MEDLINE/MEDLARS, SciSearch, Research Alert, and Neuroscience Citation Index.

PROGRAM OBJECTIVE

The goal of *Neuroimaging Clinics of North America* is to keep practicing radiologists and radiology residents up to date with current clinical practice in radiology by providing timely articles reviewing the state of the art in patient care.

TARGET AUDIENCE

Practicing radiologists, radiology residents, and other healthcare professionals who utilize neuroimaging findings to provide patient care.

LEARNING OBJECTIVES

Upon completion of this activity, participants will be able to:
1. Review methods and indications for resting state fMRI.
2. Discuss applications and limitations to resting state fMRI.
3. Recognize uses of fMRI functional connectivity in traumatic brain injury and neurodegenerative diseases.

ACCREDITATION

The Elsevier Office of Continuing Medical Education (EOCME) is accredited by the Accreditation Council for Continuing Medical Education (ACCME) to provide continuing medical education for physicians.

The EOCME designates this enduring material for a maximum of 15 *AMA PRA Category 1 Credit*(s)™. Physicians should claim only the credit commensurate with the extent of their participation in the activity.

All other healthcare professionals requesting continuing education credit for this enduring material will be issued a certificate of participation.

DISCLOSURE OF CONFLICTS OF INTEREST

The EOCME assesses conflict of interest with its instructors, faculty, planners, and other individuals who are in a position to control the content of CME activities. All relevant conflicts of interest that are identified are thoroughly vetted by EOCME for fair balance, scientific objectivity, and patient care recommendations. EOCME is committed to providing its learners with CME activities that promote improvements or quality in healthcare and not a specific proprietary business or a commercial interest.

The planning committee, staff, authors and editors listed below have identified no financial relationships or relationships to products or devices they or their spouse/life partner have with commercial interest related to the content of this CME activity:

Shrutti Agarwal, PhD; Samantha Audrain, MA; Azeezat K. Azeez, BS; Alexander Barnett, MA; John M. Billings, MD; Vince D. Calhoun, PhD; Catie Chang, PhD; Jingyuan E. Chen, PhD; Elizabeth M. Davenport, PhD; Nina de Lacy, MD, MBA; Devandra Singh Dhami, MS; Donna Dierker, MS; Maxwell Eder, BS; William C. Flood, BA; Anjali Fortna; Carl D. Hacker, MD, PhD; Mudassar Kamran, MD; Kwun Kei, NG, PhD; Siwei Liu, MD, FAHA; Leah Logan; Joseph A. Maldjian, MD; Mary Pat McAndrews, PhD; John D. Medaglia, PhD; Mikhail Milchenko, PhD; Michelle M. Miller-Thomas, MD; Albert Montillo, PhD; Suresh K. Mukherji, MD, MBA, FACR; Gowtham Murugesan, MS; Sriraam Natarajan, PhD; Thomas J. O'Neill, MD; Goffrey David Pearlson, MD; Jay J. Pillai, MD; Jarod L. Roland, MD; Mikhail Rubinov, PhD; Haris I. Sair, MD; Joshua S. Shimony, MD, PhD; Abraham Z. Snyder, MD, PhD; Karthik Subramaniam; John Vassallo; Juan Wang, PhD; Christopher T. Whitlow, MD, PhD, MHA; Juan Zhou, MD, PhD.

The planning committee, staff, authors and editors listed below have identified financial relationships or relationships to products or devices they or their spouse/life partner have with commercial interest related to the content of this CME activity:

Tammie L. Benzinger, MD, PhD has research support from Avid Radiopharmaceuticals, a wholly owned subsidiary of Ely Lilly and Company.

Bharat B. Biswal, PhD has research support from Avid Radiopharmaceuticals, a wholly owned subsidiary of Ely Lilly and Company.

Eric C. Leuthardt, MD is a consultant/advisor for Monteris Medical, Inc and Alcyone Lifesciences, Inc., and has stock ownership in Neurolutions, Inc.; OsteoVantage, Inc; Inner Cosmos; and Immunovalent Therapeutics Inc.

Daniel S. Marcus, PhD has research support from Avid Radiopharmaceuticals, a wholly owned subsidiary of Ely Lilly and Company.

Jerrel Rutlin, BA has research support from Avid Radiopharmaceuticals, a wholly owned subsidiary of Ely Lilly and Company.

UNAPPROVED/OFF-LABEL USE DISCLOSURE

The EOCME requires CME faculty to disclose to the participants:
1. When products or procedures being discussed are off-label, unlabelled, experimental, and/or investigational (not US Food and Drug Administration [FDA] approved); and
2. Any limitations on the information presented, such as data that are preliminary or that represent ongoing research, interim analyses, and/or unsupported opinions. Faculty may discuss information about pharmaceutical agents that is outside of FDA-approved labelling. This information is intended solely for CME and is not intended to promote off-label use of these

medications. If you have any questions, contact the medical affairs department of the manufacturer for the most recent pre-scribing information.

TO ENROLL
To enroll in the *Neuroimaging Clinics of North America* Continuing Medical Education program, call customer service at 1-800-654-2452 or sign up online at http://www.theclinics.com/home/cme. The CME program is available to subscribers for an additional annual fee of USD 235.

METHOD OF PARTICIPATION
In order to claim credit, participants must complete the following:
1. Complete enrolment as indicated above.
2. Read the activity.
3. Complete the CME Test and Evaluation. Participants must achieve a score of 70% on the test. All CME Tests and Evaluations must be completed online.

CME INQUIRIES/SPECIAL NEEDS
For all CME inquiries or special needs, please contact elsevierCME@elsevier.com.

NEUROIMAGING CLINICS OF NORTH AMERICA

Contributors

CONSULTING EDITOR

SURESH K. MUKHERJI, MD, MBA, FACR
Professor and Chairman, Walter F. Patenge
Endowed Chair, Department of Radiology,
Michigan State University, Chief Medical
Officer and Director of Health Care Delivery,
Michigan State University Health Team,
Department of Radiology, Michigan State
University, East Lansing, Michigan, USA

EDITOR

JAY J. PILLAI, MD
Director of Functional MRI, Associate
Professor of Radiology and Neurosurgery,
Division of Neuroradiology, The Russell H.
Morgan Department of Radiology and
Radiological Science, The Johns Hopkins
University School of Medicine, The Johns
Hopkins Hospital, Baltimore, Maryland, USA

AUTHORS

SHRUTI AGARWAL, PhD
Division of Neuroradiology, The
Russell H. Morgan Department of Radiology
and Radiological Science, The Johns Hopkins
University School of Medicine, Baltimore,
Maryland, USA

SAMANTHA AUDRAIN, MA
Krembil Research Institute, University Health
Network, Department of Psychology, University
of Toronto, Toronto, Ontario, Canada

AZEEZAT K. AZEEZ, BS
Department of Biomedical Engineering,
New Jersey Institute of Technology, Newark,
New Jersey, USA

ALEXANDER BARNETT, MA
Krembil Research Institute, University Health
Network, Department of Psychology,
University of Toronto, Toronto, Ontario,
Canada

TAMMIE L. BENZINGER, MD, PhD
Mallinckrodt Institute of Radiology,
Department of Neurological Surgery,
Washington University School of Medicine
in St. Louis, St Louis, Missouri, USA

JOHN M. BILLINGS, MD
Radiology Informatics and Image Processing
Laboratory (RIIPL), Division of Neuroradiology,
Department of Radiology, Wake Forest School
of Medicine, Winston-Salem, North Carolina,
USA

BHARAT B. BISWAL, PhD
Department of Biomedical Engineering,
New Jersey Institute of Technology, Newark,
New Jersey, USA

VINCE D. CALHOUN, PhD
The Mind Research Network, Department of
ECE, The University of New Mexico,
Albuquerque, New Mexico, USA

CATIE CHANG, PhD
Advanced Magnetic Resonance Imaging Section, Laboratory of Functional and Molecular Imaging, National Institute of Neurological Disorders and Stroke, National Institutes of Health, Bethesda, Maryland, USA

JINGYUAN E. CHEN, PhD
Departments of Radiology and Electrical Engineering, Stanford University, Stanford, California, USA

ELIZABETH M. DAVENPORT, PhD
Postdoctoral Researcher, Radiology, The University of Texas Southwestern Medical Center, Dallas, Texas, USA

NINA DE LACY, MD, MBA
Department of Psychiatry and Behavioral Science, University of Washington, Seattle, Washington, USA

DEVENDRA SINGH DHAMI, MS
School of Informatics and Computing, Indiana University, Bloomington, Indiana, USA

DONNA DIERKER, MS
Mallinckrodt Institute of Radiology, Washington University School of Medicine in St. Louis, St Louis, Missouri, USA

MAXWELL EDER, BS
Radiology Informatics and Image Processing Laboratory (RIIPL), Division of Neuroradiology, Department of Radiology, Wake Forest School of Medicine, Winston-Salem, North Carolina, USA

WILLIAM C. FLOOD, BA
Radiology Informatics and Image Processing Laboratory (RIIPL), Division of Neuroradiology, Department of Radiology, Wake Forest School of Medicine, Winston-Salem, North Carolina, USA

CARL D. HACKER, MD, PhD
Department of Neurological Surgery, Washington University School of Medicine in St. Louis, St Louis, Missouri, USA

MUDASSAR KAMRAN, MD
Mallinckrodt Institute of Radiology, Washington University School of Medicine in St. Louis, St Louis, Missouri, USA

ERIC C. LEUTHARDT, MD
Departments of Neurological Surgery and Biomedical Imaging, Washington University School of Medicine in St. Louis, St Louis, Missouri, USA

SIWEI LIU, PhD
Center for Cognitive Neuroscience, Neuroscience and Behavioral Disorders Programme, Duke-NUS Medical School, Singapore, Singapore

JOSEPH A. MALDJIAN, MD
Professor and Chief of Neuroradiology, Radiology, The University of Texas Southwestern Medical Center, Dallas, Texas, USA

DANIEL S. MARCUS, PhD
Mallinckrodt Institute of Radiology, Washington University School of Medicine in St. Louis, St Louis, Missouri, USA

MARY PAT McANDREWS, PhD
Krembil Research Institute, University Health Network, Department of Psychology, University of Toronto, Toronto, Ontario, Canada

JOHN D. MEDAGLIA, PhD
Research Assistant Professor, Department of Psychology, University of Pennsylvania, Philadelphia, Pennsylvania, USA

MIKHAIL MILCHENKO, PhD
Mallinckrodt Institute of Radiology, Washington University School of Medicine in St. Louis, St Louis, Missouri, USA

MICHELLE M. MILLER-THOMAS, MD
Mallinckrodt Institute of Radiology, Washington University School of Medicine in St. Louis, St Louis, Missouri, USA

ALBERT MONTILLO, PhD
Assistant Professor, Radiology, The University of Texas Southwestern Medical Center, Dallas, Texas, USA

GOWTHAM MURUGESAN, MS
Graduate Student, Radiology, The University of Texas Southwestern Medical Center, Dallas, Texas, USA

SRIRAAM NATARAJAN, PhD
School of Informatics and Computing, Indiana University, Bloomington, Indiana, USA

KWUN KEI NG, PhD
Center for Cognitive Neuroscience, Neuroscience and Behavioral Disorders Programme, Duke-NUS Medical School, Singapore, Singapore

THOMAS J. O'NEILL, MD
Assistant Professor, Radiology, The University of Texas Southwestern Medical Center, Dallas, Texas, USA

GODFREY DAVID PEARLSON, MD
Professor, Departments of Psychiatry and Neuroscience, Yale School of Medicine, New Haven, Connecticut; Director, Olin Neuropsychiatry Research Center, Institute of Living, Hartford, Connecticut, USA

JAY J. PILLAI, MD
Director of Functional MRI, Associate Professor of Radiology and Neurosurgery, Division of Neuroradiology, The Russell H. Morgan Department of Radiology and Radiological Science, The Johns Hopkins University School of Medicine, The Johns Hopkins Hospital, Baltimore, Maryland, USA

JAROD L. ROLAND, MD
Department of Neurological Surgery, Washington University School of Medicine in St. Louis, St Louis, Missouri, USA

MIKAIL RUBINOV, PhD
Janelia Research Campus, Howard Hughes Medical Institute, Ashburn, Virginia, USA

JERREL RUTLIN, BA
Mallinckrodt Institute of Radiology, Washington University School of Medicine in St. Louis, St Louis, Missouri, USA

HARIS I. SAIR, MD
Division of Neuroradiology, The Russell H. Morgan Department of Radiology and Radiological Science, The Johns Hopkins University School of Medicine, Baltimore, Maryland, USA

JOSHUA S. SHIMONY, MD, PhD
Mallinckrodt Institute of Radiology, Washington University School of Medicine in St. Louis, St Louis, Missouri, USA

ABRAHAM Z. SNYDER, MD, PhD
Mallinckrodt Institute of Radiology, Department of Neurology, Washington University School of Medicine in St. Louis, St Louis, Missouri, USA

JUAN WANG, PhD
Center for Cognitive Neuroscience, Neuroscience and Behavioral Disorders Programme, Duke-NUS Medical School, Singapore, Singapore

CHRISTOPHER T. WHITLOW, MD, PhD, MHA
Vice Chair of Informatics and Chief of Neuroradiology, Director, Radiology Informatics and Image Processing Laboratory, Director, CTSI Translational Imaging Program, Director, Combined MD/PhD Program, Division of Neuroradiology, Department of Radiology, Department of Biomedical Engineering, Clinical and Translational Sciences Institute, Wake Forest School of Medicine, Winston-Salem, North Carolina, USA

JUAN ZHOU, PhD
Center for Cognitive Neuroscience, Neuroscience and Behavioral Disorders Programme, Duke-NUS Medical School, Singapore, Singapore; Clinical Imaging Research Centre, Agency for Science, Technology and Research, Singapore

Contents

SECTION 1: Methods of Resting State Functional Connectivity (fMRI) Analysis

Functional MR imaging (fMR imaging) studies have recently begun to examine spontaneous changes in interregional interactions (functional connectivity) over seconds to
minutes, and their relation to natural shifts in cognitive and physiologic states. This
practice opens the potential for uncovering structured, transient configurations of
coordinated brain activity whose features may provide novel cognitive and clinical biomarkers. However, analysis of these time-varying phenomena requires careful differentiation between neural and nonneural contributions to the fMR imaging signal and
thorough validation and statistical testing. In this article, the authors present an overview of methodological and interpretational considerations in this emerging field.

For more than 20 years, the powerful, flexible family of independent component analysis (ICA) techniques has been used to examine spatial, temporal, and subject variation
in functional magnetic resonance (fMR) imaging data. This article provides an overview
of 10 key principles in the basic and advanced application of ICA to resting-state fMR
imaging. ICA's core advantages include robustness to artifact; false-positives and
autocorrelation; adaptability to variant study designs; agnosticism to the temporal evolution of fMR imaging signals; and ability to extract, identify, and analyze neural networks. ICA remains in the vanguard of fMR imaging methods development.

Resting-state functional connectivity is the synchronization of brain regions with
each another. Alterations are suggestive of neurologic or psychological disorders.
This article discusses methods and approaches used to describe resting-state brain
connectivity and the results in neurotypical and diseased brains.

Graph theoretic analyses applied to examine the brain at rest have played a critical
role in clarifying the foundations of the brain's intrinsic and task-related activity.

There are many opportunities for clinical scientists to describe and predict dysfunction using a network perspective. This primer describes the theoretic basis and practical application of graph theoretic analysis to resting state functional MR imaging data. Major practices, concepts, and findings are concisely reviewed. The theoretic and practical frontiers of resting state functional MR imaging are highlighted with observations about major avenues for conceptual advances and clinical translation.

Machine learning is one of the most exciting and rapidly expanding fields within computer science. Academic and commercial research entities are investing in machine learning methods, especially in personalized medicine via patient-level classification. There is great promise that machine learning methods combined with resting state functional MR imaging will aid in diagnosis of disease and guide potential treatment for conditions thought to be impossible to identify based on imaging alone, such as psychiatric disorders. We discuss machine learning methods and explore recent advances.

SECTION 2: Clinical Applications of Resting State Functional Connectivity

This article compares resting-state functional magnetic resonance (fMR) imaging with task fMR imaging for presurgical functional mapping of the sensorimotor (SM) region. Before tumor resection, 38 patients were scanned using both methods. The SM area was anatomically defined using 2 different software tools. Overlap of anatomic regions of interest with task activation maps and resting-state networks was measured in the SM region. A paired t-test showed higher overlap between resting-state maps and anatomic references compared with task activation when using a maximal overlap criterion. Resting state–derived maps are more comprehensive than those derived from task fMR imaging.

Resting state functional MR imaging (rs-fMR imaging) has become an indispensable tool for examining brain function. The greatest opportunity to translate rs-fMR imaging from the research domain into clinical use is as a tool for examining intrinsic brain networks for preoperative planning. Many studies have demonstrated concordance of intrinsic motor networks from rs-fMR imaging data with task-fMR imaging and direct cortical stimulation. Earlier reports show concordance of language networks as well, although more recent studies with larger numbers of subjects demonstrate subject-level variability that needs to be further investigated and addressed before widespread implementation of rs-fMR imaging for preoperative planning.

Methods of image acquisition and analysis for resting-state functional MR imaging (rsfMR imaging) are still evolving. Neurovascular uncoupling and susceptibility artifact are important confounds of rsfMR imaging in the setting of focal brain lesions such as brain tumors. This article reviews the detection of these confounds using rsfMR imaging metrics in the setting of focal brain lesions. In the near future, with the wide range of ongoing research in rsfMR imaging, these issues likely will be overcome and will open new windows into brain function and connectivity.

Neurodegenerative diseases target specific large-scale neuronal networks, leading to distinct behavioral and cognitive dysfunctions. Resting-state functional magnetic resonance imaging (rsfMR imaging)–based functional connectivity method maps symptoms-associated functional network deterioration in vivo. This article summarizes accumulating functional connectivity findings supporting the network-based neurodegeneration hypothesis. Understanding of disease mechanism can further guide early detection and predictions of disease progression and inform development of more effective treatment. With better clinical phenotyping and larger samples across multiple sites, we discuss several possible future directions to further develop rsfMR imaging–based functional connectivity methods into scientifically and clinically useful assays for neurodegenerative disorders.

Traumatic brain injury (TBI) is an important public health issue. TBI includes a broad spectrum of injury severities and abnormalities. Functional MR imaging (fMR imaging), both resting state (rs) and task, has been used often in research to study the effects of TBI. Although rs-fMR imaging is not currently applicable in clinical diagnosis of TBI, computer-aided tools are making this a possibility for the future. Specifically, graph theory is being used to study the change in networks after TBI. Machine learning methods allow researchers to build models capable of predicting injury severity and recovery trajectories.

We discuss the value of resting-state functional MR imaging (rsfMR imaging) as an emerging technique to address questions about memory and language that are central in surgery for temporal-lobe epilepsy, namely the identification and characterization of eloquent cortex to avoid surgical morbidity. The emergence of a robust set of data using rsfMR imaging has opened new avenues for exploring more direct relationships between neural networks and current cognitive function and prediction of postoperative change. These techniques are also being explored for their potential to characterize epilepsy subtypes, identify epileptic foci, and monitor treatment effects.

Godfrey David Pearlson

Resting state studies in neuropsychiatric disorders have already provided much useful information, but the field is regarded as being at a relatively preliminary stage and subject to several design issues that set limits on the overall utility.

Foreword
Functional Connectivity

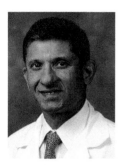

Suresh K. Mukherji, MD, MBA, FACR
Consulting Editor

The "Holy Grail" of brain imaging has been to visualize how we "think" and identify the causation of injuries or diseases that impair cognition. Functional connectivity has the promise of helping us achieve this goal. This issue of *Neuroimaging Clinics* addresses functional connectivity with a focus on resting state fMRI (rs-fMRI). There are articles that review methodology and various analytic tools. However, the majority of the issues focus on specific clinical applications that include sensorimotor and language mapping, neurodegenerative diseases, traumatic brain injury, epilepsy, and neuropsychiatric disease.

I want to thank Dr Jay Pillai for masterfully combining a state-of-the-art review of the rs-fMRI methodology with pragmatic clinical applications. I thank the article authors for their wonderful contributions with breathtaking illustrations! This issue is truly a multidisciplinary text and will benefit cognitive neuroscientists, neurologists, psychiatrists, neuroradiologists, and neurosurgeons in our quest to understand how we "think."

Suresh K. Mukherji, MD, MBA, FACR
Department of Radiology
Michigan State University
Michigan State University Health Team
Department of Radiology
Michigan State University
846 Service Road
East Lansing, MI 48824, USA

E-mail address:
mukherji@rad.msu.edu

Neuroimag Clin N Am 27 (2017) xv
http://dx.doi.org/10.1016/j.nic.2017.08.002
1052-5149/17/© 2017 Published by Elsevier Inc.

Preface
Functional Connectivity

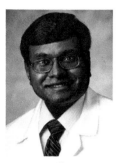

Jay J. Pillai, MD
Editor

This issue of *Neuroimaging Clinics* addresses the current state-of-the-art in human brain functional connectivity as assessed through resting-state blood oxygen level–dependent fMRI. Although other functional imaging modalities such as magnetoencephalography and task-based fMRI have been included at least in brief description, as in the case of applications to traumatic brain injury for the former, most of this issue concentrates on resting state fMRI (rs-fMRI). The issue is divided into an initial section that includes articles that focus on methodological aspects, since at this point there is little consensus in the functional imaging community as to which approaches are best for analysis of such data.

This first section includes discussion of data-driven methods such as independent component analysis, frequency domain analysis (eg, ALFF), and graph theoretic analysis. Specific inclusion of cutting-edge topics in rs-fMRI such as dynamic functional connectivity and machine learning applications (including specific applications of the latter to neuropsychiatric disease) to rs-fMRI analysis is a key feature of this section. The second section attempts to provide a broad overview of clinical applications of rs-fMRI that are prominent at the time of publication, although such applications will continue to increase exponentially in the very near future as the power harnessed via big data and deep learning initiatives continue to be realized in the era of human connectomics. Such applications include applications to sensori-motor mapping, language mapping, neurodegenerative diseases, traumatic brain injury, epilepsy, and neuropsychiatric disease, with an additional article describing potential limitations of this method in some settings such as brain tumors.

Many high-quality color illustrations are included throughout this issue to highlight important details, and an extensive list of references is included for each article in this issue, as well as a listing of key "take-home" points and a synopsis for each article. We hope that this compilation of salient articles will serve to both introduce cognitive neuroscientists, neurologists, psychiatrists, neuroradiologists, and neurosurgeons to this very rapidly evolving field that is sure to greatly enhance our understanding of brain function, as well as bring veterans in this field up-to-date via insights provided by current experts in the field. As we enter the era of big data, radiogenomics, and personalized medicine, the hope is that such new powerful methods and applications may eventually provide us with new functional "fingerprints" of normal and diseased brain to advance neuroscience and promote future physiologic imaging-based therapies based on functional as well as genotypic stratification of clinical populations and development of novel therapeutic biomarkers.

Jay J. Pillai, MD
Division of Neuroradiology
The Russell H. Morgan Department of
Radiology and Radiological Science
Johns Hopkins University School of Medicine
Johns Hopkins Hospital, 1800 Orleans Street
Baltimore, MD 21287, USA

E-mail address:
jpillai1@jhmi.edu

Neuroimag Clin N Am 27 (2017) xvii
http://dx.doi.org/10.1016/j.nic.2017.08.001
1052-5149/17/© 2017 Published by Elsevier Inc.

neuroimaging.theclinics.com

SECTION 1: Methods of Resting State Functional Connectivity (fMRI) Analysis

Methods and Considerations for Dynamic Analysis of Functional MR Imaging Data

Jingyuan E. Chen, PhD[a,b], Mikail Rubinov, PhD[c],
Catie Chang, PhD[d],*

KEYWORDS

- Functional magnetic resonance imaging ● Resting state ● Dynamics ● Networks
- Functional connectivity

KEY POINTS

- Features of spontaneous brain activity and interregional coupling (functional connectivity) have been observed to change over seconds to minutes, spontaneously and in conjunction with variation in physiologic, cognitive, and vigilance states.
- The analysis of such "dynamic" phenomena requires careful differentiation between neural and nonneural contributions to the functional MR imaging signal as well as thorough validation and statistical testing.
- Dynamic features of functional connectivity represent potentially promising biomarkers, although the specific clinical and cognitive relevance of these features remains to be established.

INTRODUCTION

Brain function emerges from the collective interactions of distributed brain regions. A central effort in the analysis of functional imaging data has been to elucidate the spatial topologies of interacting regions (referred to as functional "networks") and the strength of interactions between pairs or sets of regions (referred to as "functional connectivity", FC). In practice, FC is inferred from functional MR imaging (fMR imaging) data by quantifying statistical associations between blood-oxygen level–dependent (BOLD) signal fluctuations extracted from 2 or more brain regions. This analysis is typically conducted on data from fMR imaging scans acquired in the absence of any task or stimuli (referred to as the "resting-state" condition[1]). The resulting fMR imaging signals are attributed largely to the spontaneous, or intrinsic, activity of the brain.[2]

Most studies use the entire set of time points across a given fMR imaging scan to infer FC and thereby emphasize patterns or functional interactions that are, on average, the strongest and most stable across a range of timescales. Such an approach (often described as "static" FC) has revealed core features of spatiotemporal organization in spontaneous brain activity that exhibit remarkable stability.[3,4] For example, one can readily

Funded by: NIH; Grant number(s): P41EB15891 (NIHMS-ID: 887963).

Disclosure Statement: The authors have nothing to disclose.

[a] Department of Radiology, Stanford University, 1201 Welch Road, Stanford, CA 94305, USA; [b] Department of Electrical Engineering, Stanford University, 1201 Welch Road, Stanford, CA 94305, USA; [c] Janelia Research Campus, Howard Hughes Medical Institute, 19700 Helix Drive, Ashburn, VA 20147, USA; [d] Advanced Magnetic Resonance Imaging Section, Laboratory of Functional and Molecular Imaging, National Institute of Neurological Disorders and Stroke, National Institutes of Health, 10 Center Drive, Bethesda, MD 20892, USA

* Corresponding author.

E-mail address: catie.chang@nih.gov

Neuroimag Clin N Am 27 (2017) 547–560

http://dx.doi.org/10.1016/j.nic.2017.06.009

1052-5149/17/Published by Elsevier Inc.

identify constellations of coactivating areas that are largely conserved across individuals and different scan sessions,[5,6] and that align closely with known anatomic and functional pathways.[7–9] Nevertheless, atop this stability, the precise strength and patterns of FC within and between networks are reported to vary across different cognitive states,[10,11] conscious states,[12] and brain disorders[13,14]; as such, *variability* in FC is being heavily studied for its potential as a biomarker in health and disease.

Given the continual fluctuations in our subjective experiences and brain/body physiology during an fMR imaging scan, one might suppose that FC may also exhibit variation within the duration of a typical scan (5–15 minutes). This notion has led to the hypothesis that spontaneous variation in FC on shorter timescales (seconds to minutes) conveys information beyond that of longer, time-averaged measures. Exploring this temporal dimension of FC prompts numerous questions: could studying FC on shorter timescales uncover structured, transient configurations whose diversity and transition patterns represent novel biomarkers? Can we study dimensions of FC linked with slowly fluctuating cognitive, emotional, or autonomic function, such as mood and anxiety, arousal, and mind-wandering? Following investigations in 2010,[15,16] the area of 'dynamic' functional connectivity (DFC) for fMR imaging data has rapidly expanded to study questions such as these.[17,18]

However, there are notable difficulties in studying "dynamic" phenomena in fMR imaging data. First, it is far easier to observe variability than stability in data, especially as fMR imaging data are contaminated by noise and artifacts that are difficult to disentangle from fluctuations of neural origin. Second, various strategies for assessing DFC may induce misleading observations of variability, such as by failing to unmix overlapping signal sources or through interactions between time-windowed analysis and frequencies in the underlying signals (as discussed in Refs.[19,20] for example). Third, in parallel with static FC, increases in correlation or coherence observed across multiple regions may not arise from direct interactions between regions but rather from the common influence of a third neural source (eg, ascending arousal system) or a nonneural source (eg, head motion or breathing), as is further described in later discussion (in the section *Considerations*). Careful analysis, validation, statistical testing, and noise-reduction procedures are essential for obtaining an interpretable picture of FC dynamics,[15,19,21,22] as can concurrent monitoring of physiologic, behavioral, and neural electrical activity (such as with electroencephalogram, EEG, or, when feasible, invasive electrophysiology).[23–25]

Another notable challenge in DFC research arises from the large set of possible dynamic analyses and features (eg, Refs.[26,27]). There is no single, preferable way to interrogate DFC; ideally, whenever possible, the analysis should be guided by neuroscientific hypotheses. Furthermore, to arrive at the most faithful characterization of the data, one must take care that the DFC quantities computed are those which are most revealing of the underlying structure in the data. Functional connectivity represents projections and (typically) reductions of the original time series and may obscure the nature of the individual signals. Visualizing the time series to understand how changes in FC are shaped by the underlying temporal fluctuations is important, although the large amount of spatiotemporal data can render this effort challenging.[28] Investigation of DFC is largely exploratory, and establishing the most informative ways of characterizing dynamic properties of fMR imaging data is an active research area.

There are several existing comprehensive review articles on DFC (eg, Refs.[17,18,24,26]). Here, the authors briefly overview the range of existing methods of DFC analyses and follow with a focus on considerations involved in the analysis and in the associated interpretation.

METHODS FOR DYNAMIC FUNCTIONAL CONNECTIVITY ANALYSIS

Several classes of approaches have been proposed for examining time-varying patterns in fMR imaging data. Currently, timescales of existing DFC methodology range from a single fMR imaging timeframe (typically 1-3 seconds) to several minutes (**Fig. 1**). The temporal resolution at which to examine brain dynamics for a given neuroscience or clinical question is a consideration that depends on tradeoffs between robustness and sensitivity as well as the fact that different neural processes of interest may evolve on different timescales. Robustness entails the inclusion of sufficient numbers of time points to provide adequate statistical power and immunity to spurious fluctuations induced by the use of certain analysis methods (see later discussion), whereas sensitivity implies the capability of capturing instantaneous changes in network behavior.

Sliding Window Analysis (Temporal Resolution of Seconds to Minutes)

The simplest and most common DFC approach is the sliding window analysis (SWA), realized by dividing the entire time course into a sequence of sliding windows and estimating FC within each window. A summary of window parameters used for this approach in previous literature is presented

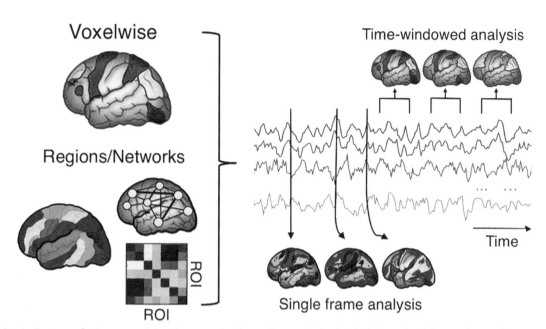

A **Spatial (node) definition**   **B**   **Time scales of analysis**

Voxelwise

Regions/Networks

ROI

ROI

Time-windowed analysis

Time

Single frame analysis

Fig. 1. Cartoon of primary spatial and temporal units serving as the basis of FC dynamics. (A) Spatial granularity at which FC dynamics are analyzed is typically voxelwise (often across the whole brain), or at the level of larger contiguous ROIs or distributed regions (networks). (B) Timescales for querying changes in the association between brain regions. Before DFC analysis, regional time series are often subdivided into overlapping or nonoverlapping windows (commonly ranging from tens of seconds to minutes). Alternatively, the multivariate BOLD signal patterns expressed at individual fMR imaging frames (commonly 1-3 seconds apart) may be considered. Other divisions at the spatial and temporal level are possible; those shown here reflect divisions that are commonly used in existing literature.

in Fig. S1 of Preti and colleagues.[26] Under such a framework, a range of FC metrics used in analyses of static connectivity (eg, correlations between regions of interest or functional networks,[15,16,29–32] regional homogeneity,[33,34] and independent component analysis, ICA[35]), as well as newly proposed metrics for dynamic analysis,[36,37] can be examined. This practice complements analyses of static connectivity in distinguishing between populations of individuals with neuropsychiatric disorders versus healthy controls.[16,38,39]

Despite its apparent simplicity, it is important to mention several technical concerns associated with SWA. One primary concern is associated with the choice of window length. Theoretically, a window should include sufficient samples to generate reliable statistical associations between time series and cover at least a full cycle of the slowest fluctuations in the signal to avoid spurious variability introduced by methodology.[19,22] However, too long a window may fail to capture sharp transitions between brain states.

An approach to circumvent such tradeoffs between robustness and sensitivity is to adaptively

adjust the window lengths to match the intrinsic timing of the underlying brain dynamics (see later discussions, *Time-frequency analysis* and *Detecting functional connectivity change points*). Apart from window lengths, other parameters such as window shapes and offsets (intervals between adjacent window onsets) may also substantially affect the results of SWA.[26,40] Notably, although there have been emerging efforts in refining SWA from a methodological perspective, they are developed with a strong emphasis on linear correlation. Thus, how the empirical or theoretic rules extend to broader FC metrics remains unclear and constitutes an open future direction. Currently, analytical approaches or nonparametric simulations are strongly recommended to establish valid null distributions for time-varying changes on a study or metric basis (see later discussion, *Statistical Testing*).

Time-Frequency Analysis (Multiscale Temporal Resolution)

Although the frequency characteristics of fMR imaging signals are thought to be inherently band limited (primarily to <0.1 Hz) because of hemodynamic smoothing, several studies have revealed heterogeneous spectral characteristics within and between various networks of resting-state functional connectivity,[41–43] the abnormality of which may inform certain pathologic conditions.[44,45] Hence, it may be important to query dynamic aspects of brain connectivity along the frequency dimension through, for instance, a joint time-frequency analysis.[15] Typically, the coherence value and phase difference between 2 time series serve as the frequency-domain counterparts to the correlation strength and temporal lag. Furthermore, in lieu of a fixed window length governed by the slowest oscillation of the time series, the temporal resolution for dynamic analysis can be adapted to each frequency scale with methods such as the wavelet transform.[15] However, one important consideration is that the signal-to-noise ratio of the fMR imaging time series is generally smaller at higher frequencies.

Point Process Analysis (Toward the Resolution of a Single fMR Imaging Timeframe)

A brief stimulus, either internally driven or task driven, may elicit BOLD responses in particular areas; conversely, the likelihood of neural activity in a region may be inferred based on its raw signal intensity. In particular, brief points at which a voxel's signal amplitude significantly deviates from baseline may correspond to "active" instances and therefore carry critical information.[46–49] Such concepts have motivated approaches to DFC that are based on point-process analysis (PPA).

Recently, Liu and Duyn[50] extended PPA by suggesting that by temporally averaging only those high-intensity events, multiple recurring but distinct spatial patterns can be obtained, which they named "coactivation patterns" (CAPs).[50] In that study, CAPs were derived by decomposing selected frames into multiple clusters based on their spatial similarity, in which each cluster characterizes distinct, multivariate patterns of activity across the brain. CAP analyses, together with subsequently developed variations and whole-brain versions,[51,52] open a novel view onto the repertoire of brain dynamics and offer diverse metrics for their quantification, for example, spatial patterns and occurrence rates of various CAPs,[27,52] and probabilities of transitioning between different CAPs.

Compared with SWA, CAP analysis promises the examination of state alternations at each individual timeframe while relying on very few model assumptions. Despite its potential to reveal elaborate details of dynamic FC, several limitations remain largely unexplored. First, the spatial patterns rendered in seed-based CAPs depend on prespecified parameters, such as the threshold that defines critical time points as well as the number of clusters (cluster number).[27,50,52,53] A second limitation relates to the low signal-to-noise ratio inherent in this single-frame–based analysis, which compromises the accuracy of allocating each time point to a specific CAP. This issue is of greater concern when attempting to learn the temporal ordering and alternation rates between different CAPs (compare, simply characterizing their spatial patterns), because of the necessity for strict temporal precision. A third limitation of CAP analysis lies in its vulnerability to temporal smoothing by intrinsic hemodynamics or by preprocessing methods, both of which may lead to prolonged above-threshold or subthreshold signals that confound true neural activities. Such concerns can be ameliorated by invoking hemodynamic response function (HRF) deconvolution before ensuing analyses.[46,47,51,54] However, existing deconvolution methods are intrinsically sensitive to noise and often assume a spatially homogeneous HRF model. Finally, although interpretations of CAPs have been commonly directed to large-scale neuronal avalanching activity,[46,50] the neurobiological underpinnings of CAPs remain poorly understood. As a relatively new approach that is gaining popularity, model validations and statistical tests of CAPs have been less thoroughly investigated than for time-windowed analyses.

Temporal Graph Analysis

Graph analysis on DFC matrices may be broadly subdivided into 2 types. The first type resembles analysis performed on groups of static FC matrices; in principle, the investigators may apply all the standard graph theory tools, including the detection of hubs,[55] the decomposition of the network into modules,[56] and the computation of global properties such as clustering and efficiency.[57] Nevertheless, despite the similarities with static graph analysis, coupling between adjacent graphs is introduced implicitly in the course of graph construction, for instance, by the use of overlapping sliding windows. The second type of analysis incorporates the temporal sequence of networks directly into the computed measures. A notable example of this approach is community detection with explicit "coupling" of temporally adjacent networks.[10,58] An advantage of this approach is the direct detection of the spatiotemporal community structure, that is, the simultaneous detection of the spatial and temporal features of each community. A disadvantage of the approach is the fairly ad hoc nature of the coupling (the addition of artificial edges between timeframes), in contrast to the more explicit assumptions underlying temporal smoothing. Robinson and colleagues[59] recently described an additional approach that does not explicitly smooth adjacent temporal windows but rather identifies temporally contiguous communities by fitting stochastic block models to distinct temporal states.

Some confusion may arise with the application and description of graph analysis measures. Many measures seeking to describe graphs acquire connotations that are not necessarily supported by the data in question. For instance, the concept of graph *efficiency* is not well defined on networks of FC. In structural graph analysis, efficiency is based on the path length with which information is putatively propagated between 2 nodes linked by causal interactions. Such an approach is not well defined on FC matrices, where the notion of paths cannot be interpreted in terms of causal interactions or information flow (and where all nodes are furthermore connected by definition, obviating the need to compute shortest paths). These problems persist and become potentially more difficult to diagnose in dynamic FC analyses.

SUMMARIZING BRAIN DYNAMICS

Upon obtaining the time-varying characteristics of FC metrics assessed across windows or frames, summary statistics of the variability, for example, standard deviation,[15,29,60] can be computed to offer a condensed view into the potential wealth of information revealed by network variability. Such metrics have been demonstrated as promising biomarkers for distinguishing between states[27,29] or between patients and healthy controls.[61–64]

By inspecting the evolution of FC snapshots over time, several groups have observed reliably recurring patterns at various timescales (eg, Refs.[30,65]), motivating the hypothesis that the dynamic repertoire evolves in a somewhat constrained manner. Under this hypothesis, a set of multivariate approaches has emerged in DFC methodology, seeking to depict the architecture of brain dynamics under the framework of transitions among a finite number of brain states, or joint expression of several spatiotemporal bases in ways that are governed by additional model assumptions. These endeavors open new views onto the way FC evolves in time, and metrics summarizing information in the temporal dimension offer new opportunities for biomarkers.

A general concern regarding multivariate methods stems from the large feature space associated with DFC and the limited number of samples that can be obtained per subject. Existing approaches to alleviate this concern essentially follow 1 of 2 main directions. One direction is to expand the sample space by collecting more time points per scan (with shortened TR or longer scan durations) or by concatenating large cohorts of subjects (collected locally or released by big data platforms[4,66–68]). The other direction is to reduce the feature space through the following: (1) shifting from voxel-wise to functional region of interest (ROI) or network-wise functional topology (see **Fig. 1**); (2) imposing sparsity constraints on the parameter space[69,70]; or (3) reducing the feature dimensionality through methods such as principal component analysis (PCA).

Temporal Clustering

The most common approach for extracting recurring FC patterns is temporal clustering, which assumes that each time instance or window is associated with a unique brain state.[30,32,33,40,71–76] The spatial patterns within each cluster, as well as the accompanying temporal information (eg, the occurrence rates of different clusters, and patterns of transitions among different patterns), can be exploited to characterize brain dynamics in clinical applications such as schizophrenia.[38,39]

Because the clustering results may heavily depend on the specified number of clusters, reanalyzing data across a range of cluster numbers to validate the robustness of major findings is strongly suggested. Alternatively, one can relax the discrete state assumptions by modeling the network pattern at each time instance as the joint expression of several functional bases, whose time course covaries freely or under constraints.[77–80] For instance, Leonardi and colleagues[79] applied PCA to the windowed correlations across functional ROIs, yielding orthogonal structured FC patterns ("eigenconnectivities"). By investigating contributions of these patterns to the overall brain dynamics at each window, the investigators were able to identify abnormality in patients with minimally disabled relapse-remitting multiple sclerosis in a specific pattern centered on the default-mode network. The authors note that community detection discussed above is another form of temporal clustering.

The Independence Assumption

ICA has been extensively used in resting-state studies to extract synchronized network patterns and to examine how they are modulated by changing cognitive states, aging, and disease.[81-83] A direct extension of ICA to the dynamic regime is implemented through SWA: by applying spatial ICA across successive windows, Kiviniemi and colleagues[35] tracked the variability of the default mode spatial patterns. However, identical resting-state networks (RSNs) do not necessarily persist over short windows, due partly to the stochastic nature of ICA; more importantly, the dependence of time series across windows is not typically accounted for when separating sources within each window. To overcome such limitations, independent vector analysis (IVA), a method which was initially introduced to enforce corresponding network patterns across subjects, was used for DFC analysis.[84] Briefly, IVA divides the entire time course into multiple windows and resolves network patterns (spatially independent sources) concurrently over all the windows while simultaneously maximizing the spatial dependence of components across windows. As such, this method enforces the correspondence of the RSNs across different windows, more readily allowing for tracking the trajectory of each RSN. Using IVA, Ma and colleagues[84] identified more variable network patterns in schizophrenia compared with a healthy population.

However, spatial ICA may be suboptimal under circumstances when distinct functional networks overlap substantially.[85] Driven by the motivation that a single brain region can be involved in multiple brain functional patterns, Smith and colleagues[20] applied temporal ICA (computed by maximizing temporal independence among components) to identify several distinct but spatially overlapping networks termed "temporal functional modes" (TFMs) during resting state.[20] TFM offers a complementary view of the dynamic architecture of brain FC (see Ref.[86] for a comprehensive discussion of concerns and interpretations regarding approaching ICA along different dimensions).

Detecting Functional Connectivity Change Points

Commonly, an FC change point is designated if the distribution of particular FC metrics exhibits salient deviation from baseline conditions, which can be achieved by comparing regional or network behavior in short snapshots preceding and following a given time point,[87] or assessing whether splitting the time course into subsegments at a given point and assuming temporal stationarity within each segment can enhance the overall modeling fitting.[69,88-90] Such an analysis directs attention to those time instances that are likely most relevant for characterizing trajectories

of brain dynamics. Further, it offers the possibility of delineating windows matching the durations of actual state changes.

Although change point analyses have lenient constraints on the temporal patterns of change instances, one should be aware that such analyses are not model free: prior assumptions on the structure of FC metrics are needed. Thus, the temporal precision of change-point analysis must be limited in order to yield reliable estimates of specified model parameters.[69] Furthermore, as these approaches generally rely on greedily searching through all the time points or partition possibilities, the anticipated computational load is massive, potentially limiting their capability to infer large-scale brain dynamics.[87,89]

Incorporating Temporal Sequence Information

Recently, temporal sequence information has been included in models characterizing brain dynamics. For instance, Majeed and colleagues[65] developed an algorithm to extract recurring spatiotemporal patterns that reveal the evolution of network structures across multiple timeframes, in contrast to a single timeframe.[65] With this proposed methodology, the investigators identified a reproducible pattern in human subjects, which spreads through regions within the default-mode network and task-positive network and accounts for a considerable proportion of low-frequency BOLD signals.

Another approach for characterizing temporal sequence information is based on the hidden Markov model (HMM).[70,91-96] Briefly, HMM extends temporal clustering by assuming that cognitive processes evolve through finite hidden states, within which the observed FC metrics obey certain distributions (eg, multivariate Gaussian distribution) instead of fixed patterns. The probability of switching between hidden states, and the occurrence rate of each state, are free parameters in the HMM, and optimized in conjunction with distributions associated with each state. Because of reduced degrees of freedom, modeling state sequence information concurrently with state patterns under a stochastic framework can presumably yield results that are less susceptible to noise (eg, motion and system noise).

HMM is most effective with large sample sizes, because of the expanded feature space inherent in the probabilistic model (eg, distribution parameters and state transition probability). Due to potential computational concerns, present HMM are mainly implemented ROI-wise, or via exerting strong sparsity constraints and dimensionality reduction. Very recently, a stochastic variational inference approach has been introduced to ease the computational load of HMM, making it applicable to very large sample sizes.[97] In the clinical realm, HMM has been applied to study the state switching patterns at rest[70,92] and identify disease-related abnormalities.[91,94] For instance, Ou and colleagues[91] applied HMM to characterize windowed correlations in healthy controls and patients with posttraumatic stress disorder (PTSD) patients and discovered that patients with PTSD tend to enter and become trapped in a negative mood state at rest.[91]

STATISTICAL TESTING

There are two issues faced by investigators when trying to determine whether observed DFC effects are meaningful. The first type involves distinguishing real fMR imaging signal from artifactual signal (see Considerations, in later discussion). The second concerns the general movement in the field from simpler static and localized descriptions of brain organization (such regional structural and activation properties) to more complex and distributed organization (structural connectivity as well as static and dynamic FC). These features of brain organization are clearly nonindependent. The challenge for DFC analyses is to show that the additional layer of complexity provided by these analyses is not captured in simpler features (such as changes in structural connectivity or static FC) and provides additional descriptive and predictive power in studies of brain organization.

Practically, analyses of significance are performed using null models. The basic idea of null models is to consider an ensemble of maximally random representations of the data in question, which preserves some basic or trivial features of the initial data. The important questions in this approach relate to the types of features the investigator wishes to control for, the choice of algorithms that preserve such features while sampling the data uniformly or in an unbiased manner, and the type of higher-order features of which the investigator wishes to test the existence. Here, some examples are considered that have been used previously in the literature for these purposes.

It is meaningful to differentiate null models based on randomizing the FC network topologies from null models based on randomizing the underlying time series. Randomization of network topologies for DFC can use methods that have been applied to static networks. For instance, algorithms may seek to preserve the total connectivity, the weight distribution, or the total connectivity associated with each node (the degree distribution), for each dynamic connectivity network.[98–100]

Null models may instead be constructed on fMR imaging time series, rather than on their network representations. These nulls have been used to test the fluctuations of graph metrics over time,[57] the significance of temporal clustering of data into dynamic patterns,[56] as well as the description of more broad properties of network organization, such as its "small-world" properties.[100] Most commonly, the nulls are constructed with random shuffling of data in the time or frequency domain. Such an approach includes the following:

- Permutations of the time series of individual nodes: preserves the temporal and autocorrelation structure but destroys all present pairwise correlations between nodes (eg, Ref.[58]).
- Permutations of the time points jointly across nodes: preserves the pairwise correlation structure but destroys all temporal properties and autocorrelation of each node (eg, Ref.[58]).
- Permutations in the frequency domain, which preserves the power spectrum but scrambles the phases of each node.[101–103]

An alternative to such permutations is to fit an autoregressive model to the time series and to generate surrogate data sets using this model (as was done in Ref.[15]).

CONSIDERATIONS
Determination of Sources Contributing to Dynamic Functional Connectivity

Numerous neural and physiologic processes, as well as nonneural effects, such as head motion, can lead to the observation of apparent brain dynamics. Determining these sources is critical to the application and interpretation of DFC metrics.

Vigilance levels
Changes in wakefulness (also referred to as arousal or vigilance) strongly impact behavior, cognition, and properties of observed brain dynamics. Several studies have linked decreases in vigilance with increases in correlated BOLD fluctuations across cortex.[104–106] In addition, fluctuations in eyelid and electrophysiological measures of vigilance across an individual scan have been found to be directly correlated with widespread synchronous modulation of cortical regions.[107,108] Decreases in vigilance have also been linked with increases in the amplitude of spontaneous signal fluctuations.[109] Thus, fluctuating vigilance states may introduce considerable temporal changes in apparent FC.[23,110] Recording markers of vigilance levels, such as eye behavior and EEG, can help to determine these effects; in the absence of such measures, recent data-driven approaches may

be valuable for detecting vigilance fluctuations in fMR imaging scans.[108,111]

Changes in signal amplitude, autocorrelation, and noise characteristics

Fluctuations in the magnitude of signal and noise levels across the scan, as well as the occurrence of nonneuronal events that generate strong, spatially correlated signal fluctuations, can give rise to variability of FC. Furthermore, inferences of DFC are based on relatively few time points, rendering the results particularly susceptible to noise.

In such cases, higher-order DFC metrics (such as correlation) may present a misleading picture of the temporal structure of brain activity. For example, an apparent increase in the sliding-window correlation between 2 regions may be driven by changes in amplitude or autocorrelation, or a sudden, common burst of activity. Therefore, the authors encourage examining and reporting whether these latter factors may comprise a more suitable characterization of the temporal behavior of observed dynamic phenomena.

Physiologic processes

FMR imaging signal fluctuations can be modulated substantially by physiologic processes linked with breathing and cardiac activity. Certain physiologic events, such as deep breaths, elicit BOLD signal changes across widespread cortical regions because of their common influence on arterial CO_2 levels and cerebral blood flow[112–115] (**Fig. 2**). Because the magnitude of this common signal change can be much higher than BOLD signals linked with neural activity, a single deep breath many manifest in increased synchrony over tens of seconds, appearing as a transient increase in FC.

Both model-based (eg, Refs.[116–118]) and data-driven (eg, Refs.[119–121]) methods have been developed for reducing such physiologic artifacts. However, given the lack of ground truth, one cannot determine the true efficacy of a noise-reduction procedure in a given dataset. In addition, physiologic changes such as heart rate variability also index neural processes related to autonomic activity. Although it is presently unclear how to best disentangle neural from artifactual physiologic effects, one promising route may involve modeling their differential dynamics.[122,123] Acquiring cardiac and respiratory recordings concurrently with the fMR imaging scan is highly recommended, because these recordings can be used to help determine whether the DFC measure

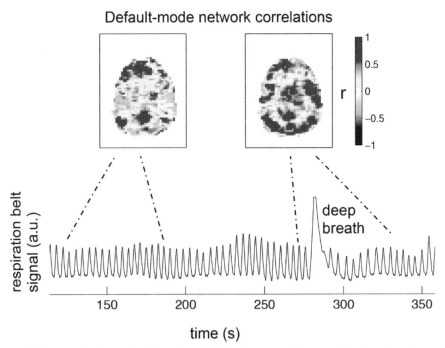

Fig. 2. Temporal changes in FC can be driven by physiologic events. For example, deep breaths are known to induce widespread modulation of BOLD signals across the brain, transiently elevating correlations between regions. Approaches for mitigating physiologic contributions in fMR imaging data (and other factors of no interest, such as head motion) may be used to diminish the influence of non-neural effects on DFC. Here, correlations are calculated between each voxel and the time series of the default-mode network, illustrated for 2 distinct windows of length 62.5 seconds for one example of an fMR imaging scan.

of interest is correlated with neural or nonneural physiologic measures.

Hemodynamic Confounds

Because BOLD fMR imaging signals are mediated by the cerebral vasculature, they inevitably contain nonneural hemodynamic effects that may present confounds for fMR imaging analyses.[124–126] Inconsistent hemodynamic responses across examined brain regions may result in time-varying intensity patterns that confound true network dynamics, especially when analyzing data in short time-windows. Several studies have attempted to disentangle hemodynamic effects via HRF deconvolution[46,47,51,127] or by measuring spatially varying hemodynamic lags using a hypercapnic challenge.[128] However, given limited knowledge regarding the spatial variation of the hemodynamic response and its variation under disease or task modulations, isolating neural dynamics from the fMR imaging signal itself is challenging. Thus, concurrent acquisitions with electrophysiological recordings (eg, EEG), as well as simulations that help quantify the sensitivity of study findings to heterogeneous HRFs, are recommended when feasible.

Issues with Short Acquisitions

Because cognitive states may fluctuate on the timescale of several minutes, a relatively short acquisition that fails to encompass full cycles of network fluctuations will not yield reliable inferences about the evolution of a subject's cognitive state. The lower bound of a sufficient scan length may be inferred, to some extent, from studies that quantify the impact of scan duration on the reliability of static network behavior. For instance, it has been reported that ROI-based FC metrics tend to saturate after 9 to 13 minutes or longer.[129,130] Nevertheless, can short acquisitions (~5 minutes or less) be harnessed for dynamic investigations through temporal concatenation? In other words, will ten 5-minute acquisitions produce functional information equivalent to one 50-minute scan? The equivalence of these cases rests upon the assumption that the probability of observing a given feature of interest is independent of the time that the subject has spent inside the scanner. The authors surmise that although this assumption may hold for certain brain network properties, others (such as relating to fluctuating vigilance states) may be dependent on scan durations.

SUMMARY

Quantification of spontaneous brain dynamics and interregional interactions in fMR imaging data has

---

> **Box 1**
> **Clinical relevance of dynamic functional connectivity**
>
> The study of DFC is burgeoning in clinical neuroscience. Investigators have pursued DFC methods in a wide variety of brain disorders, including schizophrenia,[38,131–134] bipolar disorder,[131] autism spectrum disorder,[135,136] major depression, mild cognitive impairment,[137,138] Alzheimer's disease[139] and dementia with Lewy bodies,[94] PTSD,[78] epilepsy,[61,140] and multiple sclerosis, among others.[79] Encouragingly, these studies have begun to suggest that dynamic features are more sensitive or specific than static connectivity in differentiating between healthy and control populations. However, it is somewhat premature to consider any convergence of these findings, given the relatively few studies performed on individual disorders, combined with the potentially heterogeneous nature of individual disorders and a host of confounding factors, such as systematic differences in head motion or long-term medication usage in patient populations. The promise of these measures could be evaluated in the future more directly through systematic comparisons across disorders, along with quantification of the certainty with which the presence of disease status can be predicted based on the observed properties of the signal.[141,142]

---

begun to open new possibilities for cognitive and clinical biomarkers (**Box 1**). Moving from traditional time-averaged measures toward the finer temporal variations of FC may be an important step to understanding individual differences and internal state changes, and hence for performing fMR imaging assessments at the single-subject level. This research direction also presents exciting opportunities for developing new computational methods that reveal robust, interpretable structure in the complex and high-dimensional feature space of dynamic fMR imaging data. However, there are formidable challenges involved in DFC analysis, requiring careful attention to avoiding spurious effects as well as cognizance of the hemodynamic basis of fMR imaging signals and the presence of structured, nonstationary artifacts in the data.

ACKNOWLEDGMENTS

This research was supported by NIH grant P41 EB15891 (NIHMS-ID: 887963). The authors wish to thank Jennifer Evans for figure assistance and Gary Glover for valuable comments.

REFERENCES

1. Biswal B, Yetkin FZ, Haughton VM, et al. Functional connectivity in the motor cortex of resting human brain using echo-planar MRI. Magn Reson Med 1995;34(4):537–41.

2. Fox MD, Raichle ME. Spontaneous fluctuations in brain activity observed with functional magnetic resonance imaging. Nat Rev Neurosci 2007;8(9):700–11.

3. Smith SM, Fox PT, Miller KL, et al. Correspondence of the brain's functional architecture during activation and rest. Proc Natl Acad Sci U S A 2009;106(31):13040–5.

4. Biswal BB, Mennes M, Zuo XN, et al. Toward discovery science of human brain function. Proc Natl Acad Sci U S A 2010;107(10):4734–9.

5. Van Dijk KR, Hedden T, Venkataraman A, et al. Intrinsic functional connectivity as a tool for human connectomics: theory, properties, and optimization. J Neurophysiol 2010;103(1):297–321.

6. Choe AS, Jones CK, Joel SE, et al. Reproducibility and temporal structure in weekly resting-state fMRI over a period of 3.5 years. PLoS One 2015;10(10):e0140134.

7. Damoiseaux JS, Greicius MD. Greater than the sum of its parts: a review of studies combining structural connectivity and resting-state functional connectivity. Brain Struct Funct 2009;213(6):525–33.

8. Buckner RL, Krienen FM, Castellanos A, et al. The organization of the human cerebellum estimated by intrinsic functional connectivity. J Neurophysiol 2011;106(5):2322–45.

9. Zhang D, Snyder AZ, Fox MD, et al. Intrinsic functional relations between human cerebral cortex and thalamus. J Neurophysiol 2008;100(4):1740–8.

10. Bassett DS, Wymbs NF, Porter MA, et al. Dynamic reconfiguration of human brain networks during learning. Proc Natl Acad Sci U S A 2011;108(18):7641–6.

11. Fransson P. How default is the default mode of brain function? Further evidence from intrinsic BOLD signal fluctuations. Neuropsychologia 2006;44(14):2836–45.

12. Horovitz SG, Braun AR, Carr WS, et al. Decoupling of the brain's default mode network during deep sleep. Proc Natl Acad Sci U S A 2009;106(27):11376–81.

13. Kelly C, Biswal BB, Craddock RC, et al. Characterizing variation in the functional connectome: promise and pitfalls. Trends Cogn Sci 2012;16(3):181–8.

14. Fox MD, Greicius M. Clinical applications of resting state functional connectivity. Front Syst Neurosci 2010;4:19.

15. Chang C, Glover GH. Time-frequency dynamics of resting-state brain connectivity measured with fMRI. Neuroimage 2010;50(1):81–98.

16. Sakoglu U, Pearlson GD, Kiehl KA, et al. A method for evaluating dynamic functional network connectivity and task-modulation: application to schizophrenia. MAGMA 2010;23(5–6):351–66.

17. Hutchison RM, Womelsdorf T, Allen EA, et al. Dynamic functional connectivity: promise, issues, and interpretations. Neuroimage 2013;80:360–78.

18. Calhoun VD, Miller R, Pearlson G, et al. The chronnectome: time-varying connectivity networks as the next frontier in fMRI data discovery. Neuron 2014;84(2):262–74.

19. Leonardi N, Van De Ville D. On spurious and real fluctuations of dynamic functional connectivity during rest. Neuroimage 2015;104:430–6.

20. Smith SM, Miller KL, Moeller S, et al. Temporally-independent functional modes of spontaneous brain activity. Proc Natl Acad Sci U S A 2012;109(8):3131–6.

21. Hindriks R, Adhikari MH, Murayama Y, et al. Can sliding-window correlations reveal dynamic functional connectivity in resting-state fMRI? Neuroimage 2016;127:242–56.

22. Zalesky A, Breakspear M. Towards a statistical test for functional connectivity dynamics. Neuroimage 2015;114:466–70.

23. Chang C, Liu Z, Chen MC, et al. EEG correlates of time-varying BOLD functional connectivity. Neuroimage 2013;72:227–36.

24. Keilholz SD. The neural basis of time-varying resting-state functional connectivity. Brain Connect 2014;4(10):769–79.

25. Thompson GJ, Magnuson ME, Merritt MD, et al. Short-time windows of correlation between large-scale functional brain networks predict vigilance intraindividually and interindividually. Hum Brain Mapp 2012;34:3280–98.

26. Preti MG, Bolton TA, Van De Ville D. The dynamic functional connectome: state-of-the-art and perspectives. Neuroimage 2016. [Epub ahead of print].

27. Chen JE, Chang C, Greicius MD, et al. Introducing co-activation pattern metrics to quantify spontaneous brain network dynamics. Neuroimage 2015;111:476–88.

28. Power JD. A simple but useful way to assess fMRI scan qualities. Neuroimage 2016;154:150–8.

29. Hutchison R, Womelsdorf T, Gati J, et al. Resting-state networks show dynamic functional connectivity in awake humans and anesthetized macaques. Hum Brain Mapp 2013;34(9):2154–77.

30. Allen EA, Damaraju E, Plis SM, et al. Tracking whole-brain connectivity dynamics in the resting state. Cereb Cortex 2014;24(3):663–76.

31. Handwerker DA, Roopchansingh V, Gonzalez-Castillo J, et al. Periodic changes in fMRI connectivity. Neuroimage 2012;63(3):1712–9.

32. Barttfeld P, Uhrig L, Sitt JD, et al. Signature of consciousness in the dynamics of resting-state

brain activity. Proc Natl Acad Sci U S A 2015; 112(3):887–92.

33. Hudetz AG, Liu X, Pillay S. Dynamic repertoire of intrinsic brain states is reduced in propofol-induced unconsciousness. Brain Connect 2015; 5(1):10–22.

34. Deng L, Sun J, Cheng L, et al. Characterizing dynamic local functional connectivity in the human brain. Sci Rep 2016;6:26976.

35. Kiviniemi V, Vire T, Remes J, et al. A sliding time-window ICA reveals spatial variability of the default mode network in time. Brain Connect 2011;1(4): 339–47.

36. Shine JM, Koyejo O, Bell PT, et al. Estimation of dynamic functional connectivity using multiplication of temporal derivatives. Neuroimage 2015;122: 399–407.

37. Shine JM, Koyejo O, Poldrack RA. Temporal meta-states are associated with differential patterns of time-resolved connectivity, network topology, and attention. Proc Natl Acad Sci U S A 2016;113(35): 9888–91.

38. Damaraju E, Allen EA, Belger A, et al. Dynamic functional connectivity analysis reveals transient states of dysconnectivity in schizophrenia. Neuroimage Clin 2014;5:298–308.

39. Rashid B, Damaraju E, Pearlson GD, et al. Dynamic connectivity states estimated from resting fMRI identify differences among schizophrenia, bipolar disorder, and healthy control subjects. Front Hum Neurosci 2014;8:897.

40. Shakil S, Lee CH, Keilholz SD. Evaluation of sliding window correlation performance for characterizing dynamic functional connectivity and brain states. Neuroimage 2016;133:111–28.

41. Gohel SR, Biswal BB. Functional integration between brain regions at rest occurs in multiple-frequency bands. Brain Connect 2015; 5(1):23–34.

42. Zuo XN, Di Martino A, Kelly C, et al. The oscillating brain: complex and reliable. Neuroimage 2010; 49(2):1432–45.

43. Thompson W, Fransson P. The frequency dimension of fMRI dynamic connectivity: network connectivity, functional hubs and integration in the resting brain. Neuroimage 2015;121:227–42.

44. Han Y, Wang J, Zhao Z, et al. Frequency-dependent changes in the amplitude of low-frequency fluctuations in amnestic mild cognitive impairment: a resting-state fMRI study. Neuroimage 2011;55(1): 287–95.

45. Wee CY, Yap PT, Denny K, et al. Resting-state multi-spectrum functional connectivity networks for identification of MCI patients. PLoS One 2012; 7(5):e37828.

46. Tagliazucchi E, Balenzuela P, Fraiman D, et al. Criticality in large-scale brain fMRI dynamics unveiled by a novel point process analysis. Front Physiol 2012;3.

47. Petridou N, Gaudes CC, Dryden IL, et al. Periods of rest in fMRI contain individual spontaneous events which are related to slowly fluctuating spontaneous activity. Hum Brain Mapp 2013;34(6):1319–29.

48. Tagliazucchi E, Siniatchkin M, Laufs H, et al. The voxel-wise functional connectome can be efficiently derived from co-activations in a sparse spatio-temporal point-process. Front Neurosci 2016;10:381.

49. Allan TW, Francis ST, Caballero-Gaudes C, et al. Functional connectivity in MRI is driven by spontaneous BOLD events. PLoS One 2015;10(4): e0124577.

50. Liu X, Duyn J. Time-varying functional network information extracted from brief instances of spontaneous brain activity. Proc Natl Acad Sci U S A 2013;110(11):4392–7.

51. Karahanoglu F, Van De Ville D. Transient brain activity disentangles fMRI resting-state dynamics in terms of spatially and temporally overlapping networks. Nat Commun 2015;6:7751.

52. Liu X, Chang C, Duyn JH. Decomposition of spontaneous brain activity into distinct fMRI co-activation patterns. Front Syst Neurosci 2013;7:101.

53. Di X, Biswal BB. Dynamic brain functional connectivity modulated by resting-state networks. Brain Struct Funct 2015;220(1):37–46.

54. Amico E, Gomez F, Di Perri C, et al. Posterior cingulate cortex-related co-activation patterns: a resting state fMRI study in propofol-induced loss of consciousness. PLoS One 2014;9(6).

55. Honey CJ, Kotter R, Breakspear M, et al. Network structure of cerebral cortex shapes functional connectivity on multiple time scales. Proc Natl Acad Sci U S A 2007;104(24):10240–5.

56. Betzel RF, Fukushima M, He Y, et al. Dynamic fluctuations coincide with periods of high and low modularity in resting-state functional brain networks. Neuroimage 2016;127:287–97.

57. Zalesky A, Fornito A, Cocchi L, et al. Time-resolved resting-state brain networks. Proc Natl Acad Sci U S A 2014;111(28):10341–6.

58. Bassett DS, Porter MA, Wymbs NF, et al. Robust detection of dynamic community structure in networks. Chaos 2013;23(1):013142.

59. Robinson LF, Wager TD, Lindquist MA. Change point estimation in multi-subject fMRI studies. Neuroimage 2010;49(2):1581–92.

60. Kucyi A, Davis KD. Dynamic functional connectivity of the default mode network tracks daydreaming. Neuroimage 2014;100:471–80.

61. Morgan VL, Abou-Khalil B, Rogers BP. Evolution of functional connectivity of brain networks and their dynamic interaction in temporal lobe epilepsy. Brain Connect 2015;5(1):35–44.

62. Shen H, Li Z, Zeng LL, et al. Internetwork dynamic connectivity effectively differentiates schizophrenic patients from healthy controls. Neuroreport 2014; 25(17):1344–9.

63. Laufs H, Rodionov R, Thornton R, et al. Altered FMRI connectivity dynamics in temporal lobe epilepsy might explain seizure semiology. Front Neurol 2014;5:175.

64. Falahpour M, Thompson WK, Abbott AE, et al. Underconnected, but not broken? Dynamic functional connectivity MRI shows underconnectivity in autism is linked to increased intra-individual variability across time. Brain Connect 2016;6(5): 403–14.

65. Majeed W, Magnuson M, Hasenkamp W, et al. Spatiotemporal dynamics of low frequency BOLD fluctuations in rats and humans. Neuroimage 2011;54(2):1140–50.

66. Smith S, Beckmann C, Andersson J, et al. Resting-state fMRI in the human connectome project. Neuroimage 2013;80:144–68.

67. Van Essen DC, Smith SM, Barch DM, et al. The WU-Minn Human Connectome Project: an overview. Neuroimage 2013;80:62–79.

68. Miller KL, Alfaro-Almagro F, Bangerter NK, et al. Multimodal population brain imaging in the UK Biobank prospective epidemiological study. Nat Neurosci 2016;19(11):1523–36.

69. Cribben I, Haraldsdottir R, Atlas L, et al. Dynamic connectivity regression: determining state-related changes in brain connectivity. Neuroimage 2012; 61(4):907–20.

70. Chen S, Langley J, Chen X, et al. Spatiotemporal modeling of brain dynamics using resting-state functional magnetic resonance imaging with Gaussian hidden Markov model. Brain Connect 2016;6(4):326–34.

71. Gonzalez-Castillo J, Hoy CW, Handwerker DA, et al. Tracking ongoing cognition in individuals using brief, whole-brain functional connectivity patterns. Proc Natl Acad Sci U S A 2015;112(28): 8762–7.

72. Hutchison R, Hutchison M, Manning K, et al. Isoflurane induces dose-dependent alterations in the cortical connectivity profiles and dynamic properties of the brain's functional architecture. Hum Brain Mapp 2014;35(12):5754–75.

73. Hutchison RM, Morton JB. Tracking the brain's functional coupling dynamics over development. J Neurosci 2015;35(17):6849–59.

74. Marusak HA, Calhoun VD, Brown S, et al. Dynamic functional connectivity of neurocognitive networks in children. Hum Brain Mapp 2017; 38(1):97–108.

75. Su J, Shen H, Zeng L, et al. Heredity characteristics of schizophrenia shown by dynamic functional connectivity analysis of resting-state functional MRI

scans of unaffected siblings. Neuroreport 2016; 27(11):843–8.

76. Shen H, Li Z, Qin J, et al. Changes in functional connectivity dynamics associated with vigilance network in taxi drivers. Neuroimage 2016;124(Pt A):367–78.

77. Leonardi N, Shirer W, Greicius M, et al. Disentangling dynamic networks: separated and joint expressions of functional connectivity patterns in time. Hum Brain Mapp 2014;35(12):5984–95.

78. Li X, Zhu D, Jiang X, et al. Dynamic functional connectomics signatures for characterization and differentiation of PTSD patients. Hum Brain Mapp 2014;35(4):1761–78.

79. Leonardi N, Richiardi J, Gschwind M, et al. Principal components of functional connectivity: a new approach to study dynamic brain connectivity during rest. Neuroimage 2013;83:937–50.

80. Yaesoubi M, Miller R, Calhoun V. Mutually temporally independent connectivity patterns: a new framework to study the dynamics of brain connectivity at rest with application to explain group difference based on gender. Neuroimage 2015; 107:85–94.

81. Calhoun VD, Adali T, Pearlson GD, et al. A method for making group inferences from functional MRI data using independent component analysis. Hum Brain Mapp 2001;14(3):140–51.

82. Beckmann CF, Smith SM. Probabilistic independent component analysis for functional magnetic resonance imaging. IEEE Trans Med Imaging 2004;23(2):137–52.

83. Beckmann CF, DeLuca M, Devlin JT, et al. Investigations into resting-state connectivity using independent component analysis. Philos Trans R Soc Lond B Biol Sci 2005;360(1457):1001–13.

84. Ma S, Calhoun VD, Phlypo R, et al. Dynamic changes of spatial functional network connectivity in healthy individuals and schizophrenia patients using independent vector analysis. Neuroimage 2014;90:196–206.

85. Friston KJ. Modes or models: a critique on independent component analysis for fMRI. Trends Cogn Sci 1998;2(10):373–5.

86. Calhoun VD, Eichele T, Adalı T, et al. Decomposing the brain: components and modes, networks and nodes. Trends Cogn Sci 2012;16(5):255–6.

87. Jeong S, Pae C, Park H. Connectivity-based change point detection for large-size functional networks. Neuroimage 2016;143:353–63.

88. Cribben I, Wager T, Lindquist M. Detecting functional connectivity change points for single-subject fMRI data. Front Comput Neurosci 2013;7.

89. Xu Y, Lindquist M. Dynamic connectivity detection: an algorithm for determining functional connectivity change points in fMRI data. Front Neurosci 2015;9.

90. Jia H, Hu X, Deshpande G. Behavioral relevance of the dynamics of the functional brain connectome. Brain Connect 2014;4(9):741–59.

91. Ou J, Xie L, Jin C, et al. Characterizing and differentiating brain state dynamics via hidden Markov models. Brain Topogr 2015;28(5):666–79.

92. Eavani H, Satterthwaite TD, Gur RE, et al. Unsupervised learning of functional network dynamics in resting state fMRI. Inf Process Med Imaging 2013;23:426–37.

93. Chiang S, Cassese A, Guindani M, et al. Time-dependence of graph theory metrics in functional connectivity analysis. Neuroimage 2016;125:601–15.

94. Sourty M, Thoraval L, Roquet D, et al. Identifying dynamic functional connectivity changes in dementia with lewy bodies based on product hidden Markov models. Front Comput Neurosci 2016;10:60.

95. Baker AP, Brookes MJ, Rezek IA, et al. Fast transient networks in spontaneous human brain activity. Elife 2014;3:e01867.

96. Vidaurre D, Quinn AJ, Baker AP, et al. Spectrally resolved fast transient brain states in electrophysiological data. Neuroimage 2016;126:81–95.

97. Vidaurre D, Abeysuriya R, Becker R, et al. Discovering dynamic brain networks from big data in rest and task. Neuroimage 2017. [Epub ahead of print].

98. Maslov S, Sneppen K. Specificity and stability in topology of protein networks. Science 2002; 296(5569):910–3.

99. Rubinov M, Sporns O. Complex network measures of brain connectivity: uses and interpretations. Neuroimage 2010;52(3):1059–69.

100. Zalesky A, Fornito A, Bullmore E. On the use of correlation as a measure of network connectivity. Neuroimage 2012;60(4):2096–106.

101. Prichard D, Theiler J. Generating surrogate data for time series with several simultaneously measured variables. Phys Rev Lett 1994;73(7):951–4.

102. Hindriks R, Adhikari MH, Murayama Y, et al. Corrigendum to "Can sliding-window correlations reveal dynamic functional connectivity in resting-state fMRI?" [NeuroImage 127 (2016) 242–256]. Neuroimage 2016;132:115.

103. Laumann TO, Snyder AZ, Mitra A, et al. On the stability of BOLD fMRI correlations. Cereb Cortex 2016. [Epub ahead of print].

104. Wong CW, Olafsson V, Tal O, et al. Anti-correlated networks, global signal regression, and the effects of caffeine in resting-state functional MRI. Neuroimage 2012;63(1):356–64.

105. Wong CW, Olafsson V, Tal O, et al. The amplitude of the resting-state fMRI global signal is related to EEG vigilance measures. Neuroimage 2013;83:983–90.

106. Olbrich S, Mulert C, Karch S, et al. EEG-vigilance and BOLD effect during simultaneous EEG/fMRI measurement. Neuroimage 2009;45(2):319–32.

107. Ong JL, Kong D, Chia TT, et al. Co-activated yet disconnected-neural correlates of eye closures when trying to stay awake. Neuroimage 2015;118:553–62.

108. Chang C, Leopold DA, Scholvinck ML, et al. Tracking brain arousal fluctuations with fMRI. Proc Natl Acad Sci U S A 2016;113(16):4518–23.

109. Fukunaga M, Horovitz SG, van Gelderen P, et al. Large-amplitude, spatially correlated fluctuations in BOLD fMRI signals during extended rest and early sleep stages. Magn Reson Imaging 2006; 24(8):979–92.

110. Wang C, Ong JL, Patanaik A, et al. Spontaneous eyelid closures link vigilance fluctuation with fMRI dynamic connectivity states. Proc Natl Acad Sci U S A 2016;113(34):9653–8.

111. Tagliazucchi E, Laufs H. Decoding wakefulness levels from typical fMRI resting-state data reveals reliable drifts between wakefulness and sleep. Neuron 2014;82(3):695–708.

112. Birn RM, Diamond JB, Smith MA, et al. Separating respiratory-variation-related fluctuations from neuronal-activity-related fluctuations in fMRI. Neuroimage 2006;31(4):1536–48.

113. Murphy K, Birn RM, Bandettini PA. Resting-state fMRI confounds and cleanup. Neuroimage 2013; 80:349–59.

114. Chang C, Glover GH. Relationship between respiration, end-tidal CO_2, and BOLD signals in resting-state fMRI. Neuroimage 2009;47:1381–93.

115. Nikolaou F, Orphanidou C, Wise RG, et al. Arterial CO_2 effects modulate dynamic functional connectivity in resting-state fMRI. Conf Proc IEEE Eng Med Biol Soc 2015;2015:1809–12.

116. Glover GH, Li TQ, Ress D. Image-based method for retrospective correction of physiological motion effects in fMRI: RETROICOR. Magn Reson Med 2000;44(1):162–7.

117. Chang C, Glover GH. Effects of model-based physiological noise correction on default mode network anti-correlations and correlations. Neuroimage 2009;47(4):1448–59.

118. Birn RM, Murphy K, Bandettini PA. The effect of respiration variations on independent component analysis results of resting state functional connectivity. Hum Brain Mapp 2008;29:740–50.

119. Salimi-Khorshidi G, Douaud G, Beckmann CF, et al. Automatic denoising of functional MRI data: combining independent component analysis and hierarchical fusion of classifiers. Neuroimage 2014;90:449–68.

120. Behzadi Y, Restom K, Liau J, et al. A component based noise correction method (CompCor) for BOLD and perfusion based fMRI. Neuroimage 2007;37(1):90–101.

121. Beall EB, Lowe MJ. Isolating physiologic noise sources with independently determined spatial measures. Neuroimage 2007;37(4):1286–300.

122. Chang C, Raven EP, Duyn JH. Brain-heart interactions: challenges and opportunities with functional magnetic resonance imaging at ultra-high field. Philos Trans A Math Phys Eng Sci 2016;374(2067).

123. Birn RM, Murphy K, Handwerker DA, et al. fMRI in the presence of task-correlated breathing variations. Neuroimage 2009;47(3):1092–104.

124. Menon RS. The great brain versus vein debate. Neuroimage 2012;62(2):970–4.

125. Liu TT. Neurovascular factors in resting-state functional MRI. Neuroimage 2013;80:339–48.

126. Handwerker D, Gonzalez-Castillo J, D'Esposito M, et al. The continuing challenge of understanding and modeling hemodynamic variation in fMRI. Neuroimage 2012;62(2):1017–23.

127. Gaudes CC, Petridou N, Dryden IL, et al. Detection and characterization of single-trial fMRI bold responses: paradigm free mapping. Hum Brain Mapp 2011;32(9):1400–18.

128. Chang C, Thomason ME, Glover GH. Mapping and correction of vascular hemodynamic latency in the BOLD signal. Neuroimage 2008;43(1):90–102.

129. Gonzalez-Castillo J, Handwerker DA, Robinson ME, et al. The spatial structure of resting state connectivity stability on the scale of minutes. Front Neurosci 2014;8:138.

130. Birn RM, Molloy EK, Patriat R, et al. The effect of scan length on the reliability of resting-state fMRI connectivity estimates. Neuroimage 2013;83:550–8.

131. Rashid B, Arbabshirani MR, Damaraju E, et al. Classification of schizophrenia and bipolar patients using static and dynamic resting-state fMRI brain connectivity. Neuroimage 2016;134:645–57.

132. Du Y, Pearlson GD, Yu Q, et al. Interaction among subsystems within default mode network diminished in schizophrenia patients: a dynamic connectivity approach. Schizophr Res 2016;170(1):55–65.

133. Yu Q, Erhardt EB, Sui J, et al. Assessing dynamic brain graphs of time-varying connectivity in fMRI data: application to healthy controls and patients with schizophrenia. Neuroimage 2015;107:345–55.

134. Miller RL, Yaesoubi M, Turner JA, et al. Higher dimensional meta-state analysis reveals reduced resting fMRI connectivity dynamism in schizophrenia patients. PLoS One 2016;11(3):e0149849.

135. Wee CY, Yap PT, Shen D. Diagnosis of autism spectrum disorders using temporally distinct resting-state functional connectivity networks. CNS Neurosci Ther 2016;22(3):212–9.

136. Price T, Wee CY, Gao W, et al. Multiple-network classification of childhood autism using functional connectivity dynamics. Med Image Comput Comput Assist Interv 2014;17(Pt 3):177–84.

137. Chen X, Zhang H, Gao Y, et al. High-order resting-state functional connectivity network for MCI classification. Hum Brain Mapp 2016;37(9):3282–96.

138. Wee CY, Yang S, Yap PT, et al. Alzheimer's Disease Neuroimaging I. Sparse temporally dynamic resting-state functional connectivity networks for early MCI identification. Brain Imaging Behav 2016;10(2):342–56.

139. Jones DT, Vemuri P, Murphy MC, et al. Non-stationarity in the "resting brain's" modular architecture. PLoS One 2012;7(6):e39731.

140. Liao W, Zhang Z, Mantini D, et al. Dynamical intrinsic functional architecture of the brain during absence seizures. Brain Struct Funct 2014;219(6):2001–15.

141. Kapur S, Phillips AG, Insel TR. Why has it taken so long for biological psychiatry to develop clinical tests and what to do about it? Mol Psychiatry 2012;17(12):1174–9.

142. Rubinov M, Bullmore E. Fledgling pathoconnectomics of psychiatric disorders. Trends Cogn Sci 2013;17(12):641–7.

Ten Key Observations on the Analysis of Resting-state Functional MR Imaging Data Using Independent Component Analysis

Vince D. Calhoun, PhD[a,b,*], Nina de Lacy, MD, MBA[c]

KEYWORDS

- Independent component analysis • Group ICA • fMR imaging • Dynamics • Connectivity • Brain
- Function

KEY POINTS

- Independent component analysis (ICA) is a data-driven approach for analyzing functional magnetic resonance (fMR) imaging data.
- ICA is typically used for capturing spatial and temporal signatures of brain networks within fMR imaging data as well as for separating artifactual signals from signals of interest.
- Components from an ICA analysis can be used in a wide variety of subsequent analyses, including classification, dynamic connectivity, graph theory, and dynamic causal modeling.
- The blind source separation/ICA research community continues to be vibrant and new algorithms for use with brain imaging continue to be developed.

INTRODUCTION

Since the initial prototype of a resting functional magnetic resonance (fMR) imaging analysis pipeline by Biswal and colleagues[1] in 1995, it has been known that fMR imaging data capture spontaneous fluctuations that have an interesting structure (eg, lateralization that closely corresponds with functionally known regions such as motor cortex) representing brain activity. Extant approaches typically assume little about the temporal evolution of the signal or causal circuits,

Disclosure: The authors have no commercial or financial conflicts of interest to disclose. This work was partially supported by the National Science Foundation grant 1539067, and National Institutes of Health grants R01EB006841, R01EB020407, and P20RR021938/P20GM103472 (to V.D. Calhoun) and the National Center for Advancing Translational Sciences of the National Institutes of Health under award number KL2TR000421 (to N. de Lacy). The content is solely the responsibility of the authors and does not necessarily represent the official views of the National Institutes of Health.

[a] The Mind Research Network, 1101 Yale Boulevard Northeast, Albuquerque, NM 87106, USA; [b] Department of ECE, University of New Mexico, 1 University of New Mexico, Albuquerque, NM 87131, USA; [c] Department of Psychiatry and Behavioral Science, University of Washington, Seattle, WA 98195, USA
* Corresponding author. The Mind Research Network, 1101 Yale Boulevard Northeast, Albuquerque, NM 87106.
E-mail address: vcalhoun@unm.edu

primarily looking only for evidence of coupling between time courses, instantiated in statistical correlations. In this realm, data-driven approaches are greatly needed to enabling the identification of novel relationships that were not predicted a priori. This article discusses 3 different domains: a spatial domain, a temporal domain, and a group (subject) domain, considering a spectrum of data-drivenness along temporal and spatial domains (Fig. 1). In the spatial domain, models at the most deterministic end of the spectrum define a specific region of interest or use a predetermined atlas to investigate activation. A more flexible approach is to start with an atlas and perform a constrained clustering to allow the data at hand to inform parcellation of activations. In addition, at the least predetermined end of the spectrum, fully data-driven discovery of activation patterns can be performed. In the temporal domain, a fixed time course can be assumed (as in seed-based connectivity) that is driven by the data at hand but takes a rigid approach by assuming the time course has a specific shape. Alternatively, the focus can be on an indirect measure such as amplitude of low-frequency fluctuation.[2] The most flexible approach is to perform data-driven discovery of underlying temporal covariance between brain locations. At the subject domain, assumptions can be made about subject labels (eg, diagnosis) to create a priori groups, but these may be challenged by instability within qualitative criteria,[3] poor segregation between features of interest (eg, genetic and neuropsychiatric characteristics), or subjects with overlapping phenotypes (eg, diagnostic comorbidity). Alternatively, investigators can allow for outliers by examining subjects for whom the data suggest that a different category may be more appropriate, by using available information to constrain the interpretation.[4] In addition, fully data-driven discovery of subject groups can be performed.[5,6]

One of the most widely used data-driven approaches applied to fMR imaging data is independent component analysis (ICA), which enables fully data-driven discovery of spatial patterns, temporal covariance, and even groups, as discussed in this article. ICA is exceptionally well suited to fMR imaging analysis given its robustness to artifacts, minimal assumptions on the shape of the time course or the spatial patterns, and ease of estimation.

THE BASICS OF INDEPENDENT COMPONENT ANALYSIS APPLIED TO FUNCTIONAL MAGNETIC RESONANCE IMAGING DATA

ICA of fMR imaging is most commonly implemented as spatial ICA, in which fMR imaging data are separated into a set of maximally spatially independent maps and their associated time courses. Here, "map" denotes the collective signal associated with neuronal masses with a similar activation pattern, although they may be spatially distant, and the time course of the signal from their aggregated voxels over the course of the scan. ICA is a type of matrix decomposition.

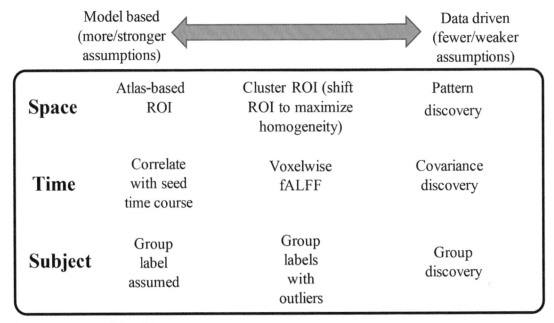

	Model based (more/stronger assumptions) ⟷ Data driven (fewer/weaker assumptions)		
Space	Atlas-based ROI	Cluster ROI (shift ROI to maximize homogeneity)	Pattern discovery
Time	Correlate with seed time course	Voxelwise fALFF	Covariance discovery
Subject	Group label assumed	Group labels with outliers	Group discovery

Fig. 1. A spectrum of data-drivenness.

Here, the fMR imaging data organized as time by voxels are represented as a matrix X, and the ICA decomposition is represented as $X = A$, where A is the unmixing matrix containing the time courses, and the rows of S contain the sources (spatial maps). There are several key benefits to this approach that have led to the widespread use of ICA. First, it does not require an assumption about the shape or nature of the time course for each component. Second, each spatial map has a value at each voxel, thus it provides a spatial filtering aspect that can be used to[1] separate artifactual signal from good signal, or[2] separate overlapping but distinct patterns arising from the same voxel,[3] identify multiple networks that may have overlapping nodes. Third, it provides a data-driven, functional parcellation of the brain, thereby reducing bias and allowing more flexibility in the consideration of subjects who may vary from standard atlases.

The multisubject extension of ICA (group ICA) was first proposed at the turn of the century[7] and has since become the dominant ICA approach for fMR imaging data.[8] Group ICA uses the fMR imaging data from all subjects to estimate aggregate components (maps that are present in all subjects), then subsequently performs an approach called back-reconstruction to estimate single-subject maps and time courses. There are multiple ways to perform back-reconstruction, ranging from regression-based approaches (eg, spatio-temporal or dual regression) to inversion-based approaches, which are discussed and compared in detail in a previous work.[9] A newer approach to back-reconstruction called group information–guided ICA (GIG-ICA), is a fully automated approach that estimates ICA first on the group level, then reoptimizes the ICA for each subject. It has been shown to be more sensitive to group differences and is better able to capture artifacts.[10,11]

There have been several more general reviews of ICA of fMR imaging over the years that discuss the basic concepts.[8,12–14] This article takes a different approach, expanding on 10 observations that highlight various aspects of the practical use of ICA in analysis that the authors think will be of use to readers. The examples provided are largely from our own work, but this article draws on other citations in order to represent the extensive amount of work performed related to ICA of fMR imaging (eg, querying "independent component" and "fMR imaging" in PubMed shows that approximately 2000 articles have been published).

One of the most scientifically appealing attributes of ICA is its ability to extract components from the mixed fMR imaging signal that represents large-scale neural networks.

These components are highly tractable to subsequent approaches examining many features of their temporal, spatial, and dynamic structures. For example, our own software platform group ICA of fMRI toolbox (GIFT) (http://mialab.mrn.org/software/gift/) makes whole-brain networks available to view and analyze on a subject, component, or multinetwork basis, including grouping into the primary neurocognitive functions (Fig. 2), as desired. A wide array of brain function measures, ranging from basic individual intranetwork integrity to averaged functional connectivity to complex features of internetwork brain dynamism, may be analyzed using the extracted components, in tandem with behavioral, psychiatric, demographic, genetic, or other subject characteristics. Tools provided in GIFT show the breadth and depth of ICA techniques for analyzing single or multiple subjects and static or dynamic connectivity, and providing more than a dozen ICA algorithms, including standard algorithms such as infomax[15] and fastICA[16]; advanced and more flexible

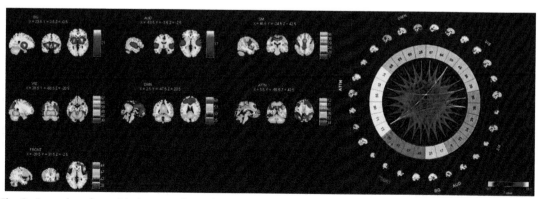

Fig. 2. Examples of graphical output from the GIFT ICA software.

algorithms, such as entropy-bound minimization[17]; and additional advanced algorithms, including independent vector analysis[18] and constrained ICA.[19,20] There are many visualization tools, including single-component or multi-component viewing tools, statistical analysis of maps and/or time courses, and toolboxes for dynamic connectivity and advanced statistical analysis.

NUMBER 1: INDEPENDENT COMPONENT ANALYSIS APPROACHES ARE ROBUST TO ARTIFACTS

One of the benefits of data-driven approaches is they fit the data better because there are more flexible. This flexibility means they fit not only signals of interest but also the artifacts. Although this can be a negative issue (eg, fitting outliers in the data better could imply overfitting to noise), in the case of blind source separation approaches like ICA, the goal is to separate the signals or sources from one another. This separation can be leveraged in several ways; for example, ICA can be used to denoise the data (for use in a subsequent analysis; eg, by a general linear model [GLM] approach) or this benefit can be exploited directly by further analyzing the good components in the context of an ICA analysis. As discussed in more detail later, there are now multiple strategies in use, including the use of single-subject[21–23] or group-level[10] ICA denoising. One of the benefits of the GIG-ICA approach is that it can robustly remove the impact of artifacts but does not require time-consuming training.[10] Another benefit is it gives researchers a second opportunity to remove motion artifact after the initial data preprocessing. An example of this approach in which ground truth maps are compared with the estimated components for several approaches in GIG-ICA is shown in Fig. 3.

Importantly, because the components have a value at every voxel, this results in a type of spatial filtering (in contrast with approaches based on hard sparsity that move voxels to zero for regions not strongly contributing). This spatial filtering enables ICA to both separate artifacts from signals of interest[10,22] and also separate task-related events that are overlapping (and in some cases may even cancel out within a single voxel).[24,25] As such, ICA is not a pure parcellation scheme in that it requires thresholding to split the brain into separate regions, hence straddling the line between lumping and 'splitting.[26] ICA can be used to evaluate the degree to which the fMR imaging response to a task is positive, negative, or neutral (Fig. 4).[24]

NUMBER 2: INDEPENDENT COMPONENT ANALYSIS IS AGNOSTIC TO THE TEMPORAL EVOLUTION OF BRAIN ACTIVITY SIGNALS

One of the early applications of ICA was to analyze task-related fMR imaging data without requiring a specific temporal model. In the early ICA studies of task-based designs, transient task-related activity was captured by independent components enabling investigators to better understand how the brain is responding in regions where activity does not perfectly temporally correspond with the task.[27,28] This property is likely one of the main reasons ICA is so widely used on resting fMR imaging data, because in this case there is no temporal model available because the subject is resting quietly without the presence of an externally controlled stimulus. ICA is free of assumptions about the temporal evolution of the data. Subject time courses can be unknown, not synchronized across individuals, and ICA extracts components that show considerable anatomic and functional structure, with some showing bilateral or anterior/posterior symmetry (Fig. 5). This benefit is a direct result of the blind source separation (BSS) approach originally motivated by the cocktail party problem, in which multiple microphones are recording sound from multiple conversations in a room: the goal of BSS is to take the multiple microphone recordings and unmix them to get to the original sources without knowing how those sources were generated. This process finds a strong parallel in resting-state fMR imaging, in which there is a mixed signal from the whole brain arising from many brain areas.

NUMBER 3: INDEPENDENT COMPONENT ANALYSIS COMPONENTS CAN BE COUPLED TO ONE ANOTHER SPATIALLY AND TEMPORALLY

Importantly, maximal independence does not remove all information about spatial coupling between different components. The linear unmixing assumption identifies components that highlight regions showing strong temporal correlation (within network connectivity); however, there can still be considerable temporal correlation between components. This correlation is known as functional network connectivity (FNC) or among network connectivity.[29] It is one of the most powerful ways to use ICA, in that it can provide information about which components are fluctuating together, which are anticorrelated with one another, and which are not correlated at all; this provides a wealth of information about the functional relationships between large-scale neural networks. The observations from an FNC analysis

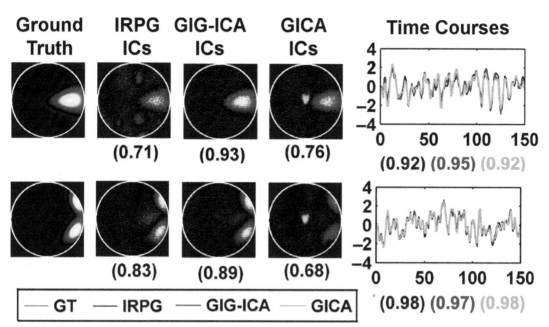

Fig. 3. GIG-ICA for artifact removal. Individual independent components (ICs) and time courses (TCs) for 1 subject obtained from Individual ICA Artifact Removal Plus Group ICA (IRPG), GIG-ICA, and standard group ICA (GICA). The values in parentheses under each estimated IC are the relevant correlation coefficients between the IC and the ground truth (GT) source. The last row shows related TCs. The correlation values under TCs from left to right correspond with IRPG, GIG-ICA, and GICA, respectively. Note that only the nonartifact ICs/TCs are shown. (*Modified from* Du YH, Allen EA, He H, et al. Artifact removal in the context of group ICA: a comparison of single-subject and group approaches. Hum Brain Mapp 2016;37(3):1005–25.)

also show face validity in that separate components with similar primary neurocognitive functions tend to be highly correlated with one another. For example, different components may be extracted that are all primarily associated with visual function, and these are highly correlated with each other, and it is similar for motor or default mode components. These attributes

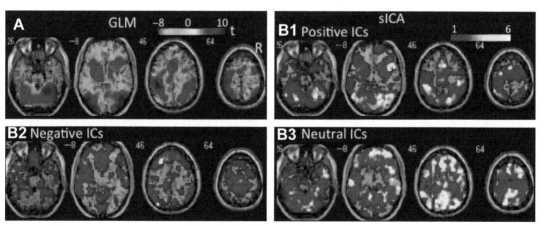

Fig. 4. Task-related modulation in blood oxygenation level-dependent (BOLD) signal during the congruent condition of the flanker task. (*A*) Color on the brain images shows task-related increases and decreases in BOLD signal as revealed by GLM-based analyses. The color bar indicates *t* values. (*B1–B3*) Color on the brain images shows regions covered by positive, negative, and neutral ICs, respectively. The color bar indicates the number of overlapping ICs. sICA, spatial independent component analysis. (*Modified from* Xu JS, Calhoun VD, Worhunsky PD, et al. Functional network overlap as revealed by fMRI using sICA and its potential relationships with functional heterogeneity, balanced excitation and inhibition, and sparseness of neuron activity. PLoS One 2015;10(2):e0117029.)

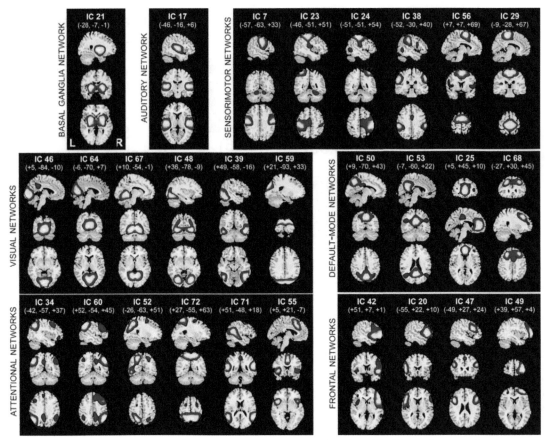

Fig. 5. Example ICA component spatial maps from rest fMR imaging data. (*Modified from* Allen EA, Erhardt EB, Damaraju E, et al. A baseline for the multivariate comparison of resting-state networks. Front Syst Neurosci 2011;5(2):2.)

open up the opportunity to examine functional connectivity patterns within neurocognitive domains containing multiple networks. In addition, default mode components tend to be seen as weakly negatively correlated with other networks, also consistent, but extending, early observations about the default mode network (**Fig. 6**). FNC has also been widely used to identify group differences or even individual subject classification,[30–32] and differences in FNC can profitably be analyzed for associations with symptoms or quantitative characteristics.

Previous work has also shown that, despite spatial independence being maximized using mutual information, spatial coupling among the components can still be identified, revealing interesting hierarchical structure to network relationships[33] even across neurocognitive domains. When working with ICA components it can be informative to evaluate not only the time courses and spatial maps but also their temporal and spatial coupling. Temporal FNC and spatial FNC, both dynamic and static, have grown to be among

the most widely used ways of querying the results from an ICA of fMR imaging analysis.

NUMBER 4: INDEPENDENT COMPONENT ANALYSIS MAY BE DATA DRIVEN BUT IT IS ALSO USEFUL FOR HYPOTHESIS-BASED STUDIES

This observation may be obvious given the large amount of work on the topic, but an important point to keep in mind is that, although ICA represents a data-driven approach for parcellating the brain into components, this does not preclude the use of ICA for hypothesis testing. In these schemata, ICA acts as an efficient, robust, and flexible way to extract brain networks and time courses to test specific, formulated hypotheses. This can be done in many ways, by generating a hypothesis to test before the analysis regarding specific widely identified networks (such as default mode[34]) or by deciding a priori to only test components that have large contributions from specific regions. Network maps can also be taken from a previous

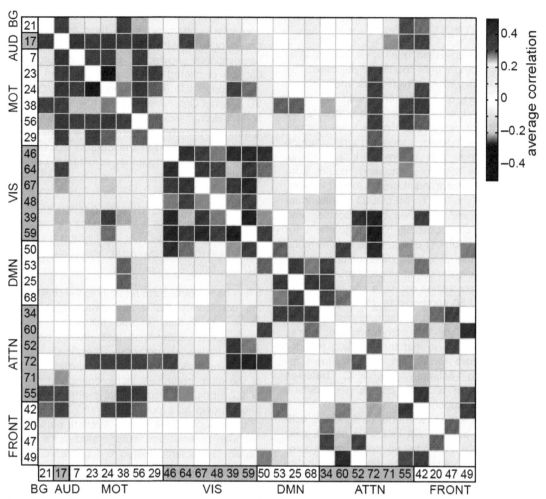

Fig. 6. Example of FNC. The component maps are ordered as shown in **Fig. 5**. Considerable modularity is observable within the matrix; for example, visual and motor regions tend to be most highly correlated with themselves and the default mode network is showing anticorrelation with multiple other networks. ATTN, attention; AUD, auditory; BG, basal ganglia; DMN, default mode network; FNC, functional network connectivity; FRONT, frontal; MOT, sensorimotor; VIS, visual. (*Modified from* Allen EA, Erhardt EB, Damaraju E, et al. A baseline for the multivariate comparison of resting-state networks. Front Syst Neurosci 2011;5(2):2.)

analysis and used to reconstruct components from a new data set.[19,20,35] These approaches are very useful when trying to use ICA for single-subject prediction, because they ensure that the data on which the analysis is predicted are completely separate from the data that were used to generate the maps and the prediction algorithm.[32]

Assumptions of Independent Component Analysis

Importantly, ICA also has several embedded assumptions. For example, ICA is most widely used in its linear form (ie, linear mixing of the components). As such, it can be mathematically

described as the multiplication of 2 matrices, exactly as in the GLM approach. In this case, after ICA has estimated the maps and time courses, it can be considered to be very similar to a seed-based approach in which the map represents the connectivity associated with the time courses (after accounting for the other component time courses),[36] with the added benefit that the ICA-derived map is data driven. Another important assumption is that the sources can be separated by assuming that they are spatially independent. This assumption, although perhaps not perfectly satisfying, has worked extremely well in fMR imaging data because networks are typically found that are not systematically overlapping.

NUMBER 5: THERE IS NO PERFECT NUMBER OF COMPONENTS

One of the often-asked questions about ICA is how many components should be selected. The choice here is between high-order models with larger numbers of components, and low-order models with fewer. Higher model orders do more splitting and produce more focal components, whereas lower model orders produce larger networks. This difference is sometimes addressed by visually comparing results from multiple component numbers.[37] Available software tools (eg, GIFT, MELODIC [multivariate exploratory linear optimized decomposition into independent components]) have algorithms for estimating the number of components and multiple articles have proposed different approaches for solving this order selection problem.[38–40] Typically, such approaches estimate somewhere between 20 and 50 components, although recently there has been a trend to estimate higher model orders (eg, 100 or 120 components or more). The benefit of this is that the resulting components are more focal, and it also allows researchers to estimate the FNC between subnodes within a given domain (eg, default mode network subnodes).

Note that a low-order model designed to estimate 20 components will include a set of good components (ie, networks) as well as noise components that will ultimately be discarded from the analysis. As a general rule, the authors typically find that 50% to 70% of components survive as networks. If the ICA produces ~10 networks, it may prove challenging to isolate specific known functional networks of interest in the study design, depending on the degree of granularity the researcher requires. For example, in a low-order model, the frontoparietal network (also called the central executive network) will be present as a single network rather than as lateralized left and right frontoparietal networks.[41] Thus, for researchers interested in the functional properties of individual networks, a higher order model may also be preferred to differentiate more networks. The authors generally find that a model order of ~75 to 100 components results in 30 to 50 networks in which the major identified networks are present as well as multiple subnetworks in neurocognitive domains such as vision, attention, or the default mode networks.

Importantly, there is a hierarchical relationship between low and high model order analyses, and this is clearly visible in the modular structure of the FNC matrix in **Fig. 6**, which shows, for example, that visual components tend to be more highly correlated to themselves. These correlated components are then more likely to group together at lower model orders. The authors have recently shown that a low model order ICA can be predicted almost perfectly from a high model order ICA (Rachakonda S, Du Y, Calhoun VD, "Model Order Prediction in ICA," in Organization for Human Brain Mapping, submitted for publication, 2017). This property makes it possible to zoom up and down in the data to see how the maps split or stay together at different levels or granularity (**Fig. 7**).

NUMBER 6: INDEPENDENT COMPONENT ANALYSIS RESULTS ARE ROBUST TO FALSE-POSITIVES AND SPATIAL AUTOCORRELATION ASSUMPTIONS COMPARED WITH GENERAL LINEAR MODEL ANALYSES

It has been pointed out recently to the brain imaging community that some data preprocessing steps can induce inflated false-positive rates when using cluster-wise tests based on parametric statistical methods. Specifically, spatial smoothing changes the autocorrelation structure of the data, potentially incrementing the number of false-positive results. This problem has long been known as a potential pitfall in the analysis of fMR imaging time series. A recent publication, although polemic and exaggerated in its claims, highlights problems related to data preprocessing and suggests that many fMR imaging studies may be affected.[42] In this circumstance, it is critical to reevaluate the methods used to preprocess and analyze neuroimaging data.

One characteristic of ICA is the goal of finding components with maximal statistical independence that tend to diminish spatial cross-correlations. Another important characteristic in ICA is the use of high-order statistics; for example, through entropy or kurtosis measures, which allows a more comprehensive estimation of independent signal sources and reduced influence of artifacts that may arise during preprocessing. Based on these characteristics, the authors argue that ICA offers advantages that might reduce the problem of inflated false-positives caused by data preprocessing. Through empirical testing, the authors evaluated the false-positive rates in the context of ICA. Results indicate false-positive rates less than 5% for P-value thresholds of .05 after false-discovery-rate correction. As anticipated, based on an argued resilience to preprocessing artifacts, ICA delivered low false-positive rates, even when using standard parametric testing. These results suggest that findings from ICA tend to be statistically conservative, providing further

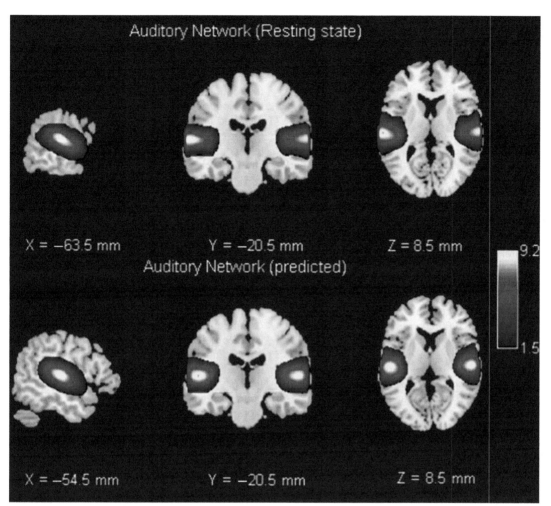

Fig. 7. The top row shows a temporal lobe component from resting-state analysis and the bottom row is a predicted temporal lobe component from a different data set.

evidence for the validity of results obtained using ICA (Fig. 8).

NUMBER 7: THE MANTRA OF "GARBAGE IN GARBAGE OUT" RINGS TRUE, BUT WITH INDEPENDENT COMPONENT ANALYSIS ONE PERSON'S GARBAGE MAY BE ANOTHER'S GOLD

The history of ICA with fMR imaging is replete with examples of studies using it to identify new and interesting aspects of the data that researchers did not know to look for before. For example, the initial use of ICA modeled the ICA time courses using a task-based approach, but then so-called transient task-related effects were observed,[7,27,43,44] including an early example of the now widely studied default mode network.[28] The use of ICA also identified spatially structured but non–task-related components

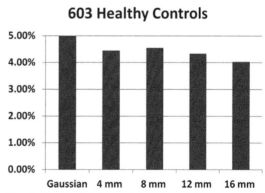

Fig. 8. Ratio of false-positives found for group ICA with 28 components on a population of 603 healthy subjects. One million iterations were performed to estimate the false-positive ratio by randomly assigning healthy subjects to 1 of 2 groups.

within task-fMR imaging data and shortly thereafter in resting-state fMR imaging data.

Another interesting example of this is in results that advance the important research topic of how resting-state and task-based networks and activation patterns relate to each other. Here, ICA was used to identify structure in covariation among task activation maps, again yielding intrinsic networks that look very similar to those now widely studied in resting fMR imaging data.[45] The goal was to explicitly compare the networks obtained from a first-level ICA (ICA on the spatiotemporal fMR imaging data) with those from a second-level ICA (ICA on computed features or second-level maps rather than on the first-level fMR imaging data). Convergent results from simulations, task-fMR imaging data, and resting-state fMR imaging data show that a second-level analysis, although slightly noisier than the first-level analysis, yields strikingly similar patterns of intrinsic networks (spatial correlations as high as 0.85 for task data and 0.65 for rest data, considerably greater than the empirical null). Second-level ICA results also largely preserve the relationship of these networks with other variables, such as age (eg, default mode network regions tended to show decreased low-frequency power for first-level analyses and decreased loading parameters for second-level analyses). Results comparing the 2 approaches are shown in **Fig. 9**. The feature-based ICA approach has also been used on smoothed peaks from a meta-analytical database, again revealing results that resemble the widely identified resting networks.[41]

More intriguingly, an ICA analysis of the (typically discarded) variance captured by motion covariates in an fMR imaging study also yields similar functional network patterns, suggesting that the noise removal process also captures variance of interest.[46] Regression of noise and motion is aggressive for fMR imaging, for good reason, but such studies highlight that there is a cost when using such a strategy. Future studies should continue to focus on improving ways of separating artifact from noise in a more precise manner.

One of the reasons ICA is so widely used is that it pushes many of the stronger assumptions to later in the analytical pipeline. ICA benefits from many existing approaches that have strong assumptions. For example, GLM approaches are often used to perform testing on the data-driven component time courses or maps (eg, to identify task-related components[47–49]). In essence, ICA is used to extract spatial maps and time courses from the data that can act as a fertile analytical substrate to be evaluated or tested in multiple

ways using preferred frameworks. Testing on the time course is perhaps the most common, including performing GLM analysis on the time courses.[50,51] Other approaches for analyzing the time courses include graph theory[52–55] and effective connectivity analysis using dynamic causal modeling.[56–58] The spatial maps can also be analyzed in several ways, including performing a GLM analysis on individual components,[8,51] but ICA component maps have also been used as input into classification algorithms.[59]

NUMBER 8: LABELING THE INDEPENDENT COMPONENT ANALYSIS COMPONENTS IS STILL LARGELY MANUAL, BUT AUTOMATION APPROACHES CONTINUE TO IMPROVE

One of the challenges with working with ICA is labeling/identifying the components. Perhaps the most important category is whether the components are artifacts (non–blood oxygenation level dependent [BOLD]) or should be considered intrinsic networks. Many investigators, ourselves among them, have used a semimanual approach in which visual inspection of the spatial maps, time course signal, and component spectra are combined with calculation of the low-frequency/high-frequency power ratio. Intrinsic networks tend to have anatomically reasonable activation patterns, smoother signals and spectra, and higher power ratios. **Fig. 10** compares an intrinsic network output from ICA with a noise component as an example of this. This approach is partly reliant on experience and the human eye, and often there are a few cusp components that pose challenges. Thus, further automation to improve standardization and comparability across studies is desirable. Several approaches have been proposed to automatically identify artifacts. These approaches include models that require training and running a classifier (eg, a support vector machine)[21,22,60] as well as those based on a set of predefined metrics.[10,23,61] They can be run either at the group level or the single-subject level.[10,22] However, despite the success of such approaches, they are not perfect and there can be a cost to misclassification.[10] A more recent approach using GIG-ICA is intended to avoid this noisy categorization and focus instead on the estimation of the individual components at the group level. Results are similar in the case in which the single-subject ICA artifact removal process is perfect and are improved when (inevitable) errors are made at the single-subject level.

Beyond artifact detection, there is also the challenge of attributing specific neurocognitive functions to individual components as well as

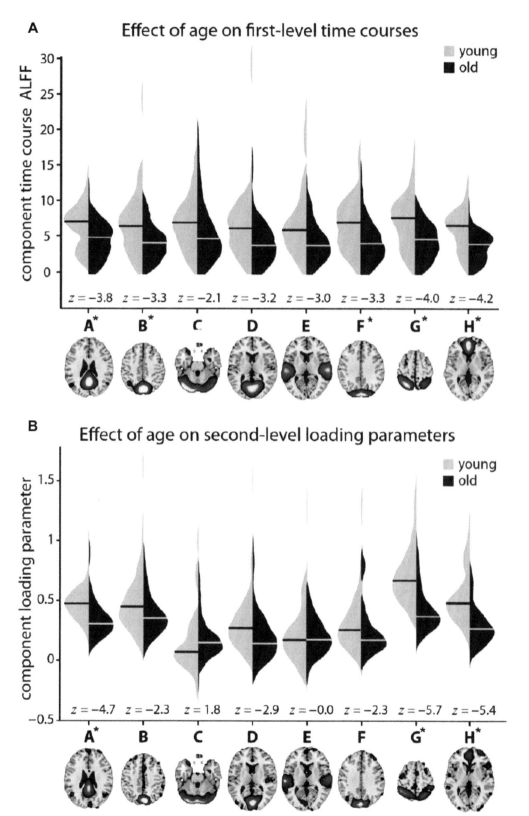

Fig. 9. Effect of age on the amplitude of low-frequency fluctuations (ALFF). Violin plots show the distributions of ALFF estimates for young (*left*) and old (*right*) subjects (40 in each group) based on the first-level (*A*) and second-level (*B*)

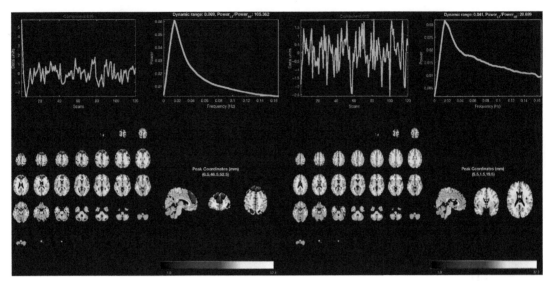

Fig. 10. Comparison of components extracted from 60 component ICA performed using GIG-ICA on resting-state data in 572 youth subjects with neurotypical development, and ADHD. On the left is an intrinsic network or 'good' component. Note the smooth shape to the power spectra (dynamic range) and high low-frequency to high-frequency power ratio. The brain activation pattern is spatially aggregated and clearly in frontal gray matter areas. On the right is a 'bad' component. Here, there is a shallow, ridged appearance to the spectra in lower frequencies and low power ratio. Activation is restricted to the ventricles. Likely this component represents artifact from cerebrospinal fluid in the brain ventricles.

gathering them into resulting functional domains. Several recent articles have shown that, when this is done, the resulting structure in the FNC matrix is highly interpretable[61,62] and suggests an ordered whole-brain functional architecture. Current strategies for automated attribution include drawing on preexisting component atlases combined with spatial regression for performing such labeling.[63] A focus on domains or groupings of regions or components is also thought provoking. For example, a focus solely on insula regions yielded multiple unique fingerprints in a dynamic connectivity analysis.[64] New methods being developed to optimize across multiple domains have yielded some interesting results.[65,66] **Fig. 11** shows an example of estimated joint functional domains compared with the static (averaged) FNC matrix. Future work should focus on the combination of these approaches with an automated and/or

dynamic labeling approach. Such work likely draw on more dynamic and flexible atlases.[67]

NUMBER 9: INDEPENDENT COMPONENT ANALYSIS CAN BE LEVERAGED TO CAPTURE DYNAMIC (TIME-VARYING) FUNCTIONAL CONNECTIVITY

In recent years there have been a large number of articles focused on the estimation of time-varying connectivity patterns. This article moves beyond consideration of averaged or static connectivity across the entire resting fMR imaging experiment (see Refs.[68–71] for reviews) and toward consideration of nonstationary functional connectivity, exploring how FNC changes over the time courses. One of the key advantages of ICA that are discussed here is that it minimizes assumptions made up front, including the nature of time

analyses. For the first-level analysis, ALFF values are calculated from the subject-specific TCs; for second-level analysis, ALFF values are the subject loading parameters from the ICA mixing matrix (matrix in **Fig. 1**B). Horizontal bars indicate the medians for each group. Because data are skewed, group differences are assessed with the nonparametric Wilcoxon rank sum test for equal medians (z-statistics are based on approximate normal distribution). Asterisks denote significantly different medians at $P<.001$, uncorrected. (*From* Calhoun VD, Allen E. Extracting intrinsic functional networks with feature-based group independent component analysis. Psychometrika 2013;78(2):243–59.)

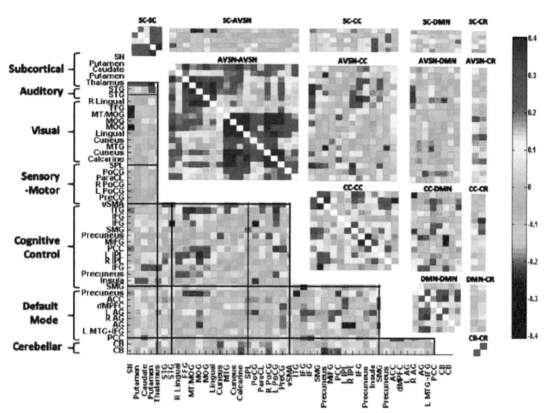

Fig. 11. Population average of static windowed functional network connectivity matrix; that is, using all 162 time points (no windowing) for 47 ICA components (networks) obtained from a group ICA decomposition. Grid lines bound 7 functional domains. Rectangular pull-outs are 15 joint functional domain connectivity blocks estimated from the ICA data using the approach described by Miller and colleagues. (*Data from* Miller RL, Vergara VM, Keator DB, et al. A method for inter-temporal functional domain connectivity analysis: application to schizophrenia reveals distorted directional information flow. IEEE Trans Biomed Eng 2016;63(12):2525–39.)

course fluctuations, allowing an ICA decomposition to provide a powerful way to further study dynamic changes among the ICA time courses. Such work can easily be done within an ICA context using a sliding-window approach to estimate the FNC,[72] other approaches including time-frequency analyses,[73] or even windowless approaches that can capture instantaneous changes and do not assume temporally smooth transitions.[74] The windowed approach consists of setting a chosen time interval (eg, a window of 20 TRs [repeat times]), computing an FNC matrix for the window and shifting the window across the time courses, and computing an FNC matrix at each point. This produces a time series of FNC matrices. Following this, clustering can be used to reduce these dynamic FNC matrices to a small number of functional connectivity states that represent connectivity patterns localized to a particular period of time.

These dynamic connectivity approaches have been shown to be a much more natural way to analyze resting fMR imaging data. They have already shown improved sensitivity to identifying group differences, brain arousal state, or diagnostic classifications from resting-state fMR imaging data.[30,62] An example of FNC states estimated from resting fMR imaging collected concurrently with electroencephalogram (EEG) data is shown in **Fig. 12**. The states are ordered according to EEG measures of drowsiness and it is apparent that the connectivity patterns are affected by the arousal state (in particular, anticorrelated connectivity, indicated in blue, diminishes with increasing drowsiness).[75,76] In terms of group differences, recent work using ICA has shown that patients schizophrenia tend to spend more time occupying a weakly connected dynamic state versus controls[62] and also that dynamic FNC estimates seem to be more sensitive for classification of bipolar patients and patients with schizophrenia[30] than static measures.

Researches can also focus on the spatial maps to identify changes in the connectivity nodes over time[77,78] or across both spatial nodes and time courses.[79] Approaches that incorporate models

Time and increased drowsiness

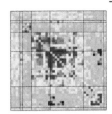 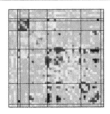 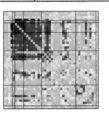 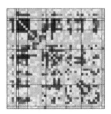

Strong antagonism between DMN and attentional networks corresponds with less low frequency power (delta, theta, and alpha)

Partial antagonism corresponds with increased alpha power

Cortical-subcortical antagonism and decreased intra-DMN connectivity corresponds with increased delta/theta power

Hypersynchronization corresponds with larger increases in delta/theta power and decreases in alpha power

Fig. 12. Example of dynamic functional network connectivity states estimated from a resting fMR imaging data set for which concurrent EEG data were also collected. Ordering the fMR imaging states according to EEG drowsiness measures reveals a striking pattern, because drowsiness increases the anticorrelated functional connectivity with the default mode network and diminishes that with other networks. DMN, default mode network.

of spatial patterns changes over time are extremely interesting, have implications for studies that attempt to create atlases of the human brain, and are currently understudied.

NUMBER 10: INDEPENDENT COMPONENT ANALYSIS ALGORITHM DEVELOPMENT IS ONGOING

New ICA and related algorithms are constantly being developed for application to brain imaging data. For example, the incorporation of multiple types of statistical diversity (such as independence and sparsity) has already been done within existing algorithms but is not yet fully understood. For example, the widely used infomax algorithm incorporates aspects of both independence and sparsity, leading to some interesting ongoing discussions.[80] The combination of both sparsity and independence (as well as other types of statistical diversity) to varying degrees may provide a more powerful toolkit for querying resting-state fMR imaging data.[81–84]

In addition, the underlying ICA algorithms that are most widely used for fMR imaging data (eg, fastICA and infomax) both make key assumptions about the underlying source distributions. For example, infomax assumes that the source distribution is unimodal and sparse. Newer algorithms with more flexible models are capable of capturing sources across a wider range of possible distributional forms, including multimodal distributions that can more effectively maximize independence.[17,85,86] In addition, constrained ICA approaches are also growing in use because they provide a way to bridge between region of interest–based and atlas-based approaches, enabling investigators to specify a region to query, and are also helpful in approaching single-subject

ICA. Blind ICA approaches can provide maps based only on the structure of the data.[10,19,20,87,88]

Another interesting direction is the development of ICA approaches that assume a linear mixing of the sources to handle the nonlinear sources that can be present in neuroimaging data and that likely represent the nature of human brain activity. The challenge here is that the parameter estimation space becomes much larger. However, there are multiple solutions proposed for solving this problem.[89,90] Most recently, deep learning approaches[91] have been combined with modifications to the concept of independence to offer interesting solutions.[92] Following an initial approach,[93] the authors can capture nonlinearities within a deep ICA model. Neuroimaging data from patients with schizophrenia and healthy controls were analyzed with 5 coupling layers each with an embedded nonlinear function composed of 2 hidden layers. Results identified significant group differences in bilateral temporal lobe activity (one of the most consistent structural abnormalities[94–96] found in schizophrenia) in addition to novel components spanning cerebellum, hippocampus, and parahippocampal gyrus. Some components showed evidence of significant nonlinearities (**Fig. 13**). Results suggest that such models can detect components that are biologically relevant that may be missed by a linear model.

Another area of active development includes the extension of the ICA BSS approach to handle multiple subspaces (eg, each subject is modeled in a personal subspace), as in the independent vector analysis (IVA) algorithm.[18,97,98] IVA has already been applied to resting-state fMR imaging in multiple studies,[18,99] yielding improved representation of intersubject variability in the spatial maps.[100] The extension of this to additional subspaces to

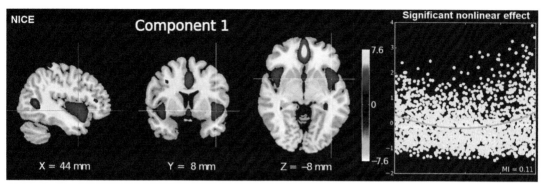

Fig. 13. Nonlinear ICA of sMRI analysis identifies significant nonlinear effects between schizophrenia and healthy controls. On the left is an example of a component captured by the nonlinear ICA approach and on the right is a plot showing the evidence of a nonlinear effect after removing the linear relationship (which only appears in certain components). MI, mutual information; NICE, nonlinear independent component estimation; sMRI, structural magnetic resonance imaging. (*Data from* Castro E, Hjelm RD, Plis SM, et al. Deep independence network analysis of structural brain imaging: application to schizophrenia. IEEE Trans Med Imaging 2016;35(7):1729–40.)

better capture other types of variability is an interesting future direction.[101]

Hybrid ICA and deep learning approaches are also showing strong potential for improved modeling of dynamic connectivity. Recent work has shown that a restricted Boltzmann machine, a basic building block for deep learning, provides results competitive with the widely used ICA approach.[102] Moving beyond this to more flexible neural network models can capture more complex relationships between spatial and temporal dynamics in fMR imaging data.[79]

SUMMARY

The application of ICA to resting fMR imaging data has been popular in large part because of the ability of ICA to capture interesting and meaningful spatiotemporal patterns in fMR imaging data while making minimal assumptions about the nature of the underlying spatial and temporal organization and being robust to artifactual effects. Although at this point ICA of fMR imaging data has been in use for almost 20 years, it continues to provide a fertile, robust basis for the development of novel extensions to further automate analysis, better capture variability, and extend into new directions, including advance prediction and indirect models capable of delineating patterns of brain dynamics via deep learning combined with subspace approaches.

ACKNOWLEDGMENTS

The corresponding author thanks Victor Vergara and Mohammad Arbabshirani for helpful discussion.

REFERENCES

1. Biswal B, Yetkin FZ, Haughton VM, et al. Functional connectivity in the motor cortex of resting human brain using echo-planar MRI. Magn Reson Med 1995;34(4):537–41.
2. Zou QH, Zhu CZ, Yang Y, et al. An improved approach to detection of amplitude of low-frequency fluctuation (ALFF) for resting-state fMRI: fractional ALFF. J Neurosci Methods 2008;172(1):137–41.
3. Insel T, Cuthbert B, Garvey M, et al. Research domain criteria (RDoC): toward a new classification framework for research on mental disorders. Am J Psychiatry 2010;167(7):748–51.
4. Clementz BA, Sweeney JA, Hamm JP, et al. Identification of distinct psychosis biotypes using brain-based biomarkers. Am J Psychiatry 2016;173(4):373–84.
5. Marquand AF, Wolfers T, Mennes M, et al. Beyond lumping and splitting: a review of computational approaches for stratifying psychiatric disorders. Biol Psychiatry Cogn Neurosci Neuroimaging 2016;1(5):433–47.
6. Du Y, Pearlson G, Liu J, et al. A group ICA based framework for evaluating resting fMRI markers when disease categories are unclear: application to schizophrenia, bipolar, and schizoaffective disorders. Neuroimage 2015;122:272–80.
7. Calhoun VD, Adali T, Pearlson GD, et al. A method for making group inferences from functional MRI data using independent component analysis. Hum Brain Mapp 2001;14(3):140–51.
8. Calhoun VD, Adali T. Multisubject independent component analysis of fMRI: a decade of intrinsic networks, default mode, and neurodiagnostic discovery. IEEE Rev Biomed Eng 2012;5:60–73.
9. Erhardt EB, Rachakonda S, Bedrick EJ, et al. Comparison of multi-subject ICA methods for analysis

of fMRI data. Hum Brain Mapp 2011;32(12): 2075–95.

10. Du YH, Allen EA, He H, et al. Artifact removal in the context of group ICA: a comparison of single-subject and group approaches. Hum Brain Mapp 2016;37(3):1005–25.

11. Salman M, Du Y, Damaraju E, et al. Group information guided ICA shows more sensitivity to group differences than dual-regression. IEEE International Symposium on Biomedical Imaging 2017. Melbourne, Australia, April 18 and 21, 2017.

12. Calhoun VD, Adali T. Unmixing fMRI with independent component analysis. IEEE Eng Med Biol Mag 2006;25(2):79–90.

13. McKeown MJ, Hansen LK, Sejnowski TJ. Independent component analysis of functional MRI: what is signal and what is noise? Curr Opin Neurobiol 2003;13(5):620–9.

14. Beckmann CF. Modelling with independent components. Neuroimage 2012;62(2):891–901.

15. Bell AJ, Sejnowski TJ. An information maximisation approach to blind separation and blind deconvolution. Neural Comput 1995;7(6):1129–59.

16. Hyvarinen A, Oja E. A fast fixed-point algorithm for independent component analysis. Neural Comput 1997;9(7):1483–92.

17. Li X, Adali T. Independent component analysis by entropy bound minimization. IEEE Trans Signal Process 2010;58(10):5151–64.

18. Lee JH, Lee TW, Jolesz FA, et al. Independent vector analysis (IVA): multivariate approach for fMRI group study. Neuroimage 2008;40(1):86–109.

19. Lin Q, Liu J, Zheng Y, et al. Semi-blind spatial ICA of fMRI using spatial constraints. Hum Brain Mapp 2010;31(7):1076–88.

20. Du Y, Fan Y. Group information guided ICA for fMRI data analysis. Neuroimage 2013;69:157–97.

21. Salimi-Khorshidi G, Douaud G, Beckmann CF, et al. Automatic denoising of functional MRI data: combining independent component analysis and hierarchical fusion of classifiers. Neuroimage 2014;90:449–68.

22. Sochat V, Supekar K, Bustillo J, et al. A robust classifier to distinguish noise from fMRI independent components. PLoS One 2014;9(4):e95493.

23. Pruim RH, Mennes M, van Rooij D, et al. ICA-AROMA: a robust ICA-based strategy for removing motion artifacts from fMRI data. Neuroimage 2015; 112:267–77.

24. Xu JS, Calhoun VD, Worhunsky PD, et al. Functional network overlap as revealed by fMRI using sICA and its potential relationships with functional heterogeneity, balanced excitation and inhibition, and sparseness of neuron activity. PLoS One 2015;10(2):e0117029.

25. Xu J, Potenza MN, Calhoun VD, et al. Large-scale functional network overlap is a general property

of brain functional organization: reconciling inconsistent fMRI findings from general-linear-model-based analyses. Neurosci Biobehav Rev 2016;71: 83–100.

26. Boles DB. The "lumping" and "splitting" of function and brain. Brain Cogn 2000;42(1):23–5.

27. McKeown MJ, Jung TP, Makeig S, et al. Spatially independent activity patterns in functional MRI data during the Stroop color-naming task. Proc Natl Acad Sci U S A 1998;95(3):803–10.

28. Calhoun VD, Pekar JJ, McGinty VB, et al. Different activation dynamics in multiple neural systems during simulated driving. Hum Brain Mapp 2002;16(3): 158–67.

29. Jafri M, Pearlson GD, Stevens M, et al. A method for functional network connectivity among spatially independent resting-state components in schizophrenia. Neuroimage 2008;39:1666–81.

30. Rashid B, Arbabshirani MR, Damaraju E, et al. Classification of schizophrenia and bipolar patients using static and dynamic resting-state fMRI brain connectivity. Neuroimage 2016;134:645–57.

31. Arbabshirani M, Kiehl KA, Pearlson G, et al. Classification of schizophrenia patients based on resting-state functional network connectivity. Front Neurosci 2013;7(133):1–16.

32. Arbabshirani MR, Plis S, Sui J, et al. Single subject prediction of brain disorders in neuroimaging: promises and pitfalls. Neuroimage 2017;145(Pt B):137–65.

33. Ma S, Correa N, Li X, et al. Automatic identification of functional clusters in fMRI data using spatial information. IEEE Trans Biomed Eng 2011;58(12): 3406–17.

34. Ongur D, Lundy M, Greenhouse I, et al. Default mode network abnormalities in bipolar disorder and schizophrenia. Psychiatry Res 2010;183(1):59–68.

35. Lu W, Rajapakse JC. Approach and applications of constrained ICA. IEEE Trans Neural Netw 2005; 16(1):203–12.

36. Joel SE, Caffo BS, van Zijl PC, et al. On the relationship between seed-based and ICA-based measures of functional connectivity. Magn Reson Med 2011;66(3):644–57.

37. Abou-Elseoud A, Starck T, Remes J, et al. The effect of model order selection in group PICA. Hum Brain Mapp 2010;31(8):1207–16.

38. Li YO, Adali T, Calhoun VD. Estimating the number of independent components for functional magnetic resonance imaging data. Hum Brain Mapp 2007;28(11):1251–66.

39. Hui M, Li J, Wen X, et al. An empirical comparison of information-theoretic criteria in estimating the number of independent components of fMRI data. PLoS One 2011;6(12):e29274.

40. Douglas PK, Harris S, Yuille A, et al. Performance comparison of machine learning algorithms and

number of independent components used in fMRI decoding of belief vs. disbelief. Neuroimage 2011;56(2):544–53.

41. Smith SM, Fox PT, Miller KL, et al. Correspondence of the brain's functional architecture during activation and rest. Proc Natl Acad Sci U S A 2009; 106(31):13040–5.

42. Eklund A, Nichols TE, Knutsson H. Cluster failure: why fMRI inferences for spatial extent have inflated false-positive rates. Proc Natl Acad Sci U S A 2016; 113(28):7900–5.

43. Konishi S, Donaldson DI, Buckner RL. Transient activation during block transition. Neuroimage 2001;13(2):364–74.

44. Calhoun VD, Adali T, Pekar JJ. A method for comparing group fMRI data using independent component analysis: application to visual, motor and visuomotor tasks. Magn Reson Imaging 2004;22(9):1181–91.

45. Calhoun VD, Allen E. Extracting intrinsic functional networks with feature-based group independent component analysis. Psychometrika 2013;78(2): 243–59.

46. Bright MG, Murphy K. Is fMRI "noise" really noise? Resting state nuisance regressors remove variance with network structure. Neuroimage 2015;114: 158–69.

47. McKeown MJ. Detection of consistently task-related activations in fMRI data with hybrid independent component analysis. Neuroimage 2000; 11(1):24–35.

48. Calhoun VD, Adali T, Pearlson GD, et al. Spatial and temporal independent component analysis of functional MRI data containing a pair of task-related waveforms. Hum Brain Mapp 2001;13(1):43–53.

49. van den Bosch GE, El Marroun H, Schmidt MN, et al. Brain connectivity during verbal working memory in children and adolescents. Hum Brain Mapp 2014;35(2):698–711.

50. Xu J, Calhoun VD, Potenza MN. Spatial ICA reveals functional activity hidden from traditional fMRI GLM-based analyses. Front Neurosci 2013; 7:154.

51. Calhoun VD, Adali T, McGinty V, et al. fMRI activation in a visual-perception task: network of areas detected using the general linear model and independent component analysis. Neuroimage 2001; 14(5):1080–8.

52. Laney J, Westlake KP, Ma S, et al. Capturing subject variability in fMRI data: a graph-theoretical analysis of GICA vs. IVA. J Neurosci Methods 2015;247:32–40.

53. Anderson A, Cohen MS. Decreased small-world functional network connectivity and clustering across resting state networks in schizophrenia: an fMRI classification tutorial. Front Hum Neurosci 2013;7:520.

54. Yu Q, Sui J, Rachakonda S, et al. Altered topological properties of functional network connectivity in schizophrenia during resting state: a small-world brain network study. PLoS One 2011;6(9): 1–12.

55. Yu Q, Allen EA, Sui J, et al. Brain connectivity networks in schizophrenia underlying resting state functional magnetic resonance imaging. Curr Top Med Chem 2012;12(21):2415–25. Special issue on "Neurochemistry of schizophrenia and psychosis: the contribution of neuroimaging".

56. Stevens M, Kiehl KA, Pearlson GD, et al. Functional neural circuits for mental timekeeping. Hum Brain Mapp 2007;28(5):394–408.

57. Stevens M, Calhoun VD, Pearlson GD, et al. Brain network dynamics during error commission. Hum Brain Mapp 2009;30(1):24–37.

58. Havlicek M, Friston K, Jan J, et al. Dynamic modeling of neuronal responses in fMRI using cubature Kalman filtering. Neuroimage 2011; 56(4):2109–28.

59. Calhoun VD, Pearlson GD, Maciejewski P, et al. Temporal lobe and 'default' hemodynamic brain modes discriminate between schizophrenia and bipolar disorder. Hum Brain Mapp 2008;29(11): 1265–75.

60. De Martino F, Gentile F, Esposito F, et al. Classification of fMRI independent components using IC-fingerprints and support vector machine classifiers. Neuroimage 2007;34(1):177–94.

61. Allen EA, Erhardt EB, Damaraju E, et al. A baseline for the multivariate comparison of resting-state networks. Front Syst Neurosci 2011;5(2):2.

62. Damaraju E, Allen EA, Belger A, et al. Dynamic functional connectivity analysis reveals transient states of dysconnectivity in schizophrenia. Neuroimage Clin 2014;5:298–308.

63. Calhoun VD. Group ICA of fMRI toolbox (GIFT). 2004. Available at: http://mialab.mrn.org/software/gift.

64. Nomi JS, Farrant K, Damaraju E, et al. Dynamic functional network connectivity reveals unique and overlapping profiles of insula subdivisions. Hum Brain Mapp 2016;37(5):1770–87.

65. Vergara V, Miller R, Van Erp T, et al. The functional dynamics of brain domains in schizophrenia. Human Brain Mapp 2016. Geneva, Switzerland, June 26–30, 2016.

66. Miller RL, Vergara VM, Keator DB, et al. A method for inter-temporal functional domain connectivity analysis: application to schizophrenia reveals distorted directional information flow. IEEE Trans Biomed Eng 2016;63(12):2525–39.

67. Yarkoni T, Poldrack RA, Nichols TE, et al. Large-scale automated synthesis of human functional neuroimaging data. Nat Methods 2011;8(8): 665–70.

68. Calhoun VD, Miller R, Pearlson G, et al. The chronnectome: time-varying connectivity networks as the next frontier in fMRI data discovery. Neuron 2014; 84(2):262–74.

69. Hutchison RM, Womelsdorf T, Allen EA, et al. Dynamic functional connectivity: promises, issues, and interpretations. Neuroimage 2013;80: 360–78.

70. Keilholz SD. The neural basis of time-varying resting state functional connectivity [review]. Brain Connect 2014;4(10):769–79.

71. Preti MG, Bolton TA, Van De Ville D. The dynamic functional connectome: state-of-the-art and perspectives. Neuroimage 2016. [Epub ahead of print].

72. Allen E, Damaraju E, Plis SM, et al. Tracking whole-brain connectivity dynamics in the resting state. Cereb Cortex 2014;24(3):663–76.

73. Yaesoubi M, Allen EA, Miller RL, et al. Dynamic coherence analysis of resting fMRI data to jointly capture state-based phase, frequency, and time-domain information. Neuroimage 2015;120: 133–42.

74. Yaesoubi M, Calhoun V. Window-less estimation of dynamic functional connectivity. Keystone Symposia - Connectomics. Santa Fe, NM, March 5–8, 2017.

75. Allen E, Eichele T, Wu L, et al. EEG signature of functional connectivity states. Proc HBM. Seattle, WA, June 16–20, 2013.

76. Damaraju E, Allen E, Wu L, et al. EEG signatures of dynamic functional network connectivity states. Brain Topogr 2017. [Epub ahead of print].

77. Kiviniemi V, Vire T, Remes J, et al. A sliding time-window ICA reveals spatial variability of the default mode network in time. Brain Connect 2011;1(4): 339–47.

78. Ma S, Calhoun VD, Phlypo R, et al. Dynamic changes of spatial functional network connectivity in healthy individuals and schizophrenia patients using independent vector analysis. Neuroimage 2014;90:196–206.

79. Hjelm D, Plis S, Calhoun VD. Recurrent neural networks for spatiotemporal dynamics of intrinsic networks from fMRI data. NIPS. Barcelona, Spain, December 9–10, 2016.

80. Calhoun VD, Potluru V, Phlypo R, et al. Independent component analysis for brain fMRI does indeed select for maximal independence. PLoS One 2013;8(8):e73309.

81. Adali T, Anderson M, Fu G. Diversity in independent component and vector analyses: identifiability, algorithms, and applications in medical imaging. IEEE Signal Process Mag 2014;31: 18–33.

82. Adali T, Anderson M, Fu G. IVA and ICA: use of diversity in independent decompositions. Proceedings of the European Signal Processing Conferences (EUSIPCO). Aug 27–31, 2012. p. 61–5.

83. Du W, Fu G, Calhoun VD, et al. Performance of complex-valued ICA algorithms for fMRI analysis: importance of taking full diversity into account. ICIP 2014. Paris, France, October 27–30, 2016.

84. Du W, Levin-Schwartz Y, Fu GS, et al. The role of diversity in complex ICA algorithms for fMRI analysis. J Neurosci Methods 2016;264:129–35.

85. Gomez-Herrero G, Rutanen K, Egiazarian K. Blind source separation by entropy rate minimization. IEEE signal processing letters 2010;17(2): 153–6.

86. Li X-L, Adali T. Complex independent component analysis by entropy bound minimization. IEEE Trans Circuits Syst 2010;57(7):1417–30.

87. Lu W, Rajapakse JC. Eliminating indeterminacy in ICA. Neurocomputing 2003;50:271–90.

88. Calhoun VD, Adali T, Stevens M, et al. Semi-blind ICA of fMRI: a method for utilizing hypothesis-derived time courses in a spatial ICA analysis. Neuroimage 2005;25(2):527–38.

89. Wu L, Calhoun V. Nonlinear ICA: applications to spatial and temporal EEG source separation. Human Brain Mapping Conference, Quebec, Canada, June 26–30, 2011.

90. Hyvarinen A, Pajunen P. Nonlinear independent component analysis: existence and uniqueness results. Neural Netw 1999;12(3):429–39.

91. Plis SM, Hjelm DR, Salakhutdinov R, et al. Deep learning for neuroimaging: a validation study. Front Neurosci 2014;8:229.

92. Castro E, Hjelm RD, Plis SM, et al. Deep independence network analysis of structural brain imaging: application to schizophrenia. IEEE Trans Med Imaging 2016;35(7):1729–40.

93. Dinh L, Krueger D, Bengio Y. NICE: non-linear independent components estimation. arXiv preprint arXiv:14108516; 2014; 2014.

94. Xu L, Groth K, Pearlson G, et al. Source based morphometry: the use of independent component analysis to identify gray matter differences with application to schizophrenia. Hum Brain Mapp 2009;30:711–24.

95. Turner J, Calhoun VD, Michael A, et al. Heritability of multivariate gray matter measures in schizophrenia. Twin Res Hum Genet 2012; 15(3):324–35.

96. Gupta CN, Calhoun VD, Rachakonda S, et al. Patterns of gray matter abnormalities in schizophrenia based on an international mega-analysis. Schizophr Bull 2015;41(5):1133–42.

97. Via J, Anderson M, Li XL, et al. A maximum likelihood approach for independent vector analysis of Gaussian data sets. Proc IEEE Workshop on Machine Learning for Signal Processing (MLSP). Beijing, China, 2011.

98. Anderson M, Fu G, Phlypo R, et al. Independent vector analysis: identification conditions and performance bounds. IEEE Trans Signal Process 2014;62(17):4399–410.

99. Michael AM, Anderson M, Miller RL, et al. Preserving subject variability in group fMRI analysis: performance evaluation of GICA vs. IVA. Front Syst Neurosci 2014;8:106.

100. Gopal S, Miller RL, Michael A, et al. Spatial variance in resting fMRI networks of schizophrenia patients: an independent vector analysis. Schizophr Bull 2016;42(1):152–60.

101. Silva RF, Plis SM, Sui J, et al. Blind source separation for unimodal and multimodal brain networks: a unifying framework for subspace modeling. IEEE J Sel Top Signal Process 2016;10(7):1134–49.

102. Hjelm RD, Calhoun VD, Salakhutdinov R, et al. Restricted Boltzmann machines for neuroimaging: an application in identifying intrinsic networks. Neuroimage 2014;96:245–60.

A Review of Resting-State Analysis Methods

Azeezat K. Azeez, BS, Bharat B. Biswal, PhD*

KEYWORDS

• Functional MR imaging • Resting-state functional connectivity • Neurologic disease

KEY POINTS

- Resting state fMRI research aims to investigate neurological processes that occur without external stimulation.
- Various methods of analysis can reveal information on resting state connectivity.
- Results which can be used to characterize specific populations.

INTRODUCTION

Functional MR imaging (fMR imaging) is a noninvasive, radiological imaging technique. Like MR imaging, it uses a series of magnetic fields, radio waves, and field gradients to generate images of inside the body. Although MR imaging captures higher resolution anatomic images, fMR imaging also captures anatomic images, albeit at lower resolution, and provides information on functional changes that occur over time. fMR imaging works with the fundamental assumption that neural activations can be measured as a function of time.

Metabolic markers that can be obtained from fMR imaging image data, including cerebral blood volume (CBV), cerebral blood flow (CBF), and blood oxygenation level–dependent (BOLD) signal. CBV refers to the amount of blood in a given amount of brain tissue. Due to physiologic limitations (perfusion and blood brain barrier), this is a relatively constant value; therefore, changes in CBF can be easily detected. CBF is tightly regulated by neuronal demands. BOLD, which is a metabolic signal that measures changes in the ratio of oxyhemoglobin to deoxyhemoglobin that are attributed to changes in neural activity, is the most commonly used measure of neurologic change. In 1990, at Bell Laboratory, Dr Seiji Ogawa and colleagues proposed that manipulations in blood oxygen could be visualized in T2-weighted MR imaging images. Ogawa's[1] 1990 pioneering paper tested this hypothesis by restricting the concentration of oxygen to the rats and examining the resulting T1-weighted image contrast. Oxygenated blood created images without distortion; however, there was significant signal loss in images from deoxygenated blood. BOLD contrast depends on the amount of deoxygenated hemoglobin present in a brain region, which is subject to the balance of oxygen supply and consumption.[2] Hemodynamic response function (HRF) refers to changes in BOLD in response to stimuli; this is the core on which fMR imaging research is based.

Changes in the BOLD signal can be best seen in task-based experimental designs. Subjects are asked to perform a task over given time periods for multiple repetitions. A common example of this is bilateral finger tapping, which activates bilateral motor areas. Subjects are asked to tap each finger to their thumb sequentially for blocks of time and then return to rest. Task activation is seen in a BOLD response that is highly correlated to the on-off task design. This type of

Funded by: NIH, Grant number(s): DA038895; MH108346 (NIHMS-ID: 888417).
Department of Biomedical Engineering, New Jersey Institute of Technology, Newark, NJ 07102, USA
* Corresponding author. Department of Biomedical Engineering, New Jersey Institute of Technology, University Heights, Newark, NJ 07102.
E-mail address: bbiswal@gmail.com

neuroimaging.theclinics.com

experimentation allows researchers to directly correlate external stimuli with neurologic activity. Although it has been commonly used, it does limit the type of research questions that can be asked, narrows the subject pool, and increases the scan time duration. Resting state is an alternative to this.

Resting-state fMR imaging research aims to investigate neurologic processes that occur without external stimulation. Unlike task-based studies that can be correlated with neurologic output, lack of task demands unburdens experimental design, increases subject compliance, and reduces training demands, making it appropriate to study children and clinical populations who are unable to complete tasks. Resting state does have its limitations, unlike task-based design, however, and questions of separating signal and noise become very important.

Resting-state functional connectivity is defined as the synchronization of brain regions with each another.[3,4] It refers to a temporal dependence of neuronal activity of regions that do not necessarily have to be physically connected.[5] Alterations in connectivity are suggestive of neurologic or psychological disorders. This article discusses methods and approaches used to describe resting-state brain connectivity.

Typically, fMR imaging has a spatial resolution of about 3 to 6 mm, but BOLD-activated images are often overlaid on higher resolution, 1 mm, anatomic MR imaging. The almost instantaneous electrochemical response to stimuli that occurs in neurons takes about 10 seconds to be seen as the metabolic or vascular analog, the HRF. Therefore, a temporal resolution of 500 to 3000 ms is sufficient to answer most research questions. BOLD hemodynamic response is a transient signal. Fundamental signal processing shows that it can be expressed in both the temporal and frequency domain, which comes with limitations.[6]

This article attempts to describe many analytical methods for resting-state functional connectivity. When research questions are posed, 1 of 2 methods is used: hypothesis-driven or data-driven investigation. The model-driven approach requires an a priori understanding of neuroanatomy or science or physiology, whereas data-driven methods make no assumptions or inquiries about the neural system. Analysis can be further divided by time, frequency, and time-frequency domains. The final differentiation is the level of analysis: single subject or group. Model type, domain, and level must be considered before using any analytical method.

Since its advent and implementation, functional imaging has helped answer the questions that have for so long perplexed humanity about the workings of the brain, the black box in our heads. Functional mapping of the brain is a complex and at times overwhelming endeavor. This may complement the actual sequencing of human genetics, which was completed in about a decade. The Human Connectome Project launched in 2010 by the National Institutes of Health has many aims, including understanding resting-state functional connectivity. Many of the techniques described here are used to aid researchers in the fulfillment of this scientific objective.

METHODS

Functional connectivity is defined as temporal correlation between spatially remote neurophysiological events. The methods of analysis by which these connections are quantified can be classified as temporal or frequency analysis. Both are useful and provide different and yet complementary information during the analysis. Temporal analysis of fMR imaging provides information on changes that can occur over a given timeseries, whereas the spectral content tells the frequency at which events occur over the same timeseries. Analysis can also be categorized into model-driven and data-driven methods, and both can include time and frequency domain analysis. Model-driven approaches are useful when experimenters have some prior knowledge of the system under investigation. In data-driven models, the data provide the information, no assumptions are made about the system, mathematical and statistical algorithms are simply applied over the whole brain, and subsequent scientific conclusions are made. Prevalent methods and potential pitfalls and limitations of each, are described. To circumvent these limitations, multiple methods should be used.

Domain	Model-Driven	Data-Driven
Temporal	Seed-based correlation, multiple regression or GLM	ICA, PCA, ReHo
Frequency	Coherence	ALFF, fALFF
Time-Frequency		Wavelet transform coherence, STFT, FOCA

Temporal Domain Methods

Temporal methods provide information on how signal changes over a specific time, and thus can indicate temporal changes. Many of the oldest and most commonly used techniques are in the temporal domain, such as the model-driven seed-based approach. Other widespread data-driven methods are regional homogeneity (ReHo), principle component analysis (PCA), and independent components analysis (ICA).

Seed-based correlation

Seed-based correlation is among the oldest and simplest functional connectivity analytical methods. It is used with the assumption that if regions are temporally correlated they should be functionally connected. Usually, a region of interest (ROI) or seed is chosen, the timeseries of the seed is correlated with all other voxels in the brain.[7,8] A connectivity map of the correlations is produced. Selection of the seed does require a priori knowledge of the system. Some of the pitfalls of this method are in the selection of the seed, which needs to be very spatially specific. This requires much prior knowledge of neuroscience, which ultimately introduces experimental bias. Selection of the same ROI across subjects requires training for reduced intersubject variability.

Regional homogeneity

ReHo analysis, much unlike ROI analysis, does not require prior knowledge of fundamental neurologic systems and anatomy. Like ROI analysis, ReHo is a method for mapping underlying connectivity activations; however, instead of quantifying spatial-temporal correlations between ROIs, ReHo assesses interconnectivity from the distances of voxels with its neighbors, using Kendall's statistical correlation. First proposed by Zang and colleagues[9] in 2004, ReHo works with the assumptions that a given voxel is temporally homogenous to its neighbor and modulations in cognitive tasks can been seen as changes in ReHo. It is a voxel-by-voxel data-driven approach. The timeseries of a voxel is correlated with its immediate neighbors, and this is performed simultaneously for each voxel. Spatial extent of its neighbors can be defined by the cluster size, typically 27 voxels. Kendall's correlation coefficient (KCC) is used to measure the correlation between a given voxel and its neighbors. A whole brain map is created that shows underling connectivity activations of clusters. Results of ReHo can be affected by the extent of spatial smoothing applied to functional image, as well as the cluster size used in KCC. Large smoothing and cluster size can yield false positives and, therefore, image quality is important

in this analysis. Despite this, ReHo is robust against noise (Equation 1).[10]

$$W = \frac{\sum (R_i)^2 - n(\overline{R})^2}{\frac{1}{12}K^2(n^3 - n)} \qquad (1)$$

W is the KCC among given voxels, ranging from 0 to 1; R_i is the sum rank of the ith time point, where the mean of the R_i is; K is the number of timeseries within a measured cluster (here, K = 7, 19, and 27, respectively; 1 given voxel plus the number of its neighbors); and n is the number of ranks.

Four-dimensional consistency of local neural activities

Four-dimensional consistency of local neural activities (FOCA) is a recent method proposed by Dong and colleagues[10] in 2014 that is both a frequency and a temporal analytical method. It is a derivative of ReHo and, as such, aims to circumvent its limitations. Whereas ReHo and other methods rely solely on temporal correlations, FOCA incorporates both temporal and spatial correlates into the analysis. A mean cross-correlation of the voxel of interest with its 27 neighbors is calculated in both temporal, Ct and spatial, Cs domain. The convolution of these means is the FOCA value of the voxel. A FOCA value for each voxel can be calculated creating a whole brain map. To reduce subject variability, the map is normalized by the whole brain mean FOCA, producing a FOCA norm for each subject. Because FOCA is derived from correlations in the temporal and spatial realms, it is influenced by temporal filtering and spatial smoothing, respectively. To get around this, these steps can be removed from the preprocessing pipeline, but this requires imaging data to be of high quality, restricting data sets. For data of poorer quality, Dong and colleagues[10] suggest that correlation Cs be calculated from unfiltered smooth data and Ct from unsmoothed filtered data. FOCA quantifies local spatial-temporal homogenous patterns, which can indicate neural connectivity.

Principle component analysis

A signal processing technique of data reduction where large amounts of high-dimensional data are reduced to components that retain most of the variability of the original data.[2] The first components are identified that that account for most of the variability in the dataset, and subsequent components are attributed to less and less of the variability, until no components remain. This iterative approach creates orthogonal relations between components. When applied to resting-state fMR imaging data, components should be representative of activation patterns that can be interpreted as intrinsic resting-state connectivity networks. These networks are produced without any prior assumptions. Limitations of PCA are that, orthogonality, a component is not independent of the next and, therefore, if a signal of interest is very small it will likely be misrepresented. Additionally there is no clear statistical evaluation of the significance of each component, making it difficult to determine noise from data.[2] To circumvent some of these issues, independent component analysis (ICA) can be used.

Independent components analysis

ICA is a temporal, data-driven approach that looks for the existence of statistically independent spatial-temporal maps across the brain. PCA is the precursor to ICA because this approach extracts the common components across the data; unlike PCA it does not assume Gaussian distribution. One of the major challenges in ICA is the assignment of spatial maps to neurologic function (Fig. 1).

Frequency Domain Methods

Frequency domain methods of analysis allow researchers to understand the spectral content of a signal. Information on period signals can reveal underlying connectives that cannot be captured in the time domain. Commonly used methods are the model-driven, coherence, and data-driven amplitude of low-frequency fluctuations (ALFFs), as well as its more refined counterpart, fractional ALLF (fALFF).

Coherence analysis

Coherence analysis is the frequency analog to seed-based correlation. Correlation maps are sensitive to the hemodynamic response function, which can vary across subjects and brain regions, as well as to high levels of biological noise. Cardiac, vasculature, and respiratory fluctuations can produce false positives in correlation maps. Coherences, $Coh_{x,y}(\lambda)$, are the spectral representation of the correlation in the frequency domain.[11] It is defined as the square of the cross-spectrum over the product of 1 timeseries power spectrum times the other. This allows for the study of time course because known artifacts can be easily filtered from the data (Equation 2).

$$Coh_{x,y}(\lambda) = \frac{|F_{x,y}(\lambda)|^2}{F_{x,x}(\lambda)F_{y,y}(\lambda)}$$

$$F_{x,y}(\lambda) = \sum_u Cov_{x,y}(u) \times e^{-j\lambda u}$$

$$F_{x,x}(\lambda) = \sum_u Cov_{x,x}(u) \times e^{-j\lambda u}$$

(2)

$$F_{y,y}(\lambda) = \sum_u Cov_{y,y}(u) \times e^{-j\lambda u}$$

Fxy is the cross-spectrum, the Fourier transform of the cross-covariance of Fx and Fy. Fxx and Fyy are the power spectrum of time series Fx and Fy respectively.[11]

Amplitude of low-frequency fluctuation or fractional amplitude of low-frequency fluctuation

The phenomenon of spontaneous resting-state low-frequency BOLD fluctuations (0.01–0.08 Hz)

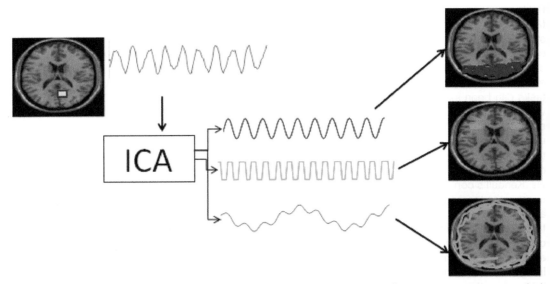

Fig. 1. Schematic flow of ICA analysis. A single timeseries of one voxel extracts the common components, which can be mapped to brain networks.

was shown to be correlated with functionally related regions.[7] The analytical method for investigating this phenomena is ALFF, which works with the assumption that all the relevant neurologic information in the BOLD signal can be represented by a single parameter. This parameter is calculated by averaging the square root of the power of low-frequency BOLD signals, and standardizing the values to a global mean ALFF value. ALFF is highly influenced by background noise, and a high value can be produced around vasculature and the edges of the brain.

To account for some of the limitations of ALFF, a more refined technique, known as fALFF, has been developed. fALFF is defined as the ratio of the power at each frequency to the integrated power of the entire frequency range across the frequency of interest 0.01 to 0.08 Hz range, then dividing by the amplitude sum across a more inclusive range of 0 to 0.25 Hz. This approach does not include band pass filtering and, like its predecessor, concerns about biological artifacts still remain.[12]

Time-Frequency Domain Methods

These methods combine the techniques of time and frequency domains, allowing researchers to study a signal simultaneously in both domains. Often, signals and their transforms are closely related; therefore, studying a signal as a whole rather than 2 separate parts can yield greater insight into the temporal fluctuations in resting-state connectivity. The more prevalent analytical methods are short-time Fourier transform (STFT), wavelet analysis, and the previously noted, more recent, FOCA.

Short-time Fourier transform
STFT is used to observe the frequency and phase content of large sinusoidal signals. The signal is divided into shorter segments of equal length and a discrete Fourier transform is applied, over a window length.[13] The changing spectral content is plotted as a function of time, thus providing information on observed frequency changes and the time-locked corresponding stimuli. This analysis is highly subjective to the size of the window length over which the signal is transformed.

Wavelet transform coherence
Wavelet transform coherence (WTC) measures coherence in the time-frequency domain, and the phase lag between 2 signals as a function of both time and frequency.[14] This is particularly useful in observing nonstationary changes between timeseries. Convolution of the timeseries

with scaled and translated versions of the wavelet function, ψ_o, result in the decomposition of the fMR imaging timeseries into time-frequency domain. This transform, W^x, expresses the amount of power in a signal as a function of time and frequency, where its angle represents the local phase shift (Equation 3).[15]

$$\psi_o(\eta) = \pi^{-1/4} e^{i\omega_0\eta} e^{-\eta^2/2}$$

$$W^x(n,\ s) = \sqrt{\frac{\Delta t}{s}} \sum_{n'=1}^{N} x_n \psi_o^* \left[(n'-n)\left(\frac{\Delta t}{s}\right)\right]$$

(3)

ψ_o is the wavelet function to be convolved with the fMR imaging timeseries. The wavelet W^x is the transform of the timeseries.

Single-Subject Analysis

The analytical methods should all be performed after preprocessing, which can be performed with various software; Statistical Parametric Mapping (SPM), FMRIB Software Library (FSL), Brain Voyager, and Analysis of Functional NeuroImages (AFNI) are commonly used. The standard preprocessing pipeline of functional images involves realignment of images to a particular slice; coregistration to anatomic image, if available, normalized into standard Montreal Neurologic Institute Talairach and Tournoux (MNI/TT) space; and application of a Gaussian spatial smoothing, regression out of motion parameters, and temporal filtering. In many software packages, the first stage in all fMR imaging studies is often referred to as first-level analysis. Many of the methods mentioned can be used for subject level analysis, including seed-based or ROI, ReHo, FOCA, and ICA or PCA. Subsequent descriptive statistics are often used to demonstrate the efficacy of the fMR imaging task design.

GROUP-LEVEL ANALYSIS

These different analytical approaches can be used on an individual subject level; however, like many research questions, answers can be found on a group level. Some of these include the very popular general linear model (GLM) regression analysis, dual regression, and the more complex graph theory.

Regression Analysis

Regression analysis works with the core assumption that the data can be explained by a combination of a linear model consisting of several regressors and residual noise. Each known regressor is given a weight, beta (β), value that represents how much weight the regressor contributed to the timeseries. For fMR imaging data (Y), the regressors are convolved with known HRFs with subsequent evaluation of the statistical significance of the regressor and its ability to explain the residual noise (ε), which is known as GLM. GLM uses cost functions (X) to evaluate how close the modeled data fit the actual data; ideally the error term should be negligible (Equation 4)

$$y_i = \beta_1 X_{i1} + \beta_2 X_{i2} + \beta_3 X_{i3} + ...X_{ij}\beta_j + \varepsilon_i \qquad (4)$$

y_i is observation i; X_{ij} is value i for predictor variable j, β_j is parameter estimate for predictor variable j, and ε_i is error for observation i.

$$Y = \beta X + \varepsilon \qquad (5)$$

GLM regressions for a single timeseries (Equation 4) and whole brain (Equation 5).[16]

Dual Regression

Dual regression is a combination of seed-based regression and multisubject ICA that can be used when comparing group-level spatial maps. Group-level ICA maps are generated and used as spatial regressors in the GLM, a normalized time course is extracted from each group-level map, which is also regressed out to find subject-specific differences.

Graph Theory

Graph theory is a large-world level of analysis that attempts to link the many brain networks into 1 complex system. It lays down the theoretic framework for these complex topographic networks to be examined. It can provide a better understanding of local and global organization of resting-state networks.[5] In graph theory, functional networks can be defined as (Equation 6)

$$G = (V, E) \qquad (6)$$

Where G is functional brain networks; V, nodes for each brain region; and E, functional connections between those regions.

A node or ROI can be defined using any of the various functional analytical methods previously described, and all functional connections with in the node (V) and other areas of the brain can be found. Subsequently functional connections between various nodes (E) can also be found. The choosing of nodes is model-driven, much like seed-based analysis. Connections between nodes can be weighted by various coefficients, including path length, clustering coefficient, node degree, degree of node distribution, centrality, and modularity. Path length is the average of how close a node is connected to every other node. Clustering coefficients describe local connectivity, that is, how close neighboring nodes are connected to each other. Node degree describes the number of connections to it; highly connected nodes are known as Hubs. Hubs with a high level of centrality have key roles in the overall efficiency of the network; likewise those with high modularity indicate increase within network connections, subnetworks.

Many studies have shown that the brain has a small-world organization, defined as high levels of local connectedness with short travel distances between nodes. All in all, the human brain is optimized to have high levels of local and global efficiency. Studying this can be helpful in understanding pathologic conditions that are thought to alter efficiency of connections.

RESULTS

The methods previously described have been implemented and reported in many notable publications, expanding the knowledge of resting-state connectivity in both healthy and diseased cohorts. Changes in connectivity have typically been seen in neurodegenerative disorders such as Alzheimer disease (AD), dementia, multiple sclerosis, and amyotrophic lateral sclerosis; behavioral disorders such as attention-deficit hyperactivity disorder, attention deficit disorder, and autism spectrum disorder; and psychiatric disorders such as schizophrenia, depression, bipolar disorder, and addictions.

Healthy Subjects

Typical neurologically developing healthy control populations are essential to resting-state research. Any insight uncovered about groups must be compared with controls. Many of the resting-state functional networks were first described in healthy subjects. For accurate assessment of the degree of deviation from the norm, it is imperative that the norm be accurately represented, especially in neuroscience research in which there are many degrees of variability: age, gender, race or ethnicity, education, and individual brain morphology. When conducting research, it is important to reduce as much variability as possible between subject pools so that any results obtained are true of the particular differences under investigation, and not noise. Statistical test are important when making such scientific claims.

Following analysis, parametric statistical tests are performed. Typical fMR images can have upwards of 300,000 voxels and 200 timeseries for each, in which each voxel is a gross approximation of 1 mm of cubic brain matter. These large numbers provide researchers greater spatial resolution, ultimately granting less refutability of the results. Because the changes in activation are on a neural level, and smaller than the voxel sizes, multiple comparison corrections are used to reduce the risk of detecting pseudoactivation (false-positives, type II error). Examples include family-wise error rate, false discovery rate, Bonferroni correction, and Monte Caro simulation. For all tests, the standard level of significance is usually set at $P<.05$, in which P is probability of type II error being less than 5%. Following these tests, common parametric hypothesis testing is done to observe whether there are significant differences between groups. The type of test used depends on the research questions posed and number of groups. The most common in fMR imaging data are the t-test, comparing differences between 2 groups; the F-test; and analysis of variance (ANOVA) for multiple group comparison, followed by post hoc test.

In healthy populations, the strength and weakness of analytical approaches can be tested and compared. A 2012 paper by Rosazza and colleagues[17] compared the results of ICA and its temporal analog, seed-based correlation, on 40 healthy subjects, and they found that ICA with 20 components yielded the most significant correspondence between the 2 techniques, suggesting that both methods are valid and, typically, both are used.

Diseased Populations

Degenerative and psychological neurologic disorders are explored, each with different clinical pathologic features and demographics. Publications about these atypical populations using the analytical methods have yielded significant results related to resting-state connectivity in diseased populations, particularly changes in known resting-state networks.

Alzheimer Disease

AD is a neurodegenerative disease that typically affects older (>65 years) populations. It is the progressive loss of memory and cognition, characterized clinically as the atrophy of brain matter. There are currently no treatments that can reverse the disease or alter prognosis once diagnoses has been made. With little to be done on the treatment end, neuroscientists have delved into understanding the mechanism of the disease.[18]

In a paper using a cohort of 14 subjects with AD and 14 age-matched and gender-matched healthy controls, a ReHo analysis was performed, followed by a t-test.[19] Results showed that AD patients had significant ReHo decreases in the posterior cingulate cortex and precuneus (PCC-PCu), as well as increases in the occipital and temporal lobes, including the bilateral cuneus, right lingual gyrus, and left fusiform gyrus. PCC-PCu is a major hub of the default mode network (DMN) and these decreases are correlated with cognitive scores, decreases in hypometabolism, and increased tissue atrophy.[19] Early-stage AD patients have been noted to have decreases in metabolism and perfusion in the medial parietal cortex, which encompasses PCC and PCu.[20–22] Occipital and temporal lobe increases have been observed in other studies that show activation during visual spatial processing.[23] This suggests that in the early stages of AD there is a compensatory mechanism for cognitive tasks.[24]

In 2008, Supekar and colleagues[25] used WTC applied to 90 ROIs for each subject. The transformation was computed by calculating the coefficient between the transformed signals and frequency band (0.01–0.05 Hz). Graph theory metrics were applied to the frequencies that showed loss of small-world organization; low clustering and high path length were seen in AD. This study shows evidence of global reorganization of the brain in AD with loss of small-world properties, which are analogous to loss of cognitive function. What was once an efficient network becomes less so as path length has to increase to recruit other brain regions that are still healthy.[18,26,27] ReHo and WTC are both used to rationalize the clinical pathologic features of AD.

Using a sample data set from the Alzheimer Disease Neuroimaging Initiative (Azeez and Biswal, unpublished data, 2017), the authors compared subjects aged 60 and older who had early and late-onset dementia with matched neurotypical controls. We used the analytical methods ALFF or fALFF, ReHo, ICA, and simple activation maps.

Mean activation maps of patients with early-stage and late-stage dementia were compared with age-matched neurotypical controls. From the data, we concluded that, in early stages of dementia, there is much recruitment of brain areas to neurologically compensate for loss of cognitive functions. As the disease progresses, there is a loss of whole brain activation. It is restricted to the cerebellum compared with the neurotypical population who show no activations. These results parallel those of AD in the literature (Fig. 2).

On the same data set, the authors also performed analysis of ALFF and fALFF. The resulting maps show some of the pitfalls of ALFF (higher power in around the edges due to noise), but fALFF mitigates this. These results reflect that of the literature in that there is some sort of compensatory mechanism during the early stages of the disease;

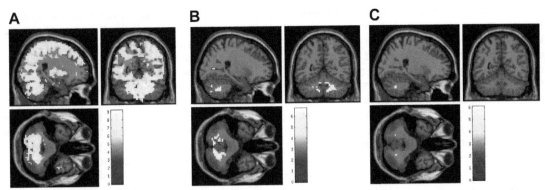

Fig. 2. Mean activation maps: (A) early-onset dementia, (B) late-onset dementia, (C) neurotypical controls.

there seems to be a recruitment of lower power frequencies (Fig. 3).

ReHo map results are less conclusive, but this is the nature of resting-state connectivity analysis, hence the need for many different analytical methods (Fig. 4).

Schizophrenia

Schizophrenia is a major psychotic disorder. First described over 100 years ago by Dr Kraepelin, it is characterized by the presence of diverse symptoms that include distorted perception of reality, disorganized behavior, avolition, and flat or inappropriate affect.[28] The clinical presentation of schizophrenia can include positive or negative symptoms. Positive symptoms are disturbances added to a patient's personality: delusions; hallucinations; and disordered thinking, speech, and behavior. Negative symptoms describe personal character traits that are lost from the patient, including emotional flattening, social withdrawal, and extreme apathy.[29,30]

In an attempt to blindly differentiate schizophrenic patients (n = 22, 24.54 ± 6.70 years) from aged matched health controls (n = 22, 26.09 ± 6.47 years), a whole brain, voxel-wise ROI correlation analysis was performed using 90 predefined regions, and known nuisance covariates were regressed out. A 90 by 90 spatial matrix was produced. Pearson correlation

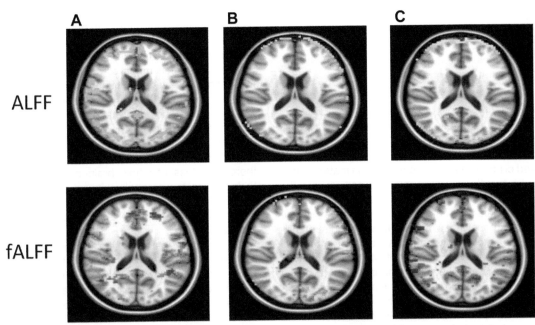

Fig. 3. ALFF and fALFF maps: (A) early-onset dementia, (B) late-onset dementia, (C) neurotypical controls.

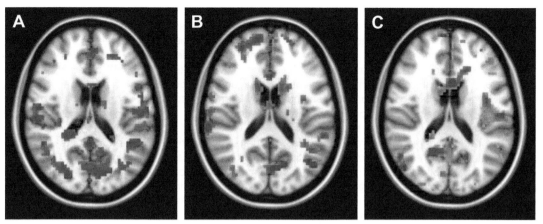

Fig. 4. ReHo maps: (*A*) early-onset dementia, (*B*) late-onset dementia, (*C*) neurotypical controls.

coefficients were used to evaluate the connectivity between pairs of ROIs. Results of the analysis showed that schizophrenic cohorts had altered functional connectivity in the visual, default mode (decrease within network), and sensorimotor networks.[31]

Arbabshirani's[32] 2013 paper also attempts to differentiate schizophrenic patients from neurotypical controls, using an ICA approach. Subjects' data were preprocessed and ICA was applied, temporally coherent networks were extracted, and corresponding maximally independent spatial maps were also extracted. A total of 20 components was extracted, excluding those of artifacts (vascular and motion). Relevant networks that remained (auditory, visual, motor, DMN, and both frontal-parietal networks) were converted into Fisher Z-maps. Functional resting-state connectivity was computed using the functional network connectivity toolbox (http://mialab.mrn.org/software/#fnc). It calculates the maximum lagged correlations across components. Results show that mean correlations between auditory and visual, and auditory and motor, was only significant in controls, and reduced within network connectivity of the DMN.

Low-amplitude frequency oscillation abnormalities were observed in schizophrenic subjects. In a cohort of 55 subjects (29 schizophrenic patients), Hoptman and colleagues[33] used both fALFF and ALFF following standard preprocessing. With fALFF, they reported reduced amplitude in the lingual gyrus, left cuneus, left insula or superior temporal gyrus, and right caudate; and increased fALFF in the medial prefrontal cortex and the right parahippocampal gyrus. ALFF reductions were noted in lingual gyrus, cuneus, and precuneus; and increases were noted in the left parahippocampal gyrus.

Resting-state analysis of schizophrenic patients has shown alterations in network connectivity and frequency oscillations. All of the methods used (ROI, ICA, and fALFF or ALFF) provide quantitative neurologic measures for a highly diverse psychological disorder. Deviations from clinical controls help explain some of the clinical symptoms of the disorder. Cognitive and emotional disturbances, abnormal filtering of visual information, dysfunctions of working memory, and motor and sensory control may all be explained by alternation in the DMN, and visual, auditory, and sensory motor networks.[31] For low-oscillatory amplitudes, areas of decrease are associated with defects in motor and sensory processing and reward sensitivity. Likewise, areas of increased frequency oscillations are linked to self-directed thought, leading to the hypotheses that deregulation and emphasis on internal stimuli results in hallucinations, all hallmarks of schizophrenia.[33]

DISCUSSION

Spontaneous synchronized fluctuations in time, despite distance, are the essence of functional connectivity. It is a concept that has only recently entered into the domain of computational neuroscience. The neurologic basis is that, if 2 (or more) regions are correlated temporally, they must working in tandem when executing neurologic functions. This postulation helped to contribute to what are now known as resting-state networks.

Resting-state functional connectivity is defined as the synchronization of brain regions with one another.[3] It refers to a temporal dependence of neuronal activity of regions which are not necessarily physically connected.[5] Alterations in connectivity suggest neurologic or psychological disorders. This article has discussed methods and approaches used to describe connectivity.

Alterations in these network indicate disease states. Many neurologic diseases, with their variety of clinical pathologic features and affected demographics, can be difficult to identify in patients, especially when the diagnostic process is subjective. Functional connectivity provides quantifiable measures for diagnosis. This, in the long term, leads to quicker and more accurate diagnoses, and, ultimately, the chance of early intervention and treatment. Publications and strides made in AD and schizophrenia, and applications of resting-state analytical approaches that have been used to make conclusions regarding these illness, were discussed.

Since the initial publication on resting-state functional connectivity,[4,34] many networks have been reported, each with its own unique neural spatial map and psychophysiological representation. In 1995, the sensorimotor network was first reported by Biswal and colleagues,[7] in which BOLD fluctuations in the left sensorimotor cortex correlated with changes in the right sensorimotor cortex, as well as the right supplementary motor area and right premotor area; all regions that automatically respond to sensorimotor stimuli. One of the most common resting-state networks is the DMN. DMN encompasses the precuneus or posterior cingulate, lateral parietal area, and mesial prefrontal cortex.[35] It has been linked to the processing and integration of cognitive, emotional, and physical information, as well as mind wandering.[5] It is most active during rest conditions, and deactivated during tasks. It is also influenced by the task performed before the network is active, suggesting some learned effects. The network has also been observed in primates. Other sensory networks include the auditory network, which covers areas involved in audition, such as the superior temporal gyrus, Heschl gyrus, insula, and postcentral gyrus.[35] The primary visual network has subnetworks, that is, mesial and lateral visual networks.[5,35] The mesial visual network encompasses the striate cortex and extrastriate regions located in the medial occipital lobe, such as lingual gyrus. These areas are closely associated with higher order visual processing, recruiting frontal lobe areas that play a role in the integration of visual spatial features.[36] The lateral visual network is involved in simpler processes, such as object recognition. Frontal parietal networks are lateralized to both hemispheres. These networks include the inferior frontal gyrus, the medial frontal gyrus, the precuneus, the inferior parietal, and the angular gyrus, which are associated with

cognition, memory, language, attention, and visual processing. Less is known about this network because its components in the prefrontal and parietal regions have overlapping cognitive functions. A study by Albert and colleagues[37] suggested that the network is affected by learned motor tasks, suggesting that effects of learning still remain. The temporal parietal network is thought to reflect the intrinsic functional connectivity between cognitive and language processing, covering areas linked with language processing and comprehension, for example, inferior frontal gyrus, medial temporal gyrus, superior temporal gyrus, and angular gyrus.[35] The executive control network is most active in working memory, recruiting regions of the medial frontal gyrus, superior frontal gyrus, and anterior cingulate cortex for these tasks. Little activation of this network is seen in the resting state, therefore it cannot be used as indication of rest.

fMR imaging data is complex and dynamic, and often it is difficult to distinguish between true positives and false positives; the different types of analytical approaches used and subsequent statistical analysis allow researchers to separate these. Model-driven methods focus on molding the data to fit a predefined model, whereas the data-driven approaches try to extract features that can have a neurologic explanation. Within the 2 approaches, analysis can be conducted in either the time or frequency domain. Each method has its strengths and weakness; ultimately it is up to the researcher to determine which method will best help to answer the questions they ask. It is important to know and understand these methods, especially when comparing findings across studies.

As neural engineering or statistical or science research evolves, researchers can reflect on the progress that has been made. In the last 20 years, the number of funded studies and publications on fMR imaging, which are noteworthy accomplishments, have skyrocketed. These are exciting times, and researchers are merely standing on the precipice of discovery with new and improved analytical techniques being invented and used daily, all for the expansion of neural connectivity knowledge. An understanding is slowly growing of the neurologic and psychological conditions that are thought to be caused or manifested by altered functional connectivity, as well as a general understanding of how things work in neurotypical control populations. The brain and its functions are elusive entities that, it can be argued, are more mysterious than the cosmos. These only began to be revealed in the last part of the twentieth century, with the help of technological advancements and human curiosity pushing the boundaries of the unknown.

REFERENCES

1. Ogawa S, Lee TM, Kay AR, et al. Brain magnetic resonance imaging with contrast dependent on blood oxygenation. Proc Natl Acad Sci U S A 1990;87(24):9868–72.
2. Huettel SA, Song AW, McCarthy G. Functional magnetic resonance imaging, vol. 1. Sunderland (MA): Sinauer Associates; 2004.
3. Shen HH. Core concept: resting-state connectivity. Proc Natl Acad Sci U S A 2015;112(46):14115–6.
4. Biswal B, Yetkin FZ, Haughton VM, et al. Functional connectivity in the motor cortex of resting human brain using echo-planar MRI. Magn Reson Med 1995;34(4):537–41.
5. van den Heuvel MP, Hulshoff Pol HE. Exploring the brain network: A review on resting-state fMRI functional connectivity. Eur Neuropsychopharmacol 2010;20(8):519–34.
6. Flandrin P. Time-frequency/time-scale analysis, vol. 10. San Diego: Academic Press; 1998.
7. Biswal B, Yetkin FZ, Haughton VM, et al. Functional connectivity in the motor cortex of resting human brain using echo-planar MRI. Magn Reson Med 1995;34:537–41.
8. Blueprint, N. Overview of the Human Connectome Project. Available at: http://www.humanconnectome.org/about/project/. Accessed August 31, 2017.
9. Zang Y, Jiang T, Lu Y, et al. Regional homogeneity approach to fMRI data analysis. Neuroimage 2004;22(1):394–400.
10. Dong L, Luo C, Cao W, et al. Spatiotemporal consistency of local neural activities: a new imaging measure for functional MRI data. J Magn Reson Imaging 2015;42(3):729–36.
11. Li K, Guo L, Nie J, et al. Review of methods for functional brain connectivity detection using fMRI. Comput Med Imaging Graph 2009;33(2):131–9.
12. Cole D, Smith S, Beckmann C. Advances and pitfalls in the analysis and interpretation of resting-state FMRI data. Front Syst Neurosci 2010;4:8.
13. Okamura S. The short time Fourier Transform and local signals. Pittsburgh (PA): Carnegie Mellon University; 2011. Available at: http://repository.cmu.edu/cgi/viewcontent.cgi?article=1065&context=dissertations.
14. Torrence C, Compo GP. A practical guide to wavelet analysis. Bull Amer Meteor Soc 1998;79(1):61–78.
15. Chang C, Glover GH. Time-frequency dynamics of resting-state brain connectivity measured with fMRI. Neuroimage 2010;50(1):81–98.
16. Kiebel S, Holmes A. The general linear model. In: Frackowiak RSJ, Friston KJ, Frith CD, et al, editors. Human brain function. 2nd edition. London: Academic Press; 2003. p. 725–60.
17. Rosazza C, Minati L, Ghielmetti F, et al. Functional Connectivity during Resting-State Functional MR Imaging: Study of the Correspondence between Independent Component Analysis and Region-of-Interest–Based Methods. AJNR Am J Neuroradiol 2012;33(1):180–7.
18. Staff, M. C. Alzheimer's disease. Available at: http://www.mayoclinic.org/diseases-conditions/alzheimers-disease/home/ovc-20167098?utm_source=Google&utm_medium=abstract&utm_content=Alzheimers-disease&utm_campaign=Knowledge-panel. Accessed August 31, 2017.
19. He Y, Wang L, Zang Y, et al. Regional coherence changes in the early stages of Alzheimer's disease: A combined structural and resting-state functional MRI study. Neuroimage 2007;35(2):488–500.
20. Liu Y, Wang K, Yu C, et al. Regional homogeneity, functional connectivity and imaging markers of Alzheimer's disease: A review of resting-state fMRI studies. Neuropsychologia 2008;46(6):1648–56.
21. NIH. Components of the Human Connectome Project. Available at: http://www.humanconnectome.org/about/project/resting-fmri.html. Accessed August 31, 2017.
22. NIH. The Human Genome Project Completion: Frequently Asked Questions. 2010. Available at: https://www.genome.gov/11006943/human-genome-project-completion-frequently-asked-questions/.
23. Prvulovic D, Hubl D, Sack A, et al. Functional imaging of visuospatial processing in Alzheimer's disease. Neuroimage 2002;17(3):1403–14.
24. Backman L, Almkvist O, Nyberg L, et al. Functional changes in brain activity during priming in Alzheimer's disease. J Cogn Neurosci 2000;12(1):134–41.
25. Supekar K, Menon V, Rubin D, et al. Network analysis of intrinsic functional brain connectivity in Alzheimer's disease. PLoS Comput Biol 2008;4(6):e1000100.
26. Bassett DS, Bullmore E. Small-world brain networks. Neuroscientist 2006;12(6):512–23.
27. Sporns O, Honey CJ. Small worlds inside big brains. Proc Natl Acad Sci 2006;103(51):19219–20.
28. Goghari VM, Sponheim SR, MacDonald AW. The functional neuroanatomy of symptom dimensions in Schizophrenia: a qualitative and quantitative review of a persistent question. Neurosci Biobehav Rev 2010;34(3):468.
29. America, M. H. Schizophrenia. Available at: http://www.mentalhealthamerica.net/conditions/schizophrenia. Accessed August 31, 2017.

30. Kasai K, Iwanami A, Yamasue H, et al. Neuro-anatomy and neurophysiology in schizophrenia. Neurosci Res 2002;43(2):93–110.

31. Tang Y, Wang L, Cao F, et al. Identify schizophrenia using resting-state functional connectivity: an exploratory research and analysis. Biomed Eng On-Line 2012;11(1):50.

32. Arbabshirani MR, Kiehl KA, Pearlson GD, et al. Classification of schizophrenia patients based on resting-state functional network connectivity. Front Neurosci 2013;7:133.

33. Hoptman MJ, Zuo X-N, Butler PD, et al. Amplitude of low-frequency oscillations in schizophrenia: a resting state fMRI study. Schizophr Res 2010; 117(1):13–20.

34. Raichle ME, MacLeod AM, Snyder AZ, et al. A default mode of brain function. Proc Natl Acad Sci U S A 2001;98(2):676–82.

35. Rosazza C, Minati L. Resting-state brain networks: literature review and clinical applications. Neurol Sci 2011;32(5):773–85.

36. Yang Y-L, Deng H-X, Xing G-Y, et al. Brain functional network connectivity based on a visual task: visual information processing-related brain regions are significantly activated in the task state. Neural Regen Res 2015;10(2):298.

37. Albert NB, Robertson EM, Miall RC. The resting human brain and motor learning. Curr Biol 2009; 19(12):1023–7.

Graph Theoretic Analysis of Resting State Functional MR Imaging

John D. Medaglia, PhD

KEYWORDS

- Resting state fMR imaging • Graph theory • Connectome • Neuroimaging • Networks
- Network analysis

KEY POINTS

- Graph theory is the mathematical basis of network science and is now widely applied to study rsfMR imaging networks.
- Several major themes have emerged in applied rsfMR imaging graph theoretic analysis.
- rsfMR imaging graph theoretic analysis has revealed several key principles of healthy and dysfunctional brain network organization.
- Open frontiers in rsfMR imaging graph theoretic analysis includes evaluating the contributions of graph theory and potential for direct clinical applications.

INTRODUCTION

Given its complexity,[1] the brain is perhaps the quintessential example of a network. Neural elements are interconnected by a large number of connections that can be studied across several orders of spatiotemporal magnitude. One is apt to seek a framework that can help describe and understand brain organization, dynamics, and cognitive-behavioral phenomena. From the perspective of network science,[2] the brain is a special case of a larger space of natural and possible networks.[3] The mathematical basis in which one can represent and study networks is graph theory, which provides fundamental mathematical knowledge and a generalizable basis in which to study networks.

In human brain networks, one can apply graph theoretic analysis to anatomic or functional networks at multiple scales to study the connectome.[4] An essential tool in the effort to understand functional brain networks is functional MR imaging (BOLD fMR imaging), which allows one to indirectly study neural activity using the hemodynamic relationship between blood flow and neural firing in the brain.[5] BOLD fMR imaging is often used to examine contrasts between different cognitive conditions to examine changes in functional signal amplitudes and connectivity associated with behavior. In addition, and the focus of the current review, it is used to understand the intrinsic[6] organization of functional brain networks to study the brain at rest[7] and its relationship with cognition and behavior.

To say that a living brain is ever at rest is potentially misleading; indeed, brains persistently bustle with complex neural and metabolic activity. Resting state fMR imaging (rsfMR imaging) is broadly used to refer to data acquired when subjects are instructed to look at a crosshair fixation or engage in no task in particular while in the scanner.[7] In contrast to studies that involve tightly controlled experimental paradigms, rsfMR imaging studies involve data that represent any number of cognitive-emotional mental activities that

Disclosure Statement: The author has no disclosures to report.
Department of Psychology, University of Pennsylvania, 306 Goddard Building, Philadelphia, PA 19104, USA
E-mail address: johnmedaglia@gmail.com

Neuroimag Clin N Am 27 (2017) 593–607
http://dx.doi.org/10.1016/j.nic.2017.06.008
1052-5149/17/© 2017 The Author(s). Published by Elsevier Inc. This is an open access article under the CC BY-NC-ND license (http://creativecommons.org/licenses/by-nc-nd/4.0/).

participants may engage in while at rest. Indeed, rsfMR imaging is used to investigate processes, such as mind-wandering,[8] introspection,[9] and imaginative thought.[10] For these reasons, it has been suggested that less leading terminology, such as intrinsic connectivity, may be preferable in referring to "resting state" data.[6] Broadly, one can examine properties of network organization observable within rsfMR imaging to identify correlates of other cognitive variables and markers of dysfunction. Although care should be applied when interpreting rsfMR imaging connectomes, it is known that rsfMR imaging networks and network statistics are overall reliable enough to afford robust analysis of connectomic organization to examine major brain systems.[11,12] Here, I review major approaches to and findings from graph theoretic analysis of rsfMR imaging data.

DATA COLLECTION AND PREPROCESSING

Data collection for rsfMR imaging typically involves asking subjects to lie in the scanner with eyes open, closed, or fixated on a target in the center of the participant's visual field over several minutes of fMR imaging data acquisition (discussed later).[13] Preprocessing techniques ensure that data meet several assumptions before analysis. The most standard steps to preprocessing rsfMR imaging data include slice timing correction,[14] motion correction,[15,16] realignment,[17] coregistration of anatomic and functional images,[18] spatial normalization,[19] and smoothing.[20] Smoothing increases signal to noise, normalizes error distributions, and accommodates anatomic and functional variation between subjects. In addition, global signal regression (GSR), which refers to the statistical removal of the average signal across all voxels in the brain, is a contentious issue in rsfMR imaging analysis.[21,22] GSR can increase the detection of localized neural signals and improve functional connectivity analysis specificity.[23,24] However, GSR introduces negative correlations mean-centered around zero and may exclude important neural signatures.[21,25–27] Finally, rsfMR imaging time series are often examined after applying a bandpass filter to BOLD data to reduce influences of nonphysiologic and physiologic nuisance signals (often between 0.01 Hz and 0.1 Hz or similar). Because no model can perfectly separate physiologic nuisance variables from neurally related signals, one must be cautious in selection of GSR and bandpassing preprocessing techniques and appropriately discuss the limitations of each selection in empirical work. Readers are encouraged to consult primary sources for in-depth empirical analysis and discussion of preprocessing issues.

GRAPH THEORETIC ANALYSIS OF RESTING STATE FUNCTIONAL MR IMAGING DATA

Once data are obtained and preprocessed, any number of techniques can be applied to examine the organization of rsfMR imaging data. The primary conceptual distinction between graph theoretic analysis of rsfMR imaging and other approaches is that the former directly links rsfMR imaging to much broader efforts with deep mathematical foundations in graph theory. This allows one to share concepts and language with investigators interested in other types of networks and encourages the potential for innovative crosstalk. In the next section, I provide basic intuition for major ideas in graph theory analysis for rsfMR imaging data and findings from applied analysis.

GRAPHS IN RESTING STATE FUNCTIONAL MR IMAGING ANALYSIS

Graph theoretic analysis is a specific approach to analyzing brain networks in which the brain network is represented in the mathematical "graph." A graph G is composed of N nodes (or vertices) and E edges (region-region relationships). The graph G is encoded in an adjacency matrix, A, whose $(i,j)^{th}$ element represents the weight of the edge between node i and node j. The edges of a graph are binary (including only 0s and 1s) or weighted (including a range of other values). Graphs are undirected, where the association between regions is bidirectional, or directed, where the association between regions may vary across directions. In rsfMR imaging analysis, the elements of the adjacency matrix A most often include full correlation coefficients representing the strength of functional communication between two regions. The elements can alternatively include covariance, partial correlation, coherence, and mutualized information shared between pairs of brain regions.

To construct A, one must define the nodes between which edges are calculated. This is typically achieved by selecting a parcellation of rsfMR imaging data voxels into coarse-grained units called parcels, which reduces the number of nodes in the system for simplicity, statistical economy, and computational efficiency. Several notable parcellations are available defined by functionally[11,28,29] or anatomically validated features. The proliferation of and continued interest in developing parcellations highlights that there is no perfect parcellation established to date. Indeed, each parcellation relies on statistical optimization or anatomically based boundary definitions paired with intuitions about what matters in brain organization. It is essential to note that the absolute value of statistics in rsfMR imaging network analysis varies depending on the parcellation.[30] Thus, caution should be used in interparcellation comparisons and one should be well aware of the nature of the parcellation selected and rationale for selecting it.

Once the adjacency matrix is defined, one can apply a rich range of concepts and tools from graph theory to examine brain networks (**Fig. 1**). In the following sections, I introduce commonly applied network statistics across scales of network organization. The reader is also referred to other excellent reviews concerning graph theoretic analysis in general[31] and specific to brain networks.[32,33]

MICROSCALE, MESOSCALE, AND MACROSCALE NETWORK ANALYSIS

One of the advantages of applying a graph theoretic perspective is that it gives the ability to study intermediate and high levels of organization across the network as a whole. This is a fundamental distinction between rsfMR imaging and other approaches to functional brain network analysis: by allowing one to examine higher level statistics, one can identify properties of networks that are not evident in any particular node or edge and potentially what cognitive-behavioral processes they may support. The scales of network analysis can coarsely be separated into microscale, mesoscale, and macroscale, representing the configuration of the elements of the network, their modular configuration, and the overall topology of the network as a whole, respectively.

Microscale

The microscale refers to the organization of nodes and edges in the network. In rsfMR imaging data, each node statistical emphasizes complementary information about brain region roles in the functional connectome. One major notion in networks is that hubs serve central roles in network organization and information processing. To represent

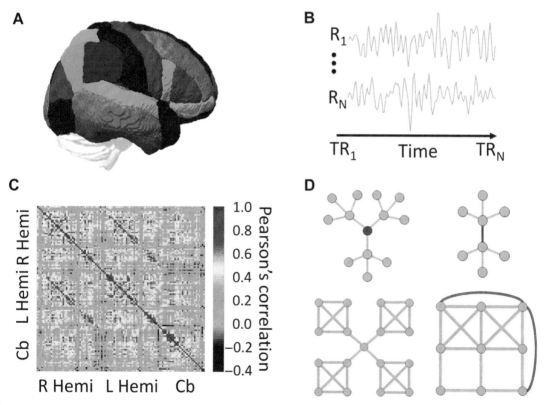

A

B

R_1

R_N

TR_1 Time TR_N

C

Cb   L Hemi   R Hemi

R Hemi   L Hemi   Cb

1.0
0.8
0.6
0.4
0.2
0.0
−0.2
−0.4

Pearson's correlation

D

Fig. 1. Schematic flow for graph theoretic analysis of rsfMR imaging data. (*A*) Nodes are established with a parcellation representing distinct parts of the brain. (*B*) After preprocessing, time series of BOLD measurements from nodes (regions; *R*) R_1 to R_N are extracted along time for time points (*TRs*) TR_1 to TR_N. (*C*) Then adjacency matrix *A* can be constructed to represent measures of connectivity, such as the Pearson correlation coefficient. (*D*) Finally, one can compute measures representing the role of nodes and edges, community organization, and global characteristics of the *A* matrix. Cb, cerebellum; Hemi, hemisphere; L, left; R, right.

this, hub coefficients[34,35] constructed from measures of node centrality have been used to quantify nodes' connectedness in the network, involvement in short paths across the network (betweenness centrality), connectedness with local neighbors (clustering coefficient or local efficiency), connectedness to important nodes in the network (eigenvector centrality), and interactions with multiple communities in the functional network (participation coefficient). Each of these statistics emphasizes a distinct aspect of nodes' varying roles in organizing information processing across the brain. In rsfMR imaging data, one can examine variation in node centrality across the brain and distinct groups to identify characteristic hub roles for nodes (Fig. 2).

Perhaps the simplest measure of node centrality is degree. In binary networks, degree is defined as the number of edges connected to a node. In weighted networks, the weighted degree (or strength) is the sum of edge weights connected to a node. Nodes of high degree or strength centrality are thought to be particularly influential on the network's function. In rsfMR imaging networks, nodes with high degree are referred to as network hubs, and are thought to be critical for general information transmission and circuit-level computing.[36,37]

Other centrality statistics capture a node's role in network organization beyond node-to-node connections. Commonly used examples include betweenness centrality, closeness centrality, and eigenvector centrality. Betweenness centrality quantifies the extent to which a node participates in shortest paths throughout the network. A shortest path is the path between node i and node j that traverses the fewest (or in weighted networks the fewest high-weight) edges. Nodes with high betweenness centrality are thought to be particularly influential across different efficient pathways of the network as a whole rather than just local direct connections. Closeness centrality quantifies the average shortest path between a given node and all other nodes in the graph. As a result, closeness centrality is used as a measure of a node's ability to communicate broadly to every node in the network. Eigenvector centrality uses the eigenspectrum of the adjacency matrix to quantify the influence of a node based on its connectedness with other high-scoring nodes in a network (Fig. 3). This statistic recursively captures the importance of a node: nodes that are connected to important nodes rank higher in eigenvector centrality. Because each of these statistics putatively identify highly central nodes, nodes that score high on these statistics are sometimes referred to as hubs given their theoretic role in network function.[38]

Some node statistics are designed to capture the role of nearby neighbors in the neighborhood (one step in topologic distance) around the node. The clustering coefficient describes how close its nearest neighbors are to being a completely connected subgraph or clique. One specific example is the local clustering coefficient, which is defined as the number of triangles in the network containing a node, divided by the number of connected triples containing that same node.[39] With this definition, the local clustering coefficient gives the density of local connections involving a given node and is often used to probe the node's ability to participate in local information integration. A complementary notion is that of node efficiency, which assesses the connectedness of the edges among neighbors of a given node, thus offering a notion of the network's local robustness to a node's removal.[40]

In addition to quantifying features of a node and its role in the network, one might also be interested in quantifying features of an edge. Perhaps the simplest statistic for an edge is its weight, which provides information about the strength of the relationship between two nodes. Moving beyond pairwise information, one can also compute something like the edge betweenness centrality, which measures the number of shortest paths between all possible pairs of nodes that pass through the edge of interest. Similar to the betweenness centrality of a node, the betweenness centrality of an edge is thought to represent its importance in efficient information transfer in networks. These are just a couple of examples of useful statistics for edges that can help one to understand the role

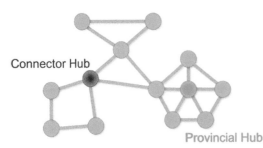

Connector Hub

Provincial Hub

Fig. 2. Notions of hubs in networks. Provincial hubs are high-degree nodes that primarily connect to nodes in the same module. This provincial hub is also a hub of high degree overall because it has a high number of connections relative to other nodes in the network and contributes to many paths through the network. Connector hubs are high-degree nodes that show a diverse connectivity profile by connecting to several different modules within the network (see also[35]).

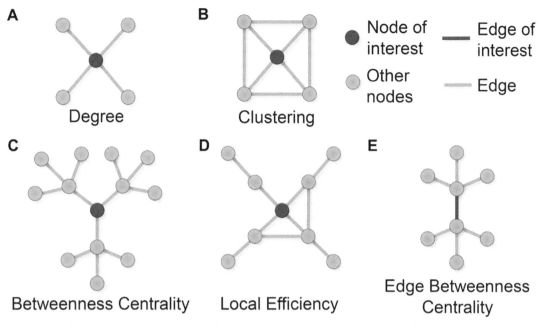

Fig. 3. Example microscale statistics. The *red node* in each image denotes the node of interest. (*A*) A node's degree is the number of edges emanating from a node. (*B*) The node has a high clustering coefficient because the node's neighbors are also connected to each other. (*C*) The *red node* has high betweenness centrality because it participates in many paths. In this case, the *red node* also has high eigenvector centrality because it is connected to three other nodes with high importance in the network. (*D*) In this illustration, the local efficiency for the node of interest is low because few connections exist among the immediate neighbors of the node of interest. (*E*) The *red edge* has high betweenness centrality because of its position along a high number of paths across the network.

of a node-node relationship in the broader network.

Mesoscale

Mesoscale organization refers to the arrangement of nodes into modules or communities. Mesoscale structure is that which is not easily characterized at either the local (node and edge) or global (entire network) scales. Networks may exhibit varying degrees and qualities of modular structure (also known as community organization), which refers to high within- and low between-module connectivity. A network exhibits a varying degree of modularity that can be quantified as the extent to which nodes exhibit nontrivial community organization relative to network null models.[41]

A contrasting mesoscale organization in networks is core-periphery structure, which refers to the tendency for a network to have a core of densely interconnected nodes surrounded by a periphery of nodes that connect to the core but not to one another. Put differently, an extreme of this is a single large module with more sparsely connected individual nodes attached to the module. More modular networks theoretically maintain

a balance of information integration within and segregation between modules, whereas core-periphery structure can offer more centralized processing.[42]

In natural networks, mesoscale networks can exhibit community organization in which individual modules have mixtures of characteristic modular, core-periphery, or assortative organization. An assortative network is one in which like-degree nodes tend to connect to one another, and a disassortative network is one in which unlike-degree nodes tend to connect to one another. In some networks, assortativity is a marker of robustness: the removal of one high-degree node is overcome by the interconnectedness of the others.[43,44] Promising techniques, such as stochastic block models,[45] allow one to identify the organization of network communities along these organizational subtypes and describe their potential diversity of network function (**Fig. 4**).

Macroscale

Another key notion in graph theory is that networks can be represented holistically, potentially described with single scalar values representing

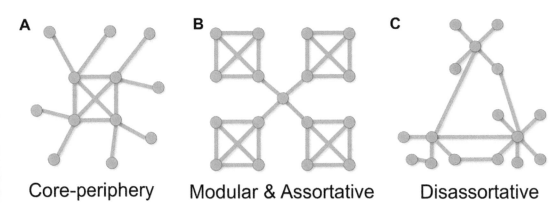

Fig. 4. Example mesoscale statistics. (*A*) A core-periphery organization involves a low number of primary modules (here marked by a single module of nodes sharing teal edges) and several sparsely connected peripheral nodes. (*B*) In contrast, a modular organization involves a few modules connected by a few intermediating nodes. In this example there is a single node that serves as a so-called "connector hub" between the modules. This network is also assortative because the highly connected nodes tend to connect to one another. (*C*) A disassorative network does not exhibit a high degree of connectivity among like nodes, and tends to be nonmodular.

a property of the network. This is a form of emergent feature of a system that is not represented in any particular part. To represent this, global statistics are important to characterize overarching network organizational principles. Perhaps the simplest statistic is a network's density: the number of existing edges relative to the number of possible edges. Many natural networks exhibit low density because edges are costly.[46] Relatedly, one often studied characteristic of a network is the shape of its degree (or strength) distribution. Long-tailed degree distributions indicate that unexpectedly large hubs exist. As within individual modules, it is often interesting to ask whether these hubs preferentially connect to one another across the entire network, forming a basis for macroscale assortativity analysis.[43]

In addition, one can examine whether a network is scale-free, which means that a network has a degree distribution that follows a power law.[47] Scale-free networks can emerge from theoretic mechanisms including preferential attachment[48] and node fitness,[49] or rules that copy a fraction of links to existent nodes.[50] Regardless of the mechanism of generation, scale-free networks are notable because they represent economical architectures for information transmission.[46] They are also robust against random damage but especially vulnerable to targeted attack to high-degree nodes.[51] Many natural networks demonstrate approximately scale-free degree distributions[52] that are characterized by power laws over some regimes of their degree distribution.[53]

Another way to describe macroscale organization is to average the values of nodal statistics. For example, a network's global clustering coefficient is equal to the average clustering coefficient of that network's nodes. High global clustering in a network indicates that nodes tend to be highly connected across all possible cliques larger than two nodes. The characteristic path length refers to the average shortest path between all pairs of nodes in the network. A short characteristic path length is thought to represent the potential for high integration across the network.[54] Global efficiency is a notion that is complementary to the characteristic path length, and is calculated as the inverse of the harmonic mean of the shortest paths in the network.[40,55] A network with a smaller characteristic path length has a higher global efficiency, indicating a theoretic ability to communicate quickly across the network as a whole.[56]

A composite statistic representing a network's tendency to exhibit higher than expected clustering and shorter than expected path lengths is famously known as small-worldness.[54] Small-world network organization theoretically supports a balance of local segregated information processing in modules in conjunction with long distance integrating processing across modules. Many small-world networks are also scale-free.[57] One problem with calling a network "small-world" is that all networks fall on a continuum of this property and it is not often robustly defined in network analysis.[58] Because small-worldness is a continuous property that is defined by the clustering and path length in networks, it is important to interpret the contribution of both of these statistics to the small-worldness of the system. A statistically rigorous definition of small-worldness for weighted networks is small world propensity, which has been validated but not yet widely applied in brain network analysis.[58]

If one is interested in studying not just the shortest path but also longer paths or walks through the network, then one might examine a generalization of network communicability.[59] Communicability describes all shortest paths and all walks (steps along the network including revisitations to nodes and edges) connecting two nodes. This accounts for the possibility that communication can occur in a network involving both the shortest path and longer and indirect paths across the network. This property may be interesting as a complement to other measures associated with network resilience. For example, nodes and networks with increased communicability may exhibit more robustness to the loss of specific edges because multiple pathways for communication exist across the nodes.

One feature of global network organization is the minimum spanning tree (MST), which is a subset of edges in a connected, weighted, undirected graph that connects all nodes together without any cycles and the minimum possible total edge weight.[60] Thus, the MST of a graph represents the least total cost architecture associating all nodes to one another with no redundancy. The size and configuration of a graph's MST is analyzed to identify efficient organization in network topology and its temporal and cross-sectional variation.

In practical network analysis, it is important to note that raw measures of global network organization are heavily influenced by the network's density (or total node strength), and it is therefore important to normalize or statistically control for graph density (strength) before making statistical inferences across networks or in relation to extrinsic variables, such as clinical status or cognition in the context of rsfMR imaging analysis. This allows one to examine the unique contributions of network topology above and beyond simple network density (**Fig. 5**).

MAJOR FINDINGS IN RESTING STATE FUNCTIONAL MR IMAGING GRAPH THEORETIC ANALYSIS

Graph theoretic analysis has been applied broadly in rsfMR imaging in healthy and clinical populations to examine intrinsic network organization and how variations in intrinsic graph properties relate to cognition and clinical syndromes. From these studies, it is known that (1) not all rsfMR imaging is created equal, (2) that human rsfMR imaging networks exhibit a complex organization that supports cognitive activity, and (3) is altered in clinical populations.

Not All Resting State Functional MR Imaging Is Equal

rsfMR imaging is a misnomer given that the brain is a persistently active system with a rich cognitive repertoire. Neurophysiologically, the link between neural field potentials and BOLD is greater in eyes closed relative to open conditions in animal models, suggesting that visual and attention-related cognitive demands modulate hemodynamic coupling.[25,61] In addition, important differences in connectivity are observed across eyes closed, eyes open, and fixation cross rsfMR imaging collection designs. In eyes closed conditions, connectivity within the auditory network is higher than the other conditions. Connectivity within default-mode, attention, and auditory networks are more reliable when eyes are fixated on a cross. In an eyes open condition without a fixation cross, visual network connectivity is most reliable.[13] This highlights that although rsfMR imaging data are thought to be

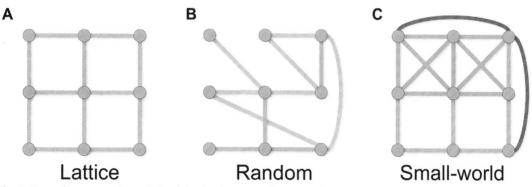

Fig. 5. Example macroscale statistics. (*A*) A lattice network is a regular network that has an example of high clustering but a long path length. (*B*) A random network tends to lack distinct modular organization but has short path lengths because of random connections across the network. (*C*) A small-world network has clustering and short path lengths because of the presence of clusters and long distance connections.

task-free, differences in how the rsfMR imaging paradigm is administered are associated with different network configurations, presumably as a function of differences in cognitive processing demands across the conditions. In addition, not all rsfMR imaging represents waking brain activity: 30% of rsfMR imaging data may be acquired during transient or sustained periods of sleep in the scanner.[13] Although eyes open and especially fixation cross designs reduce the incidence of sleep, it is an important potential confound to all rsfMR imaging analysis.[13] Thus, one should consider using fixation paradigms to help reduce the incidence of sleep in the scanner. One can also use technologies, such as eye tracking, self-report, and machine learning procedures, to identify potential sleep in the scanner.[13]

Human Brain Organization Maintains a Complex Balance Among Randomness, Small Worldness, and Modularity

In healthy humans, some major findings have resulted from rsfMR imaging network analysis. At a high level of organization, it is clear that healthy human brain networks exhibit economical sparse connectivity[46] and maintain a balance along extremes on dimensions of order, degree diversity, and heirarchy.[46,62] High order is reflected by the high clustering and modularity of brain networks, but the presence of some randomness is reflected in short path lengths that connect modules.[54,63]

rsfMR imaging networks exhibit truncated power law distributions,[30] demonstrating the presence of scale-free organization through some of the network's regime with a pronounced "rich-club" of hubs that are highly connected to one another.[64] Hubs are variably defined in the literature, but are typically characterized by an unexpectedly high number of connections given all connections observed in the entire network, within specific modules, and/or between modules,[35] and are thought to play key roles in regulating information processing across the network.[35] Step-wise functional connectivity analyses in rsfMR imaging data corroborate the view that the brain is organized hierarchically, involving connections spreading from regions in primary and secondary sensorimotor regions to multimodal integration regions and finally converging on cognitive hubs in the cortex. This suggests that classically defined neuropsychological functions across these regions are represented in a low-cost hierarchy that privileges dense communication between cognitive control and default mode regions and the rest of the brain (Fig. 6).

Resting State Networks form a Stable Organization Supporting Cognitive Function Within and Between Individuals

rsfMR imaging studies demonstrate a rich mesoscale organization involving reliably detectable intrinsic networks that are observed during rest

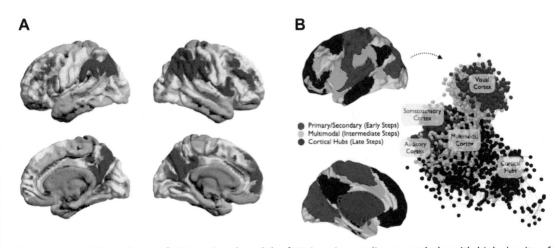

Fig. 6. Hubs and hierarchy in rsfMR imaging data. (A) rsfMR imaging studies report hubs with high density of functional connectivity in the precuneus/posterior cingulate cortex, lateral inferior parietal cortex, medial orbitofrontal cortex, and medial superior frontal cortex. (B) Step-wise functional connectivity analyses reveal a hierarchical progression of edges from primary motor and secondary sensorimotor regions to multimodal regions and finally hubs in the cortex. (Adapted from Zuo XN, Ehmke R, Mennes M, et al. Network centrality in the human functional connectome. Cereb Cortex 2012;22(8):1862–75; and Sepulcre J. Stepwise connectivity of the modal cortex reveals the multimodal organization of the human brain. J Neurosci 2012;32:10649–61.)

(Fig. 7).[28] These are often thought to represent systems with distinct cognitive roles, including frontoparietal and cingulo-opercular control networks, dorsal and ventral attention networks, a salience network, a default mode network, primary somatomotor systems, and subcortical systems. The cognitive relevance of these networks is suggested by the fact that they coactivate as units during distinct cognitive tasks.[65] Notably, connections between the frontoparietal control and other networks reconfigure most prominently across tasks, most notably in the left dorsolateral prefrontal cortex.[65] In addition, functional connections across the brain robustly predict cognitive activations among these systems during various tasks, suggesting that these systems form basic building blocks in high-level cognitive organization.[66] Patterns of connectivity can be used to accurately identify individuals and intersubject variability in intelligence from rsfMR imaging data connectivity "fingerprints,"[67] demonstrating a high information content in the brain's intrinsic profile.

Resting State Network Graph Characteristics Are Altered in Numerous Clinical Populations

Although major networks and organization are identified in healthy rsfMR imaging analyses, one can also examine whether graph theoretic analysis contributes to the characterization and understanding of clinical syndromes. A major review is outside the focus of this primer, and the reader is encouraged to consult several excellent reviews concerning graph theoretic analysis in neurologic and psychiatric syndromes.[62,68–71] So far, early studies span a wide range of syndromes with developmental, psychiatric, and neurologic mechanisms of origin. Findings indicate that rsfMR imaging analysis can indeed identify altered network topology in clinical syndromes over the lifespan. Emerging findings from rsfMR imaging analysis suggest that psychiatric and neurologic disorders across the lifespan are associated with altered intrinsic network organization. Across syndromes, disruptions in hub node activity are frequently identified, with common disruptions in cognitive control

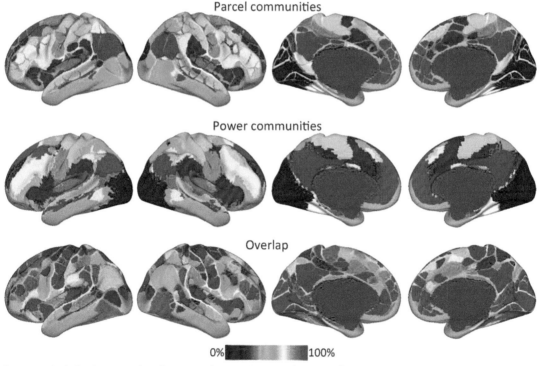

Parcel communities

Power communities

Overlap

0% ◼◼◼◼◼◼ 100%

Fig. 7. Intrinsic brain networks. The network organization of intrinsic fMR imaging networks forms a mesoscale organization replicated in two studies. (*Top*) Colors represent different communities identified with an "Infomap" community detection procedure using the boundary map-derived parcels as network nodes and an independent sample for cross-validation.[11] (*Middle*) Colors represent different communities calculated using every voxel as a network node.[28] (*Bottom*) Spatial overlap of the two community assignments demonstrates that systems demonstrate variable but generally high overlap. (*From* Gordon EM, Laumann TO, Adeyemo B, et al. Generation and evaluation of a cortical area parcellation from resting-state correlations. Cereb Cortex 2016;26(1):288–303.)

and default mode systems but notable differences in specific nodes across disorders.[62,70] Network efficiency is often disrupted via alterations of path length and mesoscale community organization.[46,70] Cognitively, general conscious activity may be supported by segregated information processing facilitated by specific functional hub organization,[72,73] and global cognitive function may depend on key long distance connections[74–76] and "connector" hubs that communicate between systems.[77] Emotionally, disrupted connectivity involving subcortical and frontal is associated with mood and anxiety syndromes and symptom profiles.[78,79] Although the number of studies for any specific disorder remains limited, it seems clear that rsfMR imaging can contribute a network-level perspective to characterize features associated with clinical diseases and disorders.

OPEN FRONTIERS IN RESTING STATE FUNCTIONAL MR IMAGING ANALYSIS

With the increase in rsfMR imaging analysis and its early promise in identifying correlates of clinical syndromes and symptoms, it is useful to clarify important theoretic frontiers and opportunities. One can potentially make great strides by studying the neural basis of rsfMR imaging graph organization, its theoretic contributions to cognitive and clinical neuroscience, its clinical utility, and integration with other techniques.

WHAT DOES RESTING STATE FUNCTIONAL MR IMAGING GRAPH ORGANIZATION REPRESENT?

It is prudent to reflect on the nature of rsfMR imaging data to evaluate its epistemologic value. Because rsfMR imaging analysis is based on the BOLD signal, there are fundamental limits to its neural interpretation from the microscale to macroscale. rsfMR imaging data are thought to represent high- and low-frequency local field potentials.[25] Beyond hemodynamic responses, how can one understand the specific network configurations observed in healthy brains? The fact that rsfMR imaging topology represents major cognitive systems may have a basis in environmental influences over development. There is evidence that rsfMR imaging network organization is a result of experience-dependent plasticity in humans following coactivation between brain regions.[80] This feature seems to persist in mature brain networks, where a simple connectivity model of activity flow among brain regions predicts network-level activation.[66] Combined with observations about the neurovascular coupling that drives widespread rsfMR imaging

activity, it is speculatively possible that intrinsic network organization is truly a robust marker of gross neurocognitive organization within and between individuals. This may be why cognitive variability is associated with intrinsic network activity. However, one must still be wary about drawing inferences about any specific cognitive activity during any particular scanning session.

One prevailing limitation in many studies is that BOLD-based graph edges are demonstrably low-dimensional when computed along entire time series and thus limited in their ability to represent brain interactions.[81] However, time-varying graph[82] and trial-wise analysis[83] are promising open areas that may add new dimensions of information to potentially link clinical nosology to brain network dynamics (Fig. 8). As these efforts develop, it will remain critical to pair rsfMR imaging analysis with good experimental designs, genetic and environmental analyses, and replication and cross-validation studies.

The unique theoretic value of graph theory rsfMR imaging analysis is at present unknown. Do the quantities afforded represent something cognitively meaningful in principle? Can they provide theoretic or predictive information one otherwise would not see? It is clear that one can continue to study brain organization and dysfunction without using graph theory. It is also possible, as it commonly done, to rely heavily on reverse inference[84,85] to interpret the graph statistics observed and previously known ideas from cognitive neuroscience. To identify specific value of graph theory, one should search for consilience between graph theoretic analysis and other neuroscientific approaches.[86]

OPTIMISM FOR CLINICAL IDENTIFICATION, PREDICTION, AND TRANSLATION

Nevertheless, a cautiously optimistic view of rsfMR imaging for some clinical purposes is justified if we maintain several priorities. The features that distinguish useful clinical research include problem base, context placement, information gain, pragmatism, patient centeredness, value for money, feasibility, and transparency.[87] Many studies do not satisfy these features and fail to provide value because of their design. It has been suggested that a major reform could address the forces that drive this problem, and the reader is strongly encouraged to consult one particularly incisive perspective.[87] As it stands, careful hypothesis testing for specific clinical end-goals should increase in general.[87]

Toward applied clinical utility, rsfMR imaging graph statistics analyzed can be combined with

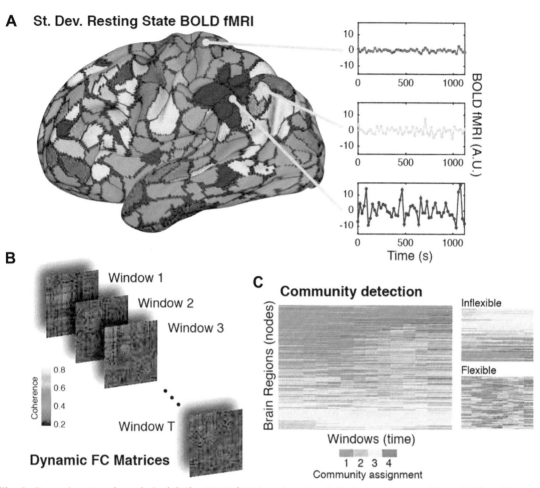

Fig. 8. Dynamic network analysis. (*A*) The BOLD fMR imaging signal displays region-specific variability. (*B*) Windowing time series and estimating the functional connectivity (FC) between pairs of regions reveals dynamic FC matrices. Each edge describes the statistical relationship (strength of connectivity) between two brain regions. The organization of FC matrices changes over time. (*C*) Dynamic FC matrices can be used as input to community detection algorithms to generate estimates of the network's modular structure at each time point. Modules, in this case, refer to collections of mutually correlated brain regions that, as a group, are weakly correlated with the rest of the network. One can characterize the dynamics of community structure in terms of individual brain regions and at the level of the whole network with the measure flexibility. Network flexibility indicates the extent to which brain regions change their community affiliation over time. A.U., arbitrary units. (*Adapted from* Mattar MG, Betzel RF, Bassett DS. The flexible brain. Brain 2016;139(8):2110–12.)

machine learning to build models that identify autism,[88] Alzheimer disease,[89,90] schizophrenia,[91] and depression,[92] relative to control subjects, in some cases with very high sensitivity and specificity. In general, the opportunities to apply machine learning to any type of neuroimaging data or derived measure are enormous and can provide novel observations.[93] The challenge in rsfMR imaging analysis is that to have clinical value, these approaches must be valid and replicable, portable to clinical environments, and either equally accurate to but cheaper than existing techniques, or demonstrably more accurate.

Integrated multimodal strategies offer potential value for treatment. For example, rsfMR imaging connectivity has been evaluated to guide or predict outcomes in neurosurgical approaches in brain injury,[94] brain tumors,[95] epilepsy,[96] and deep brain stimulation.[97] In addition, the effects of noninvasive brain stimulation have been linked to the connectivity profiles of intrinsic networks across many diseases. Specifically, suppressive transcranial magnetic stimulation is effective if the site of stimulation is positively connected with the target, whereas facilitative transcranial magnetic stimulation is effective in the opposite case.[98] Importantly, rsfMR imaging graph theoretic analyses have not been systematically linked to brain stimulation approaches to provide either neurocognitive criteria (eg, target brain network states for stimulation) or surgical or brain stimulation targeting methods. This is substantial potential for development on this front. It is possible that computer simulation models that use simplifications of neural dynamics in anatomic networks to predict rsfMR imaging connectivity[99–101] and the effects of stimulation[102] may contribute to this effort.

SUMMARY

Graph theoretic analyses in rsfMR imaging are becoming a significant tool for describing the human brain and characterizing clinical syndromes. It is becoming clear that clinical syndromes are marked by dysfunction in major brain networks and distinct hubs in intrinsic functional connectivity patterns. The specific contributions of rsfMR imaging to clinical nosology and translation will likely be understood with the benefits of hindsight. At present, the challenge is to embrace opportunities to robustly characterize network dysfunction and search for a meaningful framework to connect rsfMR imaging network analysis to clinical practice.

REFERENCES

1. Bassett DS, Gazzaniga MS. Understanding complexity in the human brain. Trends Cogn Sci 2011;15(5):200–9.
2. Lewis TG. Network science: theory and applications. Hoboken (NJ): John Wiley & Sons; 2011.
3. Bassett DS, Bullmore E. Small-world brain networks. Neuroscientist 2006;12(6):512–23.
4. Sporns O, Tononi G, Kötter R. The human connectome: a structural description of the human brain. PLoS Comput Biol 2005;1(4):e42.
5. Ogawa S, Lee TM, Kay AR, et al. Brain magnetic resonance imaging with contrast dependent on blood oxygenation. Proc Natl Acad Sci U S A 1990;87(24):9868–72.
6. Seeley WW, Menon V, Schatzberg AF, et al. Dissociable intrinsic connectivity networks for salience processing and executive control. J Neurosci 2007;27(9):2349–56.
7. Raichle ME, MacLeod AM, Snyder AZ, et al. A default mode of brain function. Proc Natl Acad Sci U S A 2001;98(2):676–82.
8. Mason MF, Norton MI, Van Horn JD, et al. Wandering minds: the default network and stimulus-independent thought. Science 2007;315(5810): 393–5.
9. Delamillieure P, Doucet G, Mazoyer B, et al. The resting state questionnaire: an introspective questionnaire for evaluation of inner experience during the conscious resting state. Brain Res Bull 2010; 81(6):565–73.
10. Beaty RE, Benedek M, Wilkins RW, et al. Creativity and the default network: a functional connectivity analysis of the creative brain at rest. Neuropsychologia 2014;64:92–8.
11. Gordon EM, Laumann TO, Adeyemo B, et al. Generation and evaluation of a cortical area parcellation from resting-state correlations. Cereb Cortex 2016;26(1):288–303.
12. Shehzad Z, Kelly AC, Reiss PT, et al. The resting brain: unconstrained yet reliable. Cereb Cortex 2009;19(10):2209–29.
13. Patriat R, Molloy EK, Meier TB, et al. The effect of resting condition on resting-state fMRI reliability and consistency: a comparison between resting with eyes open, closed, and fixated. Neuroimage 2013;78:463–73.
14. Parker D, Liu X, Razlighi QR. Optimal slice timing correction and its interaction with fMRI parameters and artifacts. Med Image Anal 2017;35:434–45.
15. Patriat R, Reynolds RC, Birn RM. An improved model of motion-related signal changes in fMRI. Neuroimage 2017;144:74–82.
16. Ciric R, Wolf DH, Power JD, et al. Benchmarking of participant-level confound regression strategies for the control of motion artifact in studies of functional connectivity. Neuroimage 2017;154:174–87.
17. Friston KJ, Holmes AP, Poline J, et al. Analysis of fMRI time-series revisited. Neuroimage 1995;2(1): 45–53.
18. Ashburner J, Friston K. Multimodal image coregistration and partitioning: a unified framework. Neuroimage 1997;6(3):209–17.
19. Ashburner J, Friston KJ. Nonlinear spatial normalization using basis functions. Hum Brain Mapp 1999;7(4):254–66.
20. Hagler DJ, Saygin AP, Sereno MI. Smoothing and cluster thresholding for cortical surface-based group analysis of fMRI data. Neuroimage 2006; 33(4):1093–103.
21. Murphy K, Birn RM, Handwerker DA, et al. The impact of global signal regression on resting state correlations: are anti-correlated networks introduced? Neuroimage 2009;44(3):893–905.
22. Murphy K, Fox MD. Towards a consensus regarding global signal regression for resting state functional connectivity MRI. Neuroimage 2017;154:169–73.
23. Fox MD, Snyder AZ, Vincent JL, et al. The human brain is intrinsically organized into dynamic, anti-correlated functional networks. Proc Natl Acad Sci U S A 2005;102(27):9673–8.
24. Smith SM, Fox PT, Miller KL, et al. Correspondence of the brain's functional architecture during

activation and rest. Proc Natl Acad Sci U S A 2009; 106(31):13040–5.

25. Schölvinck ML, Maier A, Frank QY, et al. Neural basis of global resting-state fMRI activity. Proc Natl Acad Sci U S A 2010;107(22):10238–43.

26. Saad ZS, Gotts SJ, Murphy K, et al. Trouble at rest: how correlation patterns and group differences become distorted after global signal regression. Brain Connect 2012;2(1):25–32.

27. Weissenbacher A, Kasess C, Gerstl F, et al. Correlations and anticorrelations in resting-state functional connectivity MRI: a quantitative comparison of preprocessing strategies. Neuroimage 2009; 47(4):1408–16.

28. Power JD, Cohen AL, Nelson SM, et al. Functional network organization of the human brain. Neuron 2011;72(4):665–78.

29. Shen X, Tokoglu F, Papademetris X, et al. Groupwise whole-brain parcellation from resting-state fMRI data for network node identification. Neuroimage 2013;82:403–15.

30. Wang J, Wang L, Zang Y, et al. Parcellation-dependent small-world brain functional networks: a resting-state fMRI study. Hum Brain Mapp 2009; 30(5):1511–23.

31. Newman MEJ. Networks: an introduction. Oxford: Oxford University Press; 2010.

32. Rubinov M, Sporns O. Complex network measures of brain connectivity: uses and interpretations. Neuroimage 2010;52(3):1059–69.

33. Bassett DS, Sporns O. Network neuroscience. Nat Neurosci 2017;20(3):353–64.

34. Achard S, Salvador R, Whitcher B, et al. A resilient, low-frequency, small-world human brain functional network with highly connected association cortical hubs. J Neurosci 2006;26(1):63–72.

35. van den Heuvel MP, Sporns O. Network hubs in the human brain. Trends Cogn Sci 2013;17(12): 683–96.

36. Sporns O. Networks of the brain. Cambridge (MA): MIT press; 2010.

37. Betzel RF, Gu S, Medaglia JD, et al. Optimally controlling the human connectome: the role of network topology. Sci Rep 2016;29(6):30770.

38. Sporns O, Honey CJ, Kötter R. Identification and classification of hubs in brain networks. PLoS One 2007;2(10):e1049.

39. Onnela JP, Saramäki J, Kertész J, et al. Intensity and coherence of motifs in weighted complex networks. Phys Rev E Stat Nonlin Soft Matter Phys 2005;71(6):065103.

40. Latora V, Marchiori M. Efficient behavior of small-world networks. Phys Rev Lett 2001;87(19):198701.

41. Mucha PJ, Richardson T, Macon K, et al. Community structure in time-dependent, multiscale, and multiplex networks. Science 2010;328(5980): 876–8.

42. Holme P. Core-periphery organization of complex networks. Phys Rev E Stat Nonlin Soft Matter Phys 2005;72(4):046111.

43. Newman ME. Assortative mixing in networks. Phys Rev Lett 2002;89(20):208701.

44. Newman ME. Mixing patterns in networks. Phys Rev E Stat Nonlin Soft Matter Phys 2003;67(2): 026126.

45. Martin T, Ball B, Newman ME. Structural inference for uncertain networks. Phys Rev E 2016;93(1):012306.

46. Bullmore E, Sporns O. The economy of brain network organization. Nat Rev Neurosci 2012; 13(5):336–49.

47. Barabási AL, Albert R. Emergence of scaling in random networks. Science 1999;286(5439):509–12.

48. Barabási AL, Albert R, Jeong H. Mean-field theory for scale-free random networks. Phys Stat Mech Appl 1999;272(1):173–87.

49. Albert R, Barabási AL. Statistical mechanics of complex networks. Rev Mod Phys 2002;74(1):47.

50. Kumar R, Raghavan P, Rajagopalan S, et al. Stochastic models for the web graph. Proceedings of 41st Annual Symposium on Foundations of Computer Science. Redondo Beach (CA), November 12–14, 2000, p. 57–65.

51. Albert R, Jeong H, Barabási AL. Error and attack tolerance of complex networks. Nature 2000; 406(6794):378–82.

52. Barabási AL. Scale-free networks: a decade and beyond. Science 2009;325(5939):412–3.

53. Clauset A, Shalizi CR, Newman ME. Power-law distributions in empirical data. SIAM Rev 2009;51(4): 661–703.

54. Watts DJ, Strogatz SH. Collective dynamics of 'small-world' networks. Nature 1998;393(6684): 440–2.

55. Latora V, Marchiori M. Economic small-world behavior in weighted networks. Eur Phys J B 2003;32:249–63.

56. Achard S, Bullmore E. Efficiency and cost of economical brain functional networks. PLoS Comput Biol 2007;3:e17.

57. Amaral LAN, Scala A, Barthelemy M, et al. Classes of small-world networks. Proc Natl Acad Sci U S A 2000;97(21):11149–52.

58. Muldoon SF, Bridgeford EW, Bassett DS. Small-world propensity and weighted brain networks. Sci Rep 2016;6:22057.

59. Estrada E, Hatano N. Communicability in complex networks. Phys Rev E Stat Nonlin Soft Matter Phys 2008;77(3):036111.

60. Graham RL, Hell P. On the history of the minimum spanning tree problem. Ann Hist Comput 1985; 7(1):43–57.

61. Pan WJ, Thompson GJ, Magnuson ME, et al. Infra-slow LFP correlates to resting-state fMRI BOLD signals. Neuroimage 2013;74:288–97.

62. Stam CJ. Modern network science of neurological disorders. Nat Rev Neurosci 2014;15:683–95.

63. Bassett DS, Bullmore ET. Small-world brain networks revisited. Neuroscientist 2016. [Epub ahead of print].

64. Van Den Heuvel MP, Sporns O. Rich-club organization of the human connectome. J Neurosci 2011; 31(44):15775–86.

65. Cole MW, Reynolds JR, Power JD, et al. Multi-task connectivity reveals flexible hubs for adaptive task control. Nat Neurosci 2013;16(9):1348–55.

66. Cole MW, Ito T, Bassett DS, et al. Activity flow over resting-state networks shapes cognitive task activations. Nat Neurosci 2016;19(12):1718–26.

67. Finn ES, Shen X, Scheinost D, et al. Functional connectome fingerprinting: identifying individuals using patterns of brain connectivity. Nat Neurosci 2015;18(11):1664–71.

68. Lee MH, Smyser CD, Shimony JS. Resting-state fMRI: a review of methods and clinical applications. AJNR Am J Neuroradiol 2013;34(10): 1866–72.

69. Bullmore E, Sporns O. Complex brain networks: graph theoretical analysis of structural and functional systems. Nat Rev Neurosci 2009;10(3): 186–98.

70. Bassett DS, Bullmore ET. Human brain networks in health and disease. Curr Opin Neurol 2009;22(4): 340–7.

71. Van Den Heuvel MP, Pol HEH. Exploring the brain network: a review on resting-state fMRI functional connectivity. Eur Neuropsychopharmacol 2010; 20(8):519–34.

72. Uehara T, Yamasaki T, Okamoto T, et al. Efficiency of a "small-world" brain network depends on consciousness level: a resting-state fMRI study. Cereb Cortex 2014;24(6):1529–39.

73. Achard S, Delon-Martin C, Vértes PE, et al. Hubs of brain functional networks are radically reorganized in comatose patients. Proc Natl Acad Sci U S A 2012;109(50):20608–13.

74. van den Heuvel MP, Sporns O. An anatomical substrate for integration among functional networks in human cortex. J Neurosci 2013;33(36):14489–500.

75. Markov NT, Ercsey-Ravasz M, Lamy C, et al. The role of long-range connections on the specificity of the macaque interareal cortical network. Proc Natl Acad Sci U S A 2013;110(13):5187–92.

76. Pandit AS, Expert P, Lambiotte R, et al. Traumatic brain injury impairs small-world topology. Neurology 2013;80(20):1826–33.

77. Warren DE, Power JD, Bruss J, et al. Network measures predict neuropsychological outcome after brain injury. Proc Natl Acad Sci U S A 2014; 111(39):14247–52.

78. Zhang J, Wang J, Wu Q, et al. Disrupted brain connectivity networks in drug-naive, first-episode major depressive disorder. Biol Psychiatry 2011; 70(4):334–42.

79. Ye M, Yang T, Qing P, et al. Changes of functional brain networks in major depressive disorder: a graph theoretical analysis of resting-state fMRI. PLoS One 2015;10(9):e0133775.

80. Guerra-Carrillo B, Mackey AP, Bunge SA. Resting-state fMRI: a window into human brain plasticity. Neuroscientist 2014;20(5):522–33.

81. Marrelec G, Messé A, Giron A, et al. Functional connectivity's degenerate view of brain computation. PLoS Comput Biol 2016;12(10):e1005031.

82. Mattar MG, Betzel RF, Bassett DS. The flexible brain. Brain 2016;139(8):2110–2.

83. Liu X, Chang C, Duyn JH. Decomposition of spontaneous brain activity into distinct fMRI co-activation patterns. Front Syst Neurosci 2013; 7:101.

84. Poldrack RA. Inferring mental states from neuroimaging data: from reverse inference to large-scale decoding. Neuron 2011;72(5):692–7.

85. Poldrack RA. Can cognitive processes be inferred from neuroimaging data? Trends Cogn Sci 2006; 10(2):59–63.

86. Mill RD, Ito T, Cole MW. From connectome to cognition: the search for mechanism in human functional brain networks. Neuroimage 2017.

87. Ioannidis JP. Why most clinical research is not useful. PLoS Med 2016;13(6):e1002049.

88. Zhou Y, Yu F, Duong T. Multiparametric MRI characterization and prediction in autism spectrum disorder using graph theory and machine learning. PLoS One 2014;9(6):e90405.

89. Koch W, Teipel S, Mueller S, et al. Diagnostic power of default mode network resting state fMRI in the detection of Alzheimer's disease. Neurobiol Aging 2012;33(3):466–78.

90. Khazaee A, Ebrahimzadeh A, Babajani-Feremi A. Identifying patients with Alzheimer's disease using resting-state fMRI and graph theory. Clin Neurophysiol 2015;126(11):2132–41.

91. Fekete T, Wilf M, Rubin D, et al. Combining classification with fMRI-derived complex network measures for potential neurodiagnostics. PLoS One 2013;8(5):e62867.

92. Sacchet MD, Prasad G, Foland-Ross LC, et al. Support vector machine classification of major depressive disorder using diffusion-weighted neuroimaging and graph theory. Front Psychiatry 2015;6:21.

93. Varoquaux G, Thirion B. How machine learning is shaping cognitive neuroimaging. Gigascience 2014;3(1):28.

94. Böttger J, Margulies DS, Horn P, et al. A software tool for interactive exploration of intrinsic functional connectivity opens new perspectives for brain surgery. Acta Neurochir (Wien) 2011;153(8):1561–72.

95. Sair HI, Yahyavi-Firouz-Abadi N, Calhoun VD, et al. Presurgical brain mapping of the language network in patients with brain tumors using resting-state fMRI: comparison with task fMRI. Hum Brain Mapp 2016;37(3):913–23.

96. Osipowicz K, Sperling MR, Sharan AD, et al. Functional MRI, resting state fMRI, and DTI for predicting verbal fluency outcome following resective surgery for temporal lobe epilepsy. J Neurosurg 2016;124(4):929–37.

97. Figee M, Luigjes J, Smolders R, et al. Deep brain stimulation restores frontostriatal network activity in obsessive-compulsive disorder. Nat Neurosci 2013;16(4):386–7.

98. Fox MD, Buckner RL, Liu H, et al. Resting-state networks link invasive and noninvasive brain stimulation across diverse psychiatric and neurological diseases. Proc Natl Acad Sci U S A 2014; 111(41):E4367–75.

99. Honey C, Sporns O, Cammoun L, et al. Predicting human resting-state functional connectivity from structural connectivity. Proc Natl Acad Sci U S A 2009;106(6):2035–40.

100. Hermundstad AM, Brown KS, Bassett DS, et al. Structurally-constrained relationships between cognitive states in the human brain. PLoS Comput Biol 2014;10(5):e1003591.

101. Hermundstad AM, Bassett DS, Brown KS, et al. Structural foundations of resting-state and task-based functional connectivity in the human brain. Proc Natl Acad Sci U S A 2013;110(15): 6169–74.

102. Muldoon SF, Pasqualetti F, Gu S, et al. Stimulation-based control of dynamic brain networks. PLoS Comput Biol 2016;12(9):e1005076.

Machine Learning Applications to Resting-State Functional MR Imaging Analysis

John M. Billings, MD[a,b], Maxwell Eder, BS[a,b],
William C. Flood, BA[a,b], Devendra Singh Dhami, MS[c],
Sriraam Natarajan, PhD[c],
Christopher T. Whitlow, MD, PhD, MHA[a,b,d,e,*]

KEYWORDS

- Machine learning • MR imaging • Computer science • Function MR imaging
- Resting state function MR imaging

KEY POINTS

- Machine learning is one of the most exciting and rapidly expanding fields within computer science.
- Both academic and commercial research entities are investing heavily in machine learning for personalized medicine via individual patient level classification.
- Machine learning methods combined with resting state fMRI (rs-fMRI) will aid in diagnosis of disease and guide potential treatment for a number of conditions heretofore thought to be impossible to identify based on imaging alone.

INTRODUCTION

Machine learning is broadly one of the most exciting and rapidly expanding fields within computer science that is now being applied across industries to solve problems conventionally thought of as unsolvable by computers. Academic and commercial research entities are investing heavily in machine learning methods, especially in the health care sector for personalized medicine via individual patient-level classification of disease. There is great promise that machine learning methods combined with resting state function MR imaging (rs-fMR imaging) will aid in the diagnosis of disease and guide potential treatment for a number of conditions that historically were thought to be impossible to identify based on imaging alone, such as psychiatric disorders. Additionally, these methods allow scientists to identify anatomic information and connectome-related clues that may help to direct future research efforts. Mild cognitive impairment (MCI) and Alzheimer's disease (AD) are perhaps the conditions most studied using a machine learning approach,

[a] Radiology Informatics and Image Processing Laboratory (RIIPL), Wake Forest School of Medicine, Medical Center Boulevard, Winston-Salem, NC 27157, USA; [b] Division of Neuroradiology, Department of Radiology, Wake Forest School of Medicine, Medical Center Boulevard, Winston-Salem, NC 27157, USA; [c] School of Informatics and Computing, Indiana University, Informatics East Building, Room 257, 919 E. 10th Street, Bloomington, IN 47408, USA; [d] Department of Biomedical Engineering, Wake Forest School of Medicine, Medical Center Boulevard, Winston-Salem, NC 27157, USA; [e] Clinical and Translational Sciences Institute (CTSI), Wake Forest School of Medicine, Medical Center Boulevard, Winston-Salem, NC 27157, USA
* Corresponding author. Division of Neuroradiology, Department of Radiology, Wake Forest School of Medicine, Medical Center Boulevard, Winston-Salem, NC 27157.
E-mail address: cwhitlow@wakehealth.edu

Neuroimag Clin N Am 27 (2017) 609–620
http://dx.doi.org/10.1016/j.nic.2017.06.010

because these conditions benefit from early intervention and have a significant impact on quality of life.[1] However, the application of machine learning methods to neuroimaging, and specifically rs-fMR imaging, offer significant potential across a broad range of neurologic, psychiatric, and developmental conditions. Perhaps one of the most exciting advances has been the ability for machine learning methods to go beyond group prediction based on the general linear model, with significant progress in generating inference at an individual patient level, allowing a mechanism to translate advanced neuroimaging methods, such as rs-fMR imaging, into routine clinical practice. In this article, we discuss common machine learning methods (ie, support vector machines, random forests, and artificial neural networks), and then explore recent advances that have been made in machine learning as it applies to rs-fMR imaging.

MACHINE LEARNING OVERVIEW
Support Vector Machines

Support vector machines (SVMs) are supervised machine learning algorithms that learn a model from fully annotated data and then evaluate the model using test data. Supervised models can be described as learning a function $f(x) = y$, where y is the label (also called class) of the data (0 and 1 for binary data) and x denotes the attributes of these examples (also called features). In general, there are different types of functions f learned, a direct function (f), discriminative probabilistic model ($P(y|x)$), or a generative model ($P(y,x)$). Another possible classification of these machine learning methods could be based on the type of decision boundaries that they learn between different classes, namely, linear or nonlinear.

Fig. 1 shows different functions (linear functions in this example) that can be learned for a given set of points. The lines shown in **Fig. 1** are simple classifiers that consider 2 features to separate the positive and negative classes. The best line is chosen from several possibilities according to some optimization criteria (typically training set performance). When extending this to multiple features, the lines become hyperplanes.

The specific function that is learned in SVMs is a hyperplane, which then gives rise to the concept of margins. SVM algorithms find the function (hyperplane) that returns the largest minimum distance to the examples. This distance is called a *margin*, and the examples closest to the margins are then termed "support vectors." In **Fig. 2**, the circled points are the support vectors and r is the distance of an example to the separating line. The dotted lines passing through these points represent the margin and r that is the distance between the support vectors is the width of the margin. Because the solution depends only on the support vectors, SVM models maximize the width of the margin. The SVM model defined above is the "hard margin" SVM, because the width of the margin is fixed, which is the maximum distance between the nearest examples on both sides of the linear separator, which assumes that the data are linearly separable. In the real world, the data are often nonseparable, that is, there exists no linear function that can separate the data completely. In such cases, we learn a variant of the SVM model known as "soft margin" SVMs, where misclassifications are minimized with respect to the margin by adding a loss function. The value of the loss function is 0 when there are no misclassified examples. Alternatively, the loss function is proportional to the distance of the example from the

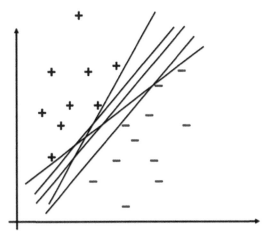

Fig. 1. Example of different linear functions for a given set of points.

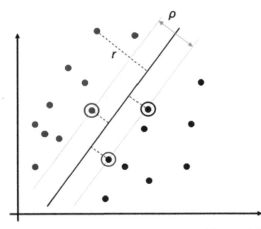

Fig. 2. Margins in an support vector machine model.

margin in case of misclassified examples. A popular way to work with nonlinear data in SVM models is by applying kernel functions, which map the data points to a higher dimension where they become linearly separable as shown in **Fig. 3**. The intuition is that the examples that are not linearly separable in the original feature space will become linearly separable in higher dimensional space, and the SVMs can then be used to classify the examples in this space (**Table 1**).

Random Forests

Random forests are popular ensemble methods that rely on the principle of combining multiple and diverse hypotheses, and can potentially lead to much more robust models than learning a single monolithic model. The key idea is that these hypotheses are themselves better than random guessing and will possibly cancel out the random errors that allow for correct decisions to be made. Random forests are 1 set of ensemble methods that learn multiple decision trees (the number of decision trees constructed is a parameter of the algorithm during the learning phase) and then combine the predictions of all the decision trees together to produce a final model (**Fig. 4**). The "random" in random forest comes from the fact that every decision tree is learned with a random subset of examples from the total examples in the data. The model combiner is the majority vote (**Table 2**).

Artificial Neural Networks

The concept of artificial neural networks is inspired by the interconnected nature of neurons in the human brain that carry electric signals back and forth from the brain. An artificial neural network has several layers of interconnected neurons that forms an artificial network consisting of 3 main types of layers (**Fig. 5**; if the "hidden layer" is absent, the model is called a perceptron). Each input node is connected by a weighted connection to every node in the hidden layer, which in turn is connected to the output layer by another set of weighted connections. The hidden layer can itself consist of a number of hidden layers, with each node connected to all the nodes in the next hidden layer. The output layer node consists of a function that converts the weights from the hidden layer into a binary value, y belonging to $\{0, 1\}$ or $\{-1, 1\}$ (as specified by the user). This final conversion is achieved by summing the weighted values according to the connections from the hidden layer(s). Recent developments have made these networks "deep" in that they have added more hidden layers and the power of computers allows them to be learned effectively (**Table 3**).

CLINICAL APPLICATIONS USING MACHINE LEARNING AND RESTING STATE FUNCTIONAL MR IMAGING
Mild Cognitive Impairment and Alzheimer's Dementia

MCI is defined as an intermediate stage along the continuum of normal age-related cognitive decline and the more severe decline of dementia. Clinically, MCI does not cause significant degradation of daily functioning; humans have significant cognitive reserve. This quality may delay diagnosis, allowing disease to progress to the point of dementia, where daily functioning is impacted, having serious ramifications on a patient's quality

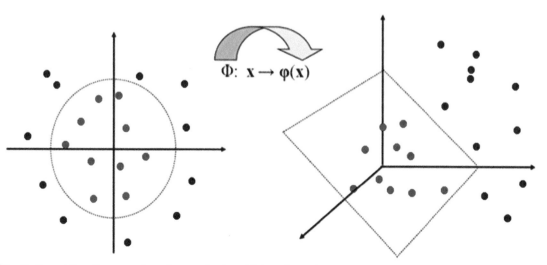

Fig. 3. Kernel function mapping of examples to a higher dimension.

Table 1
Advantages and disadvantages of SVMs

Advantages	Disadvantages
Nonlinear data types can be modeled with the use of kernel methods by SVMs. These have been very popular for many challenging tasks in the past decade.	Requires setting of many parameters and heavily dependent on choosing a good kernel for nonlinear data; typically requires a machine learning expert rather than a domain expert.
Kernels allow for flexible hypothesis.	The learned models can be difficult to interpret.

Abbreviation: SVM, support vector machine.

of life. Furthermore, MCI may predict the onset of other neurodegenerative disorders.[2] Khazaee and colleagues[3,4] have demonstrated that MCI and AD can be classified against healthy controls with an accuracy of up to 93.3%, using machine learning methods on graph measures of rs-fMR imaging. Zhu and colleagues[2] used a method where functional landmarks were identified using diffusion tensor imaging, and fused with rs-fMR imaging data to create a "connectome signature." This signature was used as a feature for machine learning, with discrimination of MCI versus healthy controls at greater than 95%. Wee and colleagues[5] produced similar results using a multimodality classification approach with discrimination exceeding 96%. Quantification of disease is also clinically important, and work done by Alahmadi and colleagues[6] demonstrates the ability to use machine learning methods using connectivity features before and after a training session are diagnostic of cognitive skills in MCI. The use of directed graph measures of fMR imaging data was shown by Khazaee and colleagues[3] to be an effective feature set for algorithms to accurately distinguish MCI, AD, and healthy controls. Using a naive Bayes classifier, they were able to achieve a classification accuracy of 93.3%. Although many studies have revolved around SVM classification algorithms, Challis and colleagues[7] were able to demonstrate the usefulness of Bayesian Gaussian process logistic regression models. Using this classification method on functional connectivity

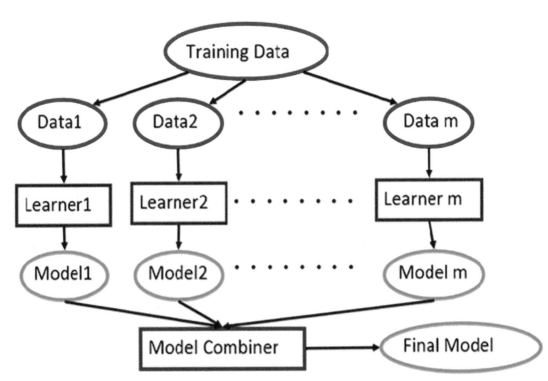

Fig. 4. An ensemble classifier. For random forest, the learners are decision trees.

Table 2	
Advantages and disadvantages of random forests	
Advantages	**Disadvantages**
The model is scalable and robust. Popular ensemble method that is inevitably the first approach taken for large datasets.	Performance can be lower in the presence of noise and outliers.
Can handle missing data. Can be extended to learning multiple types of models; there is no necessity for the base classifiers to be of the same type, that is, trees.	Interpretability is sometimes an issue because, although the individual models are interpretable, their combination is not necessarily interpretable.

data, they were able to distinguish healthy controls from those with MCI at 75% accuracy and MCI patients from those with AD at 80% accuracy on new test sets not used for training the classifier. Machine learning applied to rs-fMR imaging approaches are not the only way to differentiate AD from healthy controls.[8] In an innovative approach, Suk and colleagues[9] used sparse modeling to penalize connectivity features with large in-class variance and small between-class variance. This model allowed them to focus on high-yield connectivity coefficients with little in-class variance and high between-class variance. By applying these features to an SVM classifier they were able to achieve a classification accuracy of 89.19% for differentiating MCI from healthy controls. Ou and colleagues[10] used novel methods to generate "atomic functional connectomes,"

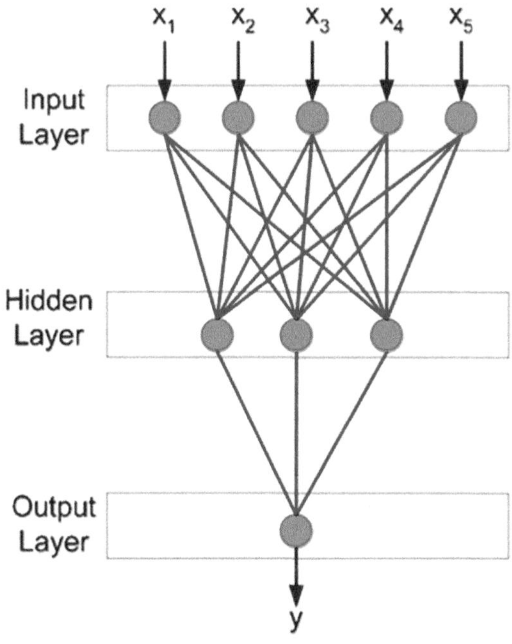

Fig. 5. An artificial neural network.

which are made of subnetwork patterns of connectivity within each connectome. They were able to find unique subnetwork connectivity patterns or "atomic functional connectomes" specific to MCI patients, creating distinct "atomic connectomics signatures" for the disease. Using these signatures, they were able to classify MCI patients from controls with greater than 83% accuracy. Severe carotid artery stenosis is a risk factor for the development of MCI and may lead to subclinical functional and structural changes. Lin and colleagues[11] examined a cohort of asymptomatic (no history of transient ischemic attack or stroke) subjects with severe unilateral carotid artery stenosis and matched healthy controls. Notably, only a subset of the unilateral carotid artery stenosis patients met the criteria for MCI. Using demographic, diffusion tensor imaging, and resting state features, an SVM classifier was able to accurately distinguish subjects with MCI from all other subjects with greater than 90% accuracy. Functional connectivity in the sensorimotor network and default mode network (DMN) were particularly discriminative rs-fMR imaging features. Li and colleagues[12] used network evolution methods on topology parameters to generate features for classification. Using SVM classification, they were able to accurately distinguish AD patients from healthy controls with greater than 93% accuracy. Suk and colleagues[13] used a combination of a deep architecture model with a state space model within the same framework with accuracies ranging from 72.58% to 81.08%.

Machine learning approaches based on rs-fMR imaging have proven beneficial in other areas of dementia research, such as frontotemporal lobar degeneration. Granulin disease represents a heterogeneous form of frontotemporal lobar degeneration where structural and functional alterations in the brain can precede overt disease by more than a decade. Premi and colleagues[14] used multivoxel pattern analysis and machine learning techniques to show that functional connectivity metrics were

Table 3
Advantages and disadvantages of artificial neural networks

Advantages	Disadvantages
The model can approximate any function, linear or nonlinear.	The models are not interpretable.
Scalable to very large problems and are recently very popular owing to their ability to handle millions of features during training.	A reasonably large amount of data is required for training.

the most accurate in distinguishing asymptomatic granulin mutation carriers from healthy controls.

Traumatic Brain Injury

Measures of resting state functional connectivity have emerged as promising biomarkers for identifying mild traumatic brain injury (TBI). Vergara and colleagues[15] used machine learning models to classify known patients into mild TBI or healthy control groups based on either fMR imaging or fractional anisotropy features. Machine learning based on fMR imaging demonstrated greater accuracy than fractional anisotropy in correctly classifying patients (84.1% accurate for fMR imaging vs 75.5% accurate for fractional anisotropy). Lui and colleagues[16] examined multiple features for the classification of TBI, including demographic, structural, rs-fMR imaging, mean kurtosis, and magnetic field correlation features. With minimal redundancy, maximal relevance feature selection, they were able to focus on 6 of the most informative features, including thalamocortical resting state networks. With the use of a multilayer perceptron classifier, they were able to discern healthy controls from TBI patients with 86% accuracy.

In addition to the diagnosis of mild TBI, machine learning approaches have been successfully used to predict outcomes. Wu and colleagues[17] examined a cohort of patients with a brain injury with consciousness levels ranging from fully alert to unresponsive wakefulness syndrome or a vegetative state, and coma. SVM classification based on functional connectivity strength features was able to predict with greater than 80% accuracy whether or not patients with unresponsive wakefulness syndrome and coma would regain consciousness at 3 months. The most predictive functional connectivity strength features were located in the posterior cingulate cortex.

Epilepsy

Currently, neuroimaging is helpful in patients with epilepsy, when an underlying lesion can be identified, targeting specific treatment. Work by Vergun

and colleagues[18] demonstrates that it is possible using rs-fMR imaging and machine learning methods to identify areas of eloquent cortex, quantify the degree of morbidity from a planned surgery, and provide the surgeon with safer maximum resection boundaries. With temporal lobe epilepsy, it is particularly important to identify the lateralization and localization of the focus of epileptogenicity, to appropriately direct surgical interventions. Using various rs-fMR imaging metrics and an SVM classifier, Yang and colleagues[19] were able to accurately predict the lateralization of temporal lobe epilepsy with 83% accuracy in a cohort of 12 patients. Using rs-fMR imaging features and a machine learning method known as computer-automated diagnosis using fMR imaging interictal graph theory, Chiang and colleagues[20] were able to lateralize temporal lobe epilepsy with 95.8% accuracy in a group of 24 patients. Notably, expert manual analysis of MR imaging data was only able to achieve 66.7% accurate lateralization, and combining computer-automated diagnosis using fMR imaging interictal graph theory with manual analysis achieved 100% accurate lateralization.

Another area of clinical interest within the field of epilepsy research is prediction of patient prognosis. Paldino and colleagues[21] investigated the application of machine learning methods on rs-fMR imaging data from patients ranging in age from 4 to 19s year old, classified into 5 global network metrics: clustering coefficient, transitivity, modularity, path length, and global efficiency. They found that 3 of these metrics (modularity, path length, and global efficiency) were independently associated with epilepsy duration, demonstrating the ability to capture the impact of epilepsy on the developing brain on an individual basis using fMR imaging data.

Schizophrenia

A potential application of machine learning in schizophrenia is enhancing early diagnosis, thereby avoiding diagnostic and therapeutic delays that may complicate treatment. Skåtun and colleagues[22] have shown the ability to discriminate between schizophrenia from healthy controls with sensitivities ranging from 63.5% to 88.2%, depending on which datasets were used for training and analysis. Interestingly, they found a correlation between reduced connectivity in the frontal, sensory, and subcortical nodes, with reduced thalamotemporal connectivity, as well as decreased connectivity between the putamen and 2 premotor nodes. These findings support the theory that aberrant sensory and perceptual processing are highly implicated in the pathophysiology of schizophrenia. Mikolas and colleagues[23] showed that salient network resting state connectivity data could be coupled with SVM models to classify patients with a first episode of schizophrenia spectrum disorder with an accuracy of 73%. Promisingly, the SVM model was able to distinguish participants independent of medication dose or the presence of psychotic symptoms. Mikolas and colleagues[23] also demonstrated that the DMN and central executive networks did not predict disease above the chance level, and that the anterior insula (salience network) also seems to be implicated. Extreme learning machine and voting extreme learning machine represent novel and fast training approaches for single-layer feedforward neural networks, with the advantage of decreased computational complexity, while typically maintaining average quality classification. Chyzhyk and colleagues[24] applied voting extreme learning machine to the classification of schizophrenia patients, achieving accuracies of nearly 90%. The anatomic localizations that they were able to validate included the hippocampus, amygdala, and parahippocampal gyrus, superior temporal gyrus, prefrontal cortex, and inferior parietal lobule. Using an unsupervised learning method, Shen and colleagues[25] have achieved sensitivities of up to 93.75%, with findings suggestive of cerebellar–frontal functional connectivity being implicated in schizophrenia, which is a novel finding relative to the extensive anatomic network described by Chyzhyk and colleagues.[24] Kim and colleagues[26] used a deep neural network approach and compared the results with 2 SVM kernels, with a significant decrease in error with deep neural network versus SVM.

Although much work has been done on the classification of disease, and understanding which networks and features are involved, Koutsouleris and colleagues[27] investigated imaging changes between prodromal patients, and those who went on to develop full psychotic symptoms. Patients were identified with an at-risk mental state, and then subclassified based on their clinical features. Gray matter volume reductions were seen within 1 group within the cerebellum, thalamus,

and prefrontal cortex bilaterally (at-risk mental state), whereas in another group there were gray matter volume reduction patterns within the anterior and posterior cingulate cortex, the orbitofrontal, and lateral prefrontal lobes, inferior temporal cortex, and the medial temporal lobe and caudate nuclei bilaterally. Using an SVM classifier, they were able to predict progression with an overall accuracy and sensitivity of approximately 80%. Other interesting work on anatomic classification continues to progress. For example, Chyzhyk and colleagues[28] looked specifically at anatomic features associated with auditory hallucinations. They compared schizophrenia patients with and without auditory hallucinations, as well as healthy controls. Using a novel lattice autoassociative memory functional connectivity algorithm (a form of single layer network), they found that seeding the algorithm from the right Heschl's gyrus (which is functionally connected to Broca's area), provided very high discrimination with sensitivities and specificities approaching 100%.

Bipolar Disorder

Bipolar disorder is a common psychiatric illness with significant morbidity, accounting for approximately 7% of all mental and substance use disorders.[29,30] Mood disorders historically have been exclusively a clinical diagnosis, with only a limited role of neuroimaging. One of the exciting possibilities for the future of neuroimaging is using differences in structural connectivity to differentiate between different mood disorders, and therefore, help to tailor individualized treatment. For example, work by Rive and colleagues[31] demonstrated the ability to differentiate between unipolar versus bipolar mood disorder, using various resting state networks, and binary gaussian process classifiers (a method similar to SVM, additionally able to predict the probability of class membership). Work by Roberts and colleagues[29] implicates the inferior frontal gyrus as having a key role in bipolar disorder, showing functional dysconnectivity from multiple regions, including the bilateral insulae, ventrolateral prefrontal gyri, superior temporal gyri, and the putamen. This work demonstrated a modest ability to discriminate between bipolar disorder and healthy controls with an accuracy of 64.3% (chance level 40.8%), and positive predictive values ranging from 49% to 54%.

Social Anxiety

The diagnosis of social anxiety disorder has relied on observed and self-reported behaviors, examinations of psychiatric symptoms, and clinical judgment. A useful objective marker for the diagnosis of social anxiety disorder has so far remained elusive. However, research into fMR imaging and machine learning methods as biomarkers for social anxiety disorder have shown potential. Zhang and colleagues[32] examined fMR imaging regional homogeneity measures from 40 patients with social anxiety disorder and matched healthy controls. SVM classification was able to achieve a diagnostic accuracy of 76.25% (sensitivity, 70%; specificity, 82.5%). Regional homogeneity alterations indicative of social anxiety disorder primarily localized to the DMN, dorsal attention network, self-referential network, and sensory network. Liu and colleagues[33] used a different approach by instead focusing on whole brain functional connectivity measures for 20 patients with social anxiety disorder and matched controls. In their paper, SVM classification was able to achieve accuracy of 82.5% (sensitivity, 85%; specificity, 80%). Informative functional connectivity features primarily localized to the DMN, sensorimotor network, affective network, and visual network. In both the work of Zhang and colleagues[32] and Liu and colleagues,[33] the orbitofrontal cortex was found to be particularly informative area distinguishing social anxiety disorder patients from healthy controls. Although both studies were somewhat limited by relatively small cohorts, these data show the potential for fMR imaging to one day be a useful biomarker for elusive conditions like social anxiety disorder.

Major Depressive Disorder

Like other mood disorders, the diagnosis of major depressive disorder is a clinical diagnosis relying primarily on subjective self-reported symptoms. Although neuroimaging research has demonstrated both structural and functional changes associated with major depressive disorder, neuroimaging currently has limited use for the diagnosis of major depressive disorder. A possible benefit of machine learning techniques based on fMR imaging is the potential to enhance the diagnosis of major depressive disorder with objective neuroimaging data.

With the use of resting state functional connectivity measures, particularly measures of community structure, Lord and colleagues[34] were able to distinguish healthy participants from those with an acute episode of major depressive disorder. This was accomplished through the use of minimum redundancy, maximum relevance algorithms to identify the most informative community structure. SVM classification based on 2 of the highest yield features achieved a classification accuracy of 90%, while increasing the amount of features to 6 allowed for accuracies of greater than 99%. Meanwhile, Cao and colleagues[35] relied on whole brain resting state functional connectivity measures and feature selection via probability density function. With SVM classification, they were able to achieve accuracies of almost 79%. Wei and colleagues[36] used the Hurst exponent, a statistical measure of the "long-term memory" of a time series, to characterize resting state networks. Using the Hurst exponent of several resting state network time series as features, SVM classification was able to distinguish major depressive disorder patients from healthy controls with 90% accuracy. Whereas previously mentioned research groups relied on supervised machine learning approaches, Zeng and colleagues[37] used an unsupervised machine learning approach known as maximized margin clustering. Maximized margin clustering based on functional connectivity measures of the perigenual cingulate was able to achieve a classification accuracy of 92.5% for distinguishing major depressive disorder from healthy controls. When supervised SVM learning methods were applied to the same dataset, similar classification accuracies were achieved. It is possible that the ability to discriminate between major depressive disorder and healthy controls may rely in part on the severity of illness. Ramasubbu and colleagues[38] demonstrated that SVM models could use rs-fMR imaging data to classify patients as very severe depression versus healthy controls at a statistically significant level. However, these machine learning techniques were unable to correctly discriminate patients with mild, moderate, and severe levels of major depressive disorder from healthy controls. Additionally, there is some evidence to suggest that rs-fMR imaging can be used to predict response to treatment. A study conducted by Sikora and colleagues[39] found that increased functional connectivity in the salience network was associated with a significantly increased response to placebo medications at an individual patient level. The authors suggested that these methods may be clinically useful for identifying patients who will benefit from reduced doses of antidepressants and/or nonpharmacologic intervention.

Attention Deficit Hyperactivity Disorder

The field of fMR imaging attention deficit hyperactivity disorder (ADHD) research has been greatly enhanced by the availability of the ADHD-200 preprocessed repository. The repository is derived from the International Neuroimaging Datasharing

Initiative ADHD-200 sample, a collection of phenotypic, rs-fMR imaging, and structural MR imaging from more than 973 participants. These data were used for the 2011 ADHD-200 competition, where various research teams competed to develop the best classification algorithm for distinguishing subtypes of ADHD and healthy controls. The competition itself has led to some interesting findings. Brown and colleagues[40] demonstrated during the ADHD-200 competition that SVM classification based only on personal characteristics such as age, gender, and IQ outperformed classification based only on fMR imaging data (62.52% vs 60.51%). This research demonstrates the importance of considering personal characteristics along with imaging data. Further research has shown that combining features from different modalities may enhance the accuracy of machine learning algorithms. Using the ADHD-200 data set, Bohland and colleagues[41] found the best overall classification accuracy was achieved when combining anatomic, functional connectivity and demographic features. Similarly, Sidhu and colleagues[42] demonstrated that classification using both fMR imaging and demographic data outperformed classification based on only imaging or demographic data.

Other methods have been used to increase the accuracy of classification based on rs-fMR imaging data. Dey and colleagues[43] used multidimensional scaling techniques to represent functional connectivity networks from the ADHD-200 set in 2-dimensional space. By applying these data to SVM classification, they were able to achieve a classification accuracy of 73.55%. Using a cohort of participants from the 1000 Functional Connectomes Project, Wang and colleagues[44] focused on ranked regional homogeneity measures as a feature set for classification. By applying these features to an SVM classifier with sequential minimal optimization, they were able to achieve a classification accuracy of 80%.

In addition to distinguishing ADHD patients from healthy controls, machine learning techniques have shown promise in distinguishing subtypes of ADHD. Sato and colleagues[45] demonstrated that regional homogeneity, resting state network, and amplitude of low-frequency fluctuation features can be combined to distinguish predominantly inattentive ADHD patients from combined inattention hyperactive ADHD patients. Machine learning methods have been used successfully to predict treatment response. Kim and colleagues[46] applied machine learning methods to rs-fMR imaging, genetic, demographic, environmental, and neuropsychosocial data. They found that SVM classification methods were able to predict treatment response with 84.6% accuracy. This study highlights the ability of machine learning techniques to integrate data from multiple modalities to answer a clinically relevant question.

Autism Spectrum Disorder

Various methods have been used with resting state fMR imaging data to distinguish patients with autism from healthy controls.[47] Using the Autism Brain Imaging Data Exchange (ABIDE) dataset, Ghiassian and colleagues[48] were able to achieve an SVM classification accuracy of up to 65%. This was accomplished by using a histogram of oriented gradients from functional imaging data and pairing it with demographic data. Heng Chen and colleagues[49] examined an adolescent cohort from the ABIDE dataset with multivariate pattern analysis. By focusing on whole brain connectivity in the low frequency, Slow-4 and Slow-5 frequency bands they were able to distinguish autism spectrum patients from healthy controls with 79% accuracy on an SVM classifier. Colleen Chen and colleagues[50] examined a cohort (ABIDE) with both SVM and random forest classification techniques. Although the SVM classification methods were able to achieve moderate accuracy between 58% and 66%, random forest classification was able to achieve 90.8% accuracy. Focusing on an ABIDE cohort of patients less than 20 years of age, Iidaka and colleagues[51] used a probabilistic neural network algorithm for classification. This method of machine learning was able to differentiate autism spectrum disorder patients from typically developed controls with 90% accuracy.

Resting state fMR imaging data paired with machine learning methods may not only offer diagnostic value, but also prognostic value. In a novel study, Plitt and colleagues[52] showed that rs-fMR imaging connectivity patterns in young adults with autism spectrum disorder held value for future autistic traits and adaptive behavior. Specifically, fMR imaging connectivity patterns predicted about 20% of the total variance in autistic traits and roughly 23% of the variance in adaptive behavior over an average time period of 2 years and 10 months. In particular, connectivity within the salience network and DMN were found to highly predictive of these outcomes.

Uddin and colleagues[53] examined both task-based fMR imaging and rs-fMR imaging in the salience network, DMN, and central executive network. They demonstrated that machine learning algorithms had an easier time distinguishing between rs-fMR imaging and task-based fMR imaging in typically developing patients than in patients with autism. Additionally, the degree of similarity between rs-fMR imaging and fMR imaging in patients with autism was predictive of symptom severity in restrictive and repetitive behaviors.

Addiction

In addiction research, Morris and colleagues[54] demonstrated the ability for machine learning methods to differentiate between patients with alcohol use disorder, binge drinking behaviors, and healthy volunteers (social drinkers). Altered subthalamic nucleus connectivity was central to differentiating pathologic drinkers from healthy controls.

Aging

As demonstrated by Meier and colleagues,[55] SVM classification can be successfully paired with rs-fMR imaging data to distinguish young and old participants. Their work shows that aging is associated with connectivity decreases within the DMN and the cinguloopercular network and is additionally associated with connectivity increases between the sensorimotor network and the frontoparietal and cingulo-opercular networks. Wang and colleagues[56] similarly developed an age prediction framework with support vector regression and rs-fMR imaging data from 137 participants aged 8 to 79 years. Their regression models were able to accurately predict participant age on the basis of rs-fMR imaging connectivity to within 10 years in 75% of participants. They observed an increase in anteroposterior functional connectivity within the DMN and task-positive network from childhood to adulthood. However, these connections decreased again in old age. Cognitive decline in memory and executive function can occur as a result of normal aging. La Corte and colleagues[57] demonstrated the ability of machine learning methods to correctly predict participant age and participant cognitive performance on the basis of fMR imaging resting state network connectivity profiles. Particularly discriminative features for age included connectivity between the salience and visual networks, and the salience network and the anterior part of the DMN. These methods were further able to predict cognitive performance on tasks of memory and executive function independent of age.

ACKNOWLEDGMENTS

Supported by the National Institutes of Health R01 NS091602 (C.T. Whitlow).

REFERENCES

1. Orrù G, Pettersson-Yeo W, Marquand AF, et al. Using support vector machine to identify imaging biomarkers of neurological and psychiatric disease: a critical review. Neurosci Biobehav Rev 2012;36(4): 1140–52.
2. Zhu D, Li K, Terry DP, et al. Connectome-scale assessments of structural and functional connectivity in MCI. Hum Brain Mapp 2014;35(7):2911–23.
3. Khazaee A, Ebrahimzadeh A, Babajani-Feremi A, Alzheimer's disease neuroimaging initiative. Classification of patients with MCI and AD from healthy controls using directed graph measures of resting-state fMRI. Behav Brain Res 2017;322(Pt B):339–50.
4. Khazaee A, Ebrahimzadeh A, Babajani-Feremi A. Application of advanced machine learning methods on resting-state fMRI network for identification of mild cognitive impairment and Alzheimer's disease. Brain Imaging Behav 2016;10(3):799–817.
5. Wee C-Y, Yap P-T, Zhang D, et al. Identification of MCI individuals using structural and functional connectivity networks. Neuroimage 2012;59(3): 2045–56.
6. Alahmadi HH, Shen Y, Fouad S, et al. Classifying cognitive profiles using machine learning with privileged information in mild cognitive impairment. Front Comput Neurosci 2016;10:117.
7. Challis E, Hurley P, Serra L, et al. Gaussian process classification of Alzheimer's disease and mild cognitive impairment from resting-state fMRI. Neuroimage 2015;112:232–43.
8. Dyrba M, Grothe M, Kirste T, et al. Multimodal analysis of functional and structural disconnection in Alzheimer's disease using multiple kernel SVM. Hum Brain Mapp 2015;36(6):2118–31.
9. Suk H-I, Wee C-Y, Lee S-W, et al. Supervised discriminative group sparse representation for mild cognitive impairment diagnosis. Neuroinformatics 2015;13(3):277–95.
10. Ou J, Xie L, Li X, et al. Atomic connectomics signatures for characterization and differentiation of mild cognitive impairment. Brain Imaging Behav 2015; 9(4):663–77.
11. Lin C-J, Tu P-C, Chern C-M, et al. Connectivity features for identifying cognitive impairment in presymptomatic carotid stenosis. PLoS One 2014;9(1) e85441.
12. Li Y, Qin Y, Chen X, et al. Exploring the functional brain network of Alzheimer's disease: based on the computational experiment. PLoS One 2013;8(9) e73186.
13. Suk HI, Wee CY, Lee SW, et al. State-space model with deep learning for functional dynamics estimation in resting-state fMRI. Neuroimage 2016;129 292–307.

14. Premi E, Cauda F, Costa T, et al. Looking for neuroimaging markers in frontotemporal lobar degeneration clinical trials: a multi-voxel pattern analysis study in granulin disease. J Alzheimers Dis 2016; 51(1):249–62.

15. Vergara VM, Mayer AR, Damaraju E, et al. Detection of mild traumatic brain injury by machine learning classification using resting state functional network connectivity and fractional anisotropy. J Neurotrauma 2017;34(5):1045–53.

16. Lui YW, Xue Y, Kenul D, et al. Classification algorithms using multiple MRI features in mild traumatic brain injury. Neurology 2014;83(14):1235–40.

17. Wu X, Zou Q, Hu J, et al. Intrinsic functional connectivity patterns predict consciousness level and recovery outcome in acquired brain injury. J Neurosci 2015;35(37):12932–46.

18. Vergun S, Gaggl W, Nair VA, et al. Classification and extraction of resting state networks using healthy and epilepsy fMRI data. Front Neurosci 2016;10:440.

19. Yang Z, Choupan J, Reutens D, et al. Lateralization of temporal lobe epilepsy based on resting-state functional magnetic resonance imaging and machine learning. Front Neurol 2015;6:184.

20. Chiang S, Levin HS, Haneef Z. Computer-automated focus lateralization of temporal lobe epilepsy using fMRI. J Magn Reson Imaging 2015;41(6):1689–94.

21. Paldino MJ, Zhang W, Chu ZD, et al. Metrics of brain network architecture capture the impact of disease in children with epilepsy. Neuroimage Clin 2017;13: 201–8.

22. Skåtun KC, Kaufmann T, Doan NT, et al. Consistent functional connectivity alterations in schizophrenia spectrum disorder: a multisite study. Schizophr Bull 2016. [Epub ahead of print].

23. Mikolas P, Melicher T, Skoch A, et al. Connectivity of the anterior insula differentiates participants with first-episode schizophrenia spectrum disorders from controls: a machine-learning study. Psychol Med 2016;46(13):2695–704.

24. Chyzhyk D, Savio A, Graña M. Computer aided diagnosis of schizophrenia on resting state fMRI data by ensembles of ELM. Neural Netw 2015;68: 23–33.

25. Shen H, Wang L, Liu Y, et al. Discriminative analysis of resting-state functional connectivity patterns of schizophrenia using low dimensional embedding of fMRI. Neuroimage 2010;49(4):3110–21.

26. Kim J, Calhoun VD, Shim E, et al. Deep neural network with weight sparsity control and pre-training extracts hierarchical features and enhances classification performance: evidence from whole-brain resting-state functional connectivity patterns of schizophrenia. Neuroimage 2016;124(Pt A):127–46.

27. Koutsouleris N, Meisenzahl EM, Davatzikos C, et al. Use of neuroanatomical pattern classification to identify subjects in at-risk mental states of psychosis and predict disease transition. Arch Gen Psychiatry 2009;66(7):700–12.

28. Chyzhyk D, Graña M, Öngür D, et al. Discrimination of schizophrenia auditory hallucinators by machine learning of resting-state functional MRI. Int J Neural Syst 2015;25(3):1550007.

29. Roberts G, Lord A, Frankland A, et al. Functional dysconnection of the inferior frontal gyrus in young people with bipolar disorder or at genetic high risk. Biol Psychiatry 2016;81(8):718–27.

30. Whiteford HA, Degenhardt L, Rehm J, et al. Global burden of disease attributable to mental and substance use disorders: findings from the Global Burden of Disease Study 2010. Lancet 2013; 382(9904):1575–86.

31. Rive MM, Redlich R, Schmaal L, et al. Distinguishing medication-free subjects with unipolar disorder from subjects with bipolar disorder: state matters. Bipolar Disord 2016;18(7):612–23.

32. Zhang W, Yang X, Lui S, et al. Diagnostic prediction for social anxiety disorder via multivariate pattern analysis of the regional homogeneity. Biomed Res Int 2015;2015:763965.

33. Liu F, Guo W, Fouche J-P, et al. Multivariate classification of social anxiety disorder using whole brain functional connectivity. Brain Struct Funct 2015; 220(1):101–15.

34. Lord A, Horn D, Breakspear M, et al. Changes in community structure of resting state functional connectivity in unipolar depression. PLoS One 2012; 7(8):e41282.

35. Cao L, Guo S, Xue Z, et al. Aberrant functional connectivity for diagnosis of major depressive disorder: a discriminant analysis. Psychiatry Clin Neurosci 2014;68(2):110–9.

36. Wei M, Qin J, Yan R, et al. Identifying major depressive disorder using Hurst exponent of resting-state brain networks. Psychiatry Res 2013; 214(3):306–12.

37. Zeng L-L, Shen H, Liu L, et al. Unsupervised classification of major depression using functional connectivity MRI. Hum Brain Mapp 2014;35(4):1630–41.

38. Ramasubbu R, Brown MRG, Cortese F, et al. Accuracy of automated classification of major depressive disorder as a function of symptom severity. Neuroimage Clin 2016;12:320–31.

39. Sikora M, Heffernan J, Avery ET, et al. Salience network functional connectivity predicts placebo effects in major depression. Biol Psychiatry Cogn Neurosci Neuroimaging 2016;1(1):68–76.

40. Brown MRG, Sidhu GS, Greiner R, et al. ADHD-200 global competition: diagnosing ADHD using personal characteristic data can outperform resting state fMRI measurements. Front Syst Neurosci 2012;6:69.

41. Bohland JW, Saperstein S, Pereira F, et al. Network, anatomical, and non-imaging measures for the

prediction of ADHD diagnosis in individual subjects. Front Syst Neurosci 2012;6:78.

42. Sidhu GS, Asgarian N, Greiner R, et al. Kernel principal component analysis for dimensionality reduction in fMRI-based diagnosis of ADHD. Front Syst Neurosci 2012;6:74.

43. Dey S, Rao AR, Shah M. Attributed graph distance measure for automatic detection of attention deficit hyperactive disordered subjects. Front Neural Circuits 2014;8:64.

44. Wang X, Jiao Y, Tang T, et al. Altered regional homogeneity patterns in adults with attention-deficit hyperactivity disorder. Eur J Radiol 2013;82(9): 1552–7.

45. Sato JR, Hoexter MQ, Fujita A, et al. Evaluation of pattern recognition and feature extraction methods in ADHD prediction. Front Syst Neurosci 2012;6:68.

46. Kim J-W, Sharma V, Ryan ND. Predicting methylphenidate response in ADHD using machine learning approaches. Int J Neuropsychopharmacol 2015; 18(11):yv052.

47. Kassraian-Fard P, Matthis C, Balsters JH, et al. Promises, pitfalls, and basic guidelines for applying machine learning classifiers to psychiatric imaging data, with autism as an example. Front Psychiatry 2016;7:177.

48. Ghiassian S, Greiner R, Jin P, et al. Using functional or structural magnetic resonance images and personal characteristic data to identify ADHD and autism. PLoS One 2016;11(12):e0166934.

49. Chen H, Duan X, Liu F, et al. Multivariate classification of autism spectrum disorder using frequency-specific resting-state functional connectivity–a multi-center study. Prog Neuropsychopharmacol Biol Psychiatry 2016;64:1–9.

50. Chen CP, Keown CL, Jahedi A, et al. Diagnostic classification of intrinsic functional connectivity highlights somatosensory, default mode, and visual regions in autism. Neuroimage Clin 2015;8: 238–45.

51. Iidaka T. Resting state functional magnetic resonance imaging and neural network classified autism and control. Cortex 2015;63:55–67.

52. Plitt M, Barnes KA, Wallace GL, et al. Resting-state functional connectivity predicts longitudinal change in autistic traits and adaptive functioning in autism. Proc Natl Acad Sci U S A 2015; 112(48):E6699–706.

53. Uddin LQ, Supekar K, Lynch CJ, et al. Brain state differentiation and behavioral inflexibility in autism. Cereb Cortex 2015;25(12):4740–7.

54. Morris LS, Kundu P, Baek K, et al. Jumping the gun: mapping neural correlates of waiting impulsivity and relevance across alcohol misuse. Biol Psychiatry 2016;79(6):499–507.

55. Meier TB, Desphande AS, Vergun S, et al. Support vector machine classification and characterization of age-related reorganization of functional brain networks. Neuroimage 2012;60(1):601–13.

56. Wang L, Su L, Shen H, et al. Decoding lifespan changes of the human brain using resting-state functional connectivity MRI. PLoS One 2012;7(8): e44530.

57. La Corte V, Sperduti M, Malherbe C, et al. Cognitive decline and reorganization of functional connectivity in healthy aging: the pivotal role of the salience network in the prediction of age and cognitive performances. Front Aging Neurosci 2016;8:204.

SECTION 2: Clinical Applications of Resting State Functional Connectivity

Resting-state Functional Magnetic Resonance Imaging in Presurgical Functional Mapping
Sensorimotor Localization

Donna Dierker, MS[a], Jarod L. Roland, MD[b],
Mudassar Kamran, MD[a], Jerrel Rutlin, BA[a],
Carl D. Hacker, MD, PhD[b], Daniel S. Marcus, PhD[a],
Mikhail Milchenko, PhD[a], Michelle M. Miller-Thomas, MD[a],
Tammie L. Benzinger, MD, PhD[a,b],
Abraham Z. Snyder, MD, PhD[a,c], Eric C. Leuthardt, MD[b,d,1],
Joshua S. Shimony, MD, PhD[a,*,1]

KEYWORDS

- Functional MR (fMR) • Resting-state fMR (RS-fMR) • Task fMR (T-MR)
- Resting-state networks (RSN) • Multilayer perceptron (MLP) • Sensorimotor network (SMN)

KEY POINTS

- Resting-state functional magnetic resonance (fMR) imaging data for mapping of functional systems is easy to acquire and does not require patient compliance.
- Resting-state fMR imaging offers unique advantages and should be considered as a primary method in patients who are unable to comply with a task paradigm.
- Resting state–derived maps are more extensive than those derived from task fMR imaging.
- Resting-state fMR imaging can localize the sensorimotor cortex reliably and automatically.
- Neurosurgeons and neuroradiologists using task and resting fMR imaging should be aware of their respective advantages and disadvantages.

Funding Source: Christopher Davidson Brain Tumor Research Fund (E.C. Leuthardt, D. Dierker); NIH R01 CA203861 (E.C. Leuthardt, J.S. Shimony); Barnes-Jewish Hospital Foundation (800-88) (T.L. Benzinger, D.S. Marcus); NIH 1P30NS09857701 NINDS Center Core for Brain Imaging (D. Dierker); NIH R25NS090978-01 (J.L. Roland); NIH U54 HD087011 Eunice Kennedy Shriver NICHD of the NIH to the Intellectual and Developmental Disabilities Research Center at Washington University (J.S. Shimony); NIH R01NS066905, P30NS048056, P30NS098577, R01 EB009352 (D.S. Marcus, A.Z. Snyder); NIA/NIH AG003991, 2UF1AG032438 (T.L. Benzinger).
[a] Mallinckrodt Institute of Radiology, Washington University School of Medicine, 4525 Scott Avenue, Saint Louis, MO 63110, USA; [b] Department of Neurological Surgery, Washington University School of Medicine, 4525 Scott Avenue, Saint Louis, MO 63110, USA; [c] Department of Neurology, Washington University School of Medicine, 4525 Scott Avenue, Saint Louis, MO 63110, USA; [d] Department of Biomedical Imaging, Washington University School of Medicine, 4525 Scott Avenue, Saint Louis, MO 63110, USA
[1] Dr J.S. Shimony and E.C. Leuthardt contributed equally to this work.
* Corresponding author. Mallinckrodt Institute of Radiology, Washington University School of Medicine, Campus Box 8131, 4525 Scott Avenue, St Louis, MO 63110.
E-mail address: shimonyj@wustl.edu

INTRODUCTION

The first demonstration of correlated spontaneous fluctuations of the blood oxygenation level–dependent (BOLD) functional magnetic resonance (fMR) imaging signal was reported in1995 by Biswal and colleagues.[1] This phenomenon currently is widely referred to as resting-state functional connectivity.[2,3] The associated topographies are known as resting-state networks (RSNs). Advances in the understanding of resting-state functional connectivity and improved data processing techniques have enabled clinical application of resting-state fMR (RS-fMR) imaging for purposes of presurgical planning.[4–16] RS-fMR imaging is efficient and robust. Nevertheless, the predominant method for presurgical mapping of brain function currently remains task-based fMR (T-fMR) imaging, using paradigms to activate the motor and language systems.

Several studies in normal cohorts have shown that RSNs and T-fMR imaging responses show similar, although not identical, topographies.[17–19] The primary advantage of functional mapping with RS-fMR imaging is that the patients are not required to comply with a task paradigm, although they must rest quietly in the scanner. RS-fMR imaging is compatible with light sedation and even sleep.[20–24] Thus, RS-fMR imaging is feasible in patients who are not candidates for T-fMR imaging, such as in young children and uncooperative or confused adults. Acquisition is simple and requires no specialized equipment or technical skills. For these reasons, use of RS-fMR imaging for presurgical mapping of function is increasing. It is therefore important to compare results obtained by these 2 methods to better understand their relative advantages and disadvantages.

This article compares and contrasts the 2 methods from the technical perspective in a series of patients with brain tumors. It focuses on the differences between the maps of the sensorimotor (SM) system, as seen with T-fMR imaging versus RS-fMR imaging. It uses the anatomic stability of the primary sensory and motor cortex within the precentral and postcentral gyri to compare fMR imaging with anatomic results, which cannot be done with the more variable language system. It also compares our results with similar literature in this area.[25–28]

METHODS
Patients

Patients were recruited from the neurosurgery brain tumor service, initially as part of an National Institutes of Health (NIH)–funded tumor database

grant (NIH 5R01NS066905). All aspects of the study were approved by the Washington University (WU) Institutional Review Board. All patients provided informed consent. The following inclusion criteria were used: new diagnosis of primary brain tumor; age more than 18 years; and clinical need for a magnetic resonance (MR) imaging scan, including fMR imaging for presurgical planning as determined by the treating neurosurgeon. In addition, it was required that the patients have both a motor paradigm T-fMR and an RS-fMR imaging scan. Exclusion criteria included prior surgery for brain tumor, inability to have an MR imaging scan, and patients referred from an outside institute with an MR imaging scan not performed at WU. Patient age, sex, and tumor characteristics are listed in **Table 1**.

Acquisition

Patients were scanned with either a Siemens 3T Trio or Skyra scanner (Erlangen, Germany) using a standard clinical presurgical tumor protocol. Anatomic imaging included T1-weighted (T1w) magnetization prepared rapid acquisition gradient echo (MPRAGE), T2-weighted (T2w) fast spin echo, FLAIR imaging, susceptibility-weighted imaging, and precontrast and postcontrast T1w fast spin echo in 3 projections. Specific sequences for presurgical mapping included diffusion tensor imaging for track tracing, T-fMR imaging for motor localization, and RS-fMR imaging.

Both the T-fMR and RS-fMR imaging was acquired using a T2* echo planar imaging sequence (voxel size $3 \times 3 \times 3$ mm; echo time = 27 milliseconds; recovery time = 2 seconds; field of view = 256 mm; flip angle = 90°). The motor T-fMR imaging used a block design in which finger tapping was repeated over 4 off/on cycles, each off and on block lasting for 20 seconds (10 frames) for a total of 80 frames (2:40 minutes total per T-fMR imaging run). For most subjects, only 1 motor task session was acquired. For 8 subjects, a second motor task session was acquired, and, for 1 subject, a third task session was acquired. If more than 1 task session was usable, the session providing the maximum overlap index, as defined later, was used for the subsequent overlap analyses. RS-fMR imaging was always acquired as two 6-minute runs (total of 360 frames = 12 minutes).

Preprocessing

Resting-state functional magnetic resonance imaging
Preprocessing of RS-fMR imaging data was performed using previously described

Table 1
Patient clinical and demographic data

Patient ID	Age	Sex	Tumor Location	Tumor Size (mL)	Tumor Pathology
RS_001	31	M	Right frontal lobe	70	Oligodendroglioma
RS_002	27	M	Left frontal lobe	11.7	Oligoastrocytoma
RS_003	44	M	Left basal ganglia	8.7	Glioblastoma
			Left temporal lobe	4.8	
RS_004	24	M	Left frontal lobe	56.2	Anaplastic glioma
RS_005	36	M	Left frontal lobe	1.2	Anaplastic mixed oligoastrocytoma
			Left frontal lobe	0.2	
RS_006	36	M	Left inferior frontal lobe	81.1	Anaplastic mixed oligoastrocytoma
RS_007	64	M	Left parieto-occipital	85.1	Glioblastoma
RS_009	65	F	Left peritrigonal area	147	Glioblastoma
RS_010	50	F	Right peritrigonal area	15.5	Anaplastic astrocytoma
RS_011	24	M	Left frontotemporal	56.4	Mixed oligoastrocytoma
RS_012	42	M	Left frontal lobe	7.8	Anaplastic oligodendroglioma
RS_013	65	F	Right frontal lobe	8.5	Oligodendroglioma
RS_014	44	M	Left frontal/insular lobe	69.2	Oligodendroglioma
RS_015	62	F	Left frontal lobe	34.7	Mixed oligoastrocytoma
RS_016	57	F	Left insula	15.2	Glioblastoma
RS_017	54	M	Left frontal lobe	64.3	Mixed oligoastrocytoma
RS_018	39	F	Left frontal lobe	13.5	Oligodendroglioma
RS_019	33	F	Right frontoparietal	207	Anaplastic oligodendroglioma
RS_021	25	M	Left frontal lobe	63.3	Mixed oligoastrocytoma
RS_022	67	M	Right frontal lobe	2.2	Metastatic lung carcinoma
RS_023	50	F	Left parietal/splenium	28.7	Oligodendroglioma
RS_024	56	M	Left frontal lobe	4.7	Anaplastic oligoastrocytoma
RS_028	64	M	Left parietal lobe	50.1	Glioblastoma
RS_029	52	M	Left frontal lobe	14.5	Oligodendroglioma
RS_030	71	M	Right basal ganglia /thalamus	16.6	Glioblastoma
RS_031	53	F	Left thalamus	5.8	Glioblastoma
RS_032	46	M	Right temporal lobe	5.7	Glioblastoma
RS_033	37	M	Left frontal lobe	185	Mixed oligoastrocytoma
RS_035	28	F	Left temporal lobe	10.1	Oligoastrocytoma
RS_036	48	M	Left frontal lobe	20.6	Glioblastoma
RS_039	25	M	Right parietal lobe	32.0	Mixed oligoastrocytoma
RS_041	40	M	Left frontal lobe	23.3	Mixed oligoastrocytoma
RS_042	60	M	Left parietal lobe	0.7	Glioblastoma
RS_043	33	M	Right temporal lobe	4.0	Low-grade glioneuronal tumor
RS_044	23	M	Left frontal lobe	0.4	Ganglioglioma
RS_045	28	F	Both frontal lobes (left>right)	118	Anaplastic astrocytoma
RS_047	55	M	Left frontal lobe	66.2	Glioblastoma
RS_048	31	F	Right insula	14.3	Oligodendroglioma

Abbreviations: F, female; ID, identification code; M, male.

techniques.[29,30] Preprocessing steps included compensation for slice-dependent time shifts, elimination of systemic odd-even slice intensity differences caused by interleaved acquisition, and rigid body correction for head movement within and across runs. Atlas transformation was achieved by composition of affine transforms connecting the fMR imaging volumes with the T2-weighted and MPRAGE structural images, resulting in a volumetric time series in $(3 \text{ mm})^3$ atlas space. Additional preprocessing included spatial smoothing (6 mm full-width half-maximum gaussian blur in each direction), voxelwise removal of linear trends over each run, and temporal low pass filtering retaining frequencies less than 0.1 Hz. Spurious variance was reduced by regression of nuisance waveforms derived from head motion correction and extraction of the time series from regions of white matter and cerebrospinal fluid. The whole-brain (global) signal was included as a nuisance regressor.[31,32] Frame censoring was performed to minimize the impact of head motion on the correlation results.[30] Thus, frames (volumes) in which the root mean square (evaluated over the whole brain) change in voxel intensity relative to the previous frame exceeded 0.5% (relative to the whole-brain mean) were excluded from the functional connectivity computations.[33] The preprocessed fMR imaging data then were analyzed by a previously trained multilayer perceptron (MLP).[34] The MLP assigns to each voxel 7 values expressing the likelihood of belonging to each of 7 RSNs. The SM network (SMN) was defined as all voxels in which the MLP identified the SMN as the most likely RSN.

Task functional magnetic resonance imaging processing

T-fMR imaging was processed using standard general linear model methods. After preprocessing, activation maps were generated from the T-fMR imaging (as described in Ref.[35]). Activation maps were smoothed with a 7-mm gaussian filter and a subject-specific intracranial mask was applied. Both MLP SM maps and smoothed/masked activation maps were resampled to 1 mm^3 for intersection with the high-resolution anatomic regions of interest (ROIs) described later.

Anatomic Regions

Two different methods were used for anatomically identifying the primary SM region. The Brodmann method is based on volumetric registration of each individual to a standard atlas; this method is robust in the sense of working all cases but does not take into account individual sulcal anatomy. The FreeSurfer[36,37] method provides more accurate localization based on sulcal anatomy; however, the FreeSurfer method has a finite failure rate, especially when brain anatomy is distorted by tumor mass effect.

Brodmann Primary Sensorimotor Region of Interest

The Brodmann SM anatomic ROI was projected to a volume ribbon 1.5 mm above and below the population atlas landmark surface (PALS)–based mean midthickness atlas surface using Caret version 5.65 as shown in **Fig. 1**,[38] then dilated to 10 mm using Connectome Workbench (wb_command).[39]

FreeSurfer Primary Sensorimotor Region of Interest

The SM region was segmented using the patient's MPRAGE image through FreeSurfer (Version 5.3.0). Owing to concerns about tumors affecting stereotaxic registration and downstream processing, we input cubic 1-mm MPRAGE images already in atlas space. The FreeSurfer surfaces and volumes were imported into Connectome Workbench (Version 1.2.3) using methods adapted from the Human Connectome Project.[40] Native mesh surfaces were used for visualization. All hemispheres were inspected to ensure quality control, using automatically generated Connectome Workbench scenes like those shown in **Fig. 2**. This display addressed the accuracy of

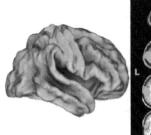
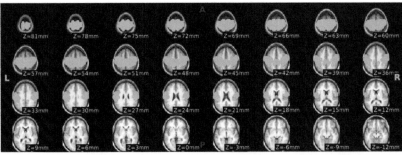

Fig. 1. B-SM anatomic ROI. Brodmann areas 1, 2, 3, and 4 surface-based labels in the PALS atlas were projected to a volume ribbon 1.5 mm above and 1.5 mm below the mean PALS midthickness surface in atlas space, and then dilated to a distance of 10 mm. This ROI requires no exclusions, but does not precisely localize the patient's primary sensorimotor.

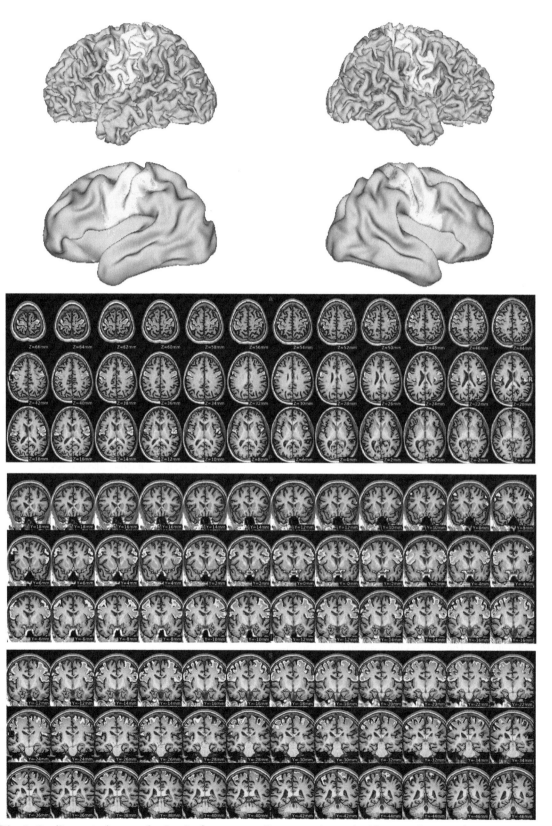

Fig. 2. Quality control scenes for FreeSurfer precentral/postcentral parcels. After creating template scenes, captures like this were generated for all patients to determine which hemispheres had usable precentral/postcentral parcellations for the overlap computations.

the FreeSurfer segmentation and parcellation in SM cortex.

Where the quality of the segmentation was poor and/or the parcellation accuracy was doubtful, the affected hemisphere was excluded from downstream analysis. No manual patching of the FreeSurfer results or other interventions was performed. The precentral and postcentral labels from the usable hemispheres were extracted from Free-Surfer's "aparc + aseg" output volume to compute the Jaccard index (JI)[41] overlap (discussed later).

Jaccard Index Overlap

To measure anatomic overlap the Jaccard index (JI) was used.[41] This index is sensitive to mismatch even when anatomic overlap is strong. For each patient, the anatomic ROI, thresholded task activation map, and thresholded MLP SMN were masked according to which hemispheres had valid anatomic ROIs. The authors define:

A_{fMR} imaging = area (number of nonzero voxels) in the thresholded T-fMR imaging or RS-fMR image

A_{anat} = area (number of nonzero voxels) in the anatomic ROI (Brodmann or FreeSurfer)

Then, the JI for either the task or MLP was computed as:

$$JI = \frac{(A_{fMRI} \cap A_{anat})}{A_{fMRI} + A_{anat} - (A_{fMRI} \cap A_{anat})},$$

where $\cap$ indicates the intersection operation. Two anatomic ROIs were used for this analysis, one minimizing subject exclusions and another more precisely addressing localization questions.

Task Threshold

To compute the overlap with the anatomic SM parcellation, methods similar to those of Sair and colleagues[16] were adopted, choosing the task threshold with the maximum JI overlap with the anatomic ROI. The authors first zeroed out all negative activations and included zero voxels when computing the percentile, then iterated task threshold from 1 to 100 percentile. Iterating percentiles rather than incrementing the intensity directly was important for comparing between subjects with varied distributions of activation intensities.

Multilayer Perceptron Threshold

The analysis was run 2 ways: first, the MLP threshold was fixed at 0.95, which has been used clinically in our institution for the last several years. Second, the MLP threshold was adjusted to maximize the JI in the anatomic ROI (FreeSurfer

primary SM [FS-SM] or B-SM), in the same manner as the task threshold.

Hemisphere Masks

To exclude hemispheres where the FS-SM ROIs were unreliable, hemisphere masks were applied to the volumes. These masks were also used for subanalysis of unaffected-only overlaps, based on which hemisphere was affected.

RESULTS

Four subjects were unable to complete the motor task. One subject was unable to complete any tasks, but completed RS-fMR imaging scanning. Another subject completed both task and RS-fMR imaging, but failed preprocessing for either T-fMR or RS-fMR imaging, owing to problems with atlas space registration. All of these subjects were excluded.

Eleven more subjects were excluded from the FS-SM analysis: 3 failed to complete FreeSurfer processing (recon-all), and the remaining 8 had problems with segmentation and labeling that rendered the FS-SM parcellation unreliable. These subjects were included in the B-SM analyses. For 2 subjects, only the left hemisphere FS-SM was reliable; for 11 subjects, only the right hemisphere FS-SM was reliable. Masks were used to exclude the unreliable hemisphere's data. The B-SM is not subject specific but does allow more subjects to be included (eg, fewer exclusions caused by FreeSurfer processing/parcellation errors, most of which are tumor related).

Fixed Multilayer Perceptron Threshold

Table 2 lists paired t-tests between the JI of T-fMR and RS-fMR imaging. Overlap is greater for task in the B-SM, whereas overlap is greater for MLP in the FS-SM. The difference is significant in the FS-SM (both unaffected and all usable hemispheres).

Maximum Jaccard Index Multilayer Perceptron Threshold

Table 3 lists paired t-tests between the JI of T-fMR and RS-fMR imaging when the MLP threshold was set to the maximum JI within the ROI. In such cases, RS-fMR imaging overlap significantly exceeded that of T-fMR except for affected hemispheres in the FS-SM. Only 14 of the affected hemispheres had usable FS-SM parcellations, compared with the 27 unaffected hemispheres.

Fig. 3 shows surface representation examples of localization of the precentral and postcentral gyri and central sulcus using maximum JI

Table 2
Paired *t*-test: task versus resting-state functional magnetic resonance imaging–Jaccard index overlap by affected/unaffected and region of interest (multilayer perceptron threshold fixed at 0.95)

Hemisphere/ROI	FS-SM Anatomic ROI	B-SM Anatomic ROI
All usable hemispheres	MLP>task: P = .0252[a] t = −2.376, n = 27 Mean task = 0.085 (SD, 0.038) Mean MLP = 0.103 (SD, 0.039)	Task>MLP: P = .1293 t = 1.551, n = 38 Mean task = 0.162 (SD, 0.043) Mean MLP = 0.144 (SD, 0.058)
Unaffected hemisphere only	MLP>task: P = .0027[a] t = −3.320, n = 27 Mean task = 0.082 (SD, 0.032) Mean MLP = 0.106 (SD, 0.041)	Task>MLP: P = .1261 t = 1.565, n = 38 Mean task = 0.166 (SD, 0.048) Mean MLP = 0.147 (SD, 0.062)
Affected hemisphere only	MLP>task: P = .2819 t = −1.123, n = 14 Mean task = 0.094 (SD, 0.049) Mean MLP = 0.108 (SD, 0.038)	Task>MLP: P = .1176 t = 1.602, n = 38 Mean task = 0.160 (SD, 0.046) Mean MLP = 0.140 (SD, 0.061)

[a] $P<.05$.

thresholds for both T-fMR and RS-fMR imaging. **Fig. 3** shows examples of a low, medium, and high overlap. Ranks are based on the FS-SM analysis using all hemispheres passing FreeSurfer quality control inspection.

Fig. 4 shows the corresponding volumetric/slice views for the same subjects and thresholds presented in **Fig. 3**.

DISCUSSION

T-fMR imaging currently is the predominant noninvasive method used for localization of eloquent cortex before neurosurgery. This technique is well established and available from most of the MR vendors. Successful T-fMR imaging mapping requires patient cooperation and depends on modest radiological expertise in acquiring and processing the data. RS-fMR imaging is an alternative method of brain mapping, with substantial and growing support in the literature.[4–16] Several publications have shown how RS-fMR imaging has been able to help individual patients in situations in which T-fMR imaging was not available.[11,42,43] RS-fMR imaging does not require active patient participation (beyond laying still during the MR imaging scan) and data acquisition is simple.[10,15] However, analysis of the acquired data depends on substantial expertise. In our hands, RS-fMR imaging is more robust, with a clinical failure rate of 13% compared with 33% with T-fMR imaging. Here, this article compares

Table 3
Paired *t*-test: task versus resting-state functional magnetic resonance imaging–Jaccard index overlap by affected/unaffected and region of interest: multilayer perceptron threshold maximizing Jaccard index

Hemisphere/ROI	FS-SM Anatomic ROI	B-SM Anatomic ROI
All usable hemispheres	MLP>task: P = .0037[a] t = −3.193, n = 27 Mean task = 0.085 (SD, 0.038) Mean MLP = 0.109 (SD, 0.037)	MLP>task: $P<.0001$[a] t = −5.030, n = 38 Mean task = 0.162 (SD, 0.043) Mean MLP = 0.219 (SD, 0.051)
Unaffected hemisphere only	MLP>task: P = .0004[a] t = −4.091, n = 27 Mean task = 0.082 (SD, 0.032) Mean MLP = 0.110 (SD, 0.039)	MLP>task: P = .0001[a] t = −4.290, n = 38 Mean task = 0.166 (SD, 0.048) Mean MLP = 0.220 (SD, 0.057)
Affected hemisphere only	MLP>task: P = .0924 t = −1.816, n = 14 Mean task = 0.094 (SD, 0.049) Mean MLP = 0.115 (SD, 0.033)	MLP>task: $P<.0001$[a] t = −5.219, n = 38 Mean task = 0.160 (SD, 0.046) Mean MLP = 0.220 (SD, 0.051)

[a] $P<.05$.

TASK   MLP

RS_022: Low Overlap (task rank 27/27; MLP rank 25/27)

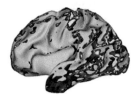 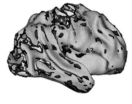 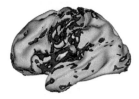 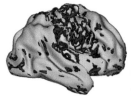

RS_041: Medium Overlap (task rank 8/27; MLP rank 10/27)

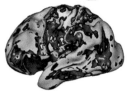 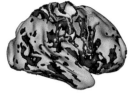 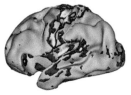 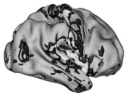

RS_045: High Overlap (task rank 1/27; MLP rank 4/27)

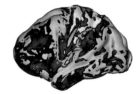 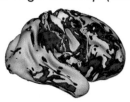 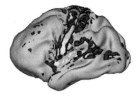 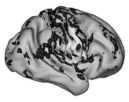

Fig. 3. Surface views across a range of Jaccard overlap indices. Task activation maps (*left*) and MLP probability maps (*right*) are shown for subjects with low, medium, and high overlap with FS-SM on the patient's native mesh inflated surface. Green borders delimit FS-SM ROI (*left and right columns*). Task (*left columns*): dark blue borders encircle regions exceeding the task threshold with maximum overlap. Task maps are scaled to 2.7, the mean of maximum overlap thresholds across patients. MLP (*right columns*): blue borders encircle regions exceeding the MLP threshold with maximum overlap. MLP probability maps are scaled 0.7 to 1.0.

results obtained by the two methods with a focus on localization of the SM system, this being an area of primary concern for surgeons.

Anatomic mapping of the SM system is facilitated by its consistency of anatomic localization to the precentral and postcentral gyri. This consistency provides the opportunity to use anatomic localization as a reference to compare results obtained by both T-fMR imaging and RS-fMR imaging. The authors used 2 complementary methods of anatomic localization, one volumetric and atlas-based (less accurate but more robust), the other based on individually computed gyral segmentation (more accurate, but less robust).

Our comparison reflects the inherent differences between T-fMR imaging and RS-fMR imaging. Although both are based on fMR imaging, they measure different aspects of brain function. T-fMR imaging imposes a behavior on the patient and yields the representation of a fixed sensory, motor, or cognitive process. RS-fMR imaging measures something different; because there is no imposed task, RS-fMR imaging reveals RSN; that is, the topography of temporally synchronous spontaneous neural activity. Although the physiologic functions of intrinsic brain activity remain uncertain (for discussion see Refs.[44,45]), RSNs are of practical interest because they topographically resemble fMR imaging responses to a wide range of cognitive, sensory, and motor tasks. Here, this article compares T-fMR imaging responses to a finger-tapping task, which recruits the hand area of SM cortex, versus the full SMN as revealed by RS-fMR imaging, which is more extensive and includes Brodmann areas 1 to 4 as well as supplementary motor cortex.

In this context, the most informative comparison measure is reliability. Our selection of the full

Task   MLP

RS_022: Low Overlap (task rank 27/27; MLP rank 25/27)

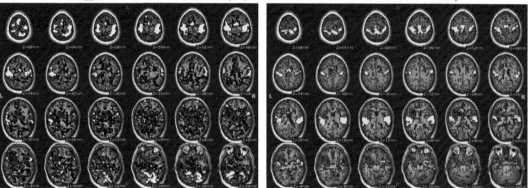

RS_041: Medium Overlap (task rank 8/27; MLP rank 10/27)

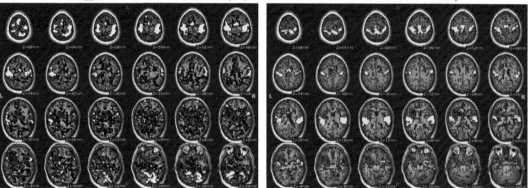

RS_045: High Overlap (task rank 1/27; MLP rank 4/27)

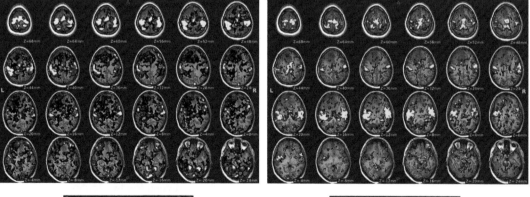

Fig. 4. Volume views across a range of overlap indices. Top row: task activation map *(left)* and MLP probability map *(right)* are shown for a patient with low FS-SM overlap laid over the patient's MPRAGE image. Task activation maps are scaled to 2.7, which is the mean maximum overlap threshold across patients. MLP probability maps *(right)* are scaled 0.7 to 1.0. Corresponding views for subjects with medium and high overlap are also shown.

anatomic extent of the SM system is based on neurosurgical considerations. Estimating the full extent of the SM system delineates all areas that contribute to motor function and, hence, should

be preserved to reduce postoperative morbidity. Finger-tapping T-fMR imaging provides a restricted estimate of the hand area, although this can be extrapolated to a more complete view of the SM system. However, that extrapolation is subjective and potentially misleading, especially when some of the cortical areas of task activation are not purely motor with regard to cognitive operations (ie, attention or sensory processes). Thus, the authors opted to make the comparison of the resting-state data at 2 different thresholds: one at a maximal overlap criteria determined by the JI and a second at a fixed threshold commonly used in our institution for presurgical planning. The RS-fMR imaging overlap index is significantly greater when using the maximal overlap criteria. The present results are more ambiguous with the fixed threshold, with T-fMR imaging showing a trend toward greater overlap when using the B-SM anatomy region, but RS-fMR imaging performing better when using the FS-SM anatomy reference. T-fMR imaging activates all regions of the brain recruited to perform a task (eg, visual system), which is what it was designed to do, but not all regions are equally relevant in a given presurgical application. The MLP maps include secondary somatosensory cortex or S2, which shows responses to tactile stimulation.[46] Although this article focused on the SMN, MLP also identifies visual, auditory/language, and other RSNs.

Interpretation of fMR imaging data is complicated by the question of potentially compromised neurovascular coupling,[47] which has been reported to lead to false-negative T-fMR imaging results in a high proportion of low-grade gliomas.[48] It has been suggested that altered RS-fMR imaging functional connectivity in the SMN can occur on the same basis in patients with brain tumors.[49] Although neurovascular uncoupling could be a contributor in the cases that fail our RS-fMR imaging analysis, our overall failure rate is low, and, in most cases, we can identify a specific cause for this failure (typically, patient motion or sedation). It is possible that neurovascular uncoupling is less of a problem in the current data set because we focused mostly on high-grade gliomas. Speculatively, MLP mapping is resistant to this phenomenon owing to its use of high-quality prior information.

Several prior articles have compared T-fMR imaging with RS-fMR in the SM system. Mannfolk and colleagues[25] compared functional data in 10 healthy volunteers and focused primarily on within-session test-retest reliability. They conclude that both methods have comparable test-retest reliability. In addition, they present comparable SM maps of the two methods side by side but do not report a numerical comparison. The resting-state analysis was done using independent components analysis, because the

investigators correctly point out that placement of a seed could be difficult in a brain distorted by tumor mass effect. Although our RS-fMR imaging method uses prior information on the expected appearance of standard RSNs (entered into the neural network during the MLP training phase[34]), it is not a classic seed-based approach. Nevertheless, the MLP has been shown to provide robust results even in brains distorted by tumors.[50] MLP RSN mapping is based not on the absolute location of a voxel (which can be shifted in patients with brain tumors) but on its connectivity pattern to the rest of the brain. This analytical design feature provides a robust prior information.[34]

Kristo and colleagues[26] also focused on test-retest reliability in 16 normal subjects, but across 2 scans spaced by 7 weeks. They report better overlap for the T-fMR imaging compared with the resting-state data, which had a less focal spatial pattern, as would be expected from our preceding discussion. Importantly, they state: "…just like task fMRI, task-free fMRI can properly identify critical brain areas for motor task performance."[26]

Rosazza and colleagues[27] compared T-fMR imaging versus RS-fMR imaging in 13 patients with lesions close to the SM. They used a preprocessing scheme that was different from ours, and analyzed several tasks that included the hand, leg, and face areas. An additional novel aspect of their study was a comparison with intraoperative electrocortical stimulation. The numerical criteria they used are not directly comparable with the present JI. We considered metrics like those used by Rosazza and colleagues[27] and Sair and colleagues,[16] but ultimately chose to compare overlap of T-fMR imaging and RS-fMR imaging with a neutral anatomic ROI. Rosazza and colleagues[27] report that RS-fMR imaging can localize the SM successfully, with partial agreement with T-fMR imaging and also describe larger areas of correlated activity defined with the RS-fMR imaging data. They conclude that, because the methods are not equivalent, RS-fMR imaging should not be an outright replacement for T-fMR imaging; however: "since there is significant agreement between the two techniques, RS-fMRI can be considered with caution as a potential alternative to T-MRI when patients are unable to perform the task."[27]

Hou and colleagues[28] compared the location of the hand motor functional areas as determined by RS-fMR imaging, T-fMR imaging, and anatomy in 10 healthy subjects and 25 patients with left hemisphere brain tumors. They determined that, for most of their tumor cases, there was too large a discrepancy between the location of the hand motor area as determined by the T-fMR imaging and the location as determined by the anatomy and RS-fMR imaging. Their conclusion was that RS-fMR imaging is an inadequate replacement for T-fMR imaging. The authors believe that the differences in methodology between our study and that of Hou and colleagues[28] explain our discrepant conclusions. Hou and colleagues[28] used a classic seed-based approach in single subjects with a small seed size. Although the authors have used a similar approach in the past, we no longer do so because the signal to noise ratio (SNR) is poor and can lead to erroneous results. Our current approach using the MLP overcomes limited SNR by using prior information obtained from a large sample of control subjects. Hou and colleagues[28] also focused exclusively on the hand motor area, whereas we focus on the full extent of the SM system.

When taken together and considered clinically, there are advantages to the RS-fMR imaging approach that go beyond the task-independent nature of the imaging acquisition. In this study, RS-fMR imaging covered a larger portion of the SM system, rather than the more focal region identified with T-fMR imaging. From a neurosurgical standpoint, this is of high importance. Lesions that are to be resected can be in proximity to any portion of the motor system. In the case of task-based localization, this either requires customized tasks to best assess motor location relevant to that lesion or, if the same task is used consistently (ie, finger tapping), requires the surgeon to extrapolate the area of activation to other areas presumed to be motor and thus introduces the potential for error. Having a more comprehensive representation is fundamentally better from a neurosurgical standpoint. Because of the unique anatomic nature of motor organization, a focal activation and associated anatomic extrapolations are still usable, but this does not hold true for other functional systems, such a language. As an example, a focal activation of language task does not necessarily identify the full language system, nor can those locations be anatomically inferred from the focal activations. Thus, although this study used the anatomic nature of motor systems as a ground truth, it highlights that resting-state imaging approaches capture a more capacious assessment of the functional system, which has important implications for other functional systems in which there are fewer anatomic cues for localization and task only provides a more restricted localization.

SUMMARY

Localization of the SM system was compared in 38 patients with brain tumors using finger-tapping T-fMR imaging versus RS-fMR imaging. Our reference comparison was anatomic information obtained from 2 different registration schemes. Because T-fMR imaging and RS-fMR imaging measure a different aspect of brain function (task activation vs synchronous intrinsic activity), identical results were not expected; however, as expected and in agreement with prior publications, both methods provided accurate representation of the SM region, with the resting-state representation covering a larger portion of the SM system. The authors conclude that either method can provide the information necessary for appropriate presurgical planning, provided that the differences between the two methods are appropriately considered. In addition, RS-fMR imaging offers the logistical advantage of simple acquisition without the need for patient cooperation. However, effective RSN mapping requires considerable sophistication in preprocessing of RS-fMR imaging data as well as in the application of advanced numerical techniques (ie, MLP regression) to analyze the preprocessed data.

REFERENCES

1. Biswal B, Yetkin FZ, Haughton VM, et al. Functional connectivity in the motor cortex of resting human brain using echo-planar MRI. Magn Reson Med 1995;34(4):537–41.
2. Raichle ME. Two views of brain function. Trends Cogn Sci 2010;14(4):180–90.
3. Raichle ME. The restless brain: how intrinsic activity organizes brain function. Philos Trans R Soc Lond B Biol Sci 2015;370(1668):20140172.
4. Kokkonen SM, Nikkinen J, Remes J, et al. Preoperative localization of the sensorimotor area using independent component analysis of resting-state fMRI. Magn Reson Imaging 2009;27(6):733–40.
5. Shimony JS, Zhang D, Johnston JM, et al. Resting-state spontaneous fluctuations in brain activity: a new paradigm for presurgical planning using fMRI. Acad Radiol 2009;16(5):578–83.
6. Liu H, Buckner RL, Talukdar T, et al. Task-free presurgical mapping using functional magnetic resonance imaging intrinsic activity. J Neurosurg 2009; 111(4):746–54.
7. Zhang D, Johnston JM, Fox MD, et al. Preoperative sensorimotor mapping in brain tumor patients using spontaneous fluctuations in neuronal activity imaged with functional magnetic resonance imaging: initial experience. Neurosurgery 2009;65(6 Suppl):226–36.
8. Bottger J, Margulies DS, Horn P, et al. A software tool for interactive exploration of intrinsic functional connectivity opens new perspectives for brain surgery. Acta Neurochir (Wien) 2011;153(8):1561–72.

9. Lee MH, Smyser CD, Shimony JS. Resting-state fMRI: a review of methods and clinical applications. AJNR Am J Neuroradiol 2013;34(10):1866–72.

10. Lang S, Duncan N, Northoff G. Resting-state functional magnetic resonance imaging: review of neurosurgical applications. Neurosurgery 2014;74(5): 453–64 [discussion: 464–5].

11. Kamran M, Hacker CD, Allen MG, et al. Resting-state blood oxygen level-dependent functional magnetic resonance imaging for presurgical planning. Neuroimaging Clin North Am 2014;24(4): 655–69.

12. Tie Y, Rigolo L, Norton IH, et al. Defining language networks from resting-state fMRI for surgical planning–a feasibility study. Hum Brain Mapp 2014; 35(3):1018–30.

13. Leuthardt EC, Allen M, Kamran M, et al. Resting-state blood oxygen level-dependent functional MRI: a paradigm shift in preoperative brain mapping. Stereotact Funct Neurosurg 2015;93(6): 427–39.

14. Hart MG, Price SJ, Suckling J. Functional connectivity networks for preoperative brain mapping in neurosurgery. J Neurosurg 2017;126(6): 1941–50.

15. Lee MH, Miller-Thomas MM, Benzinger TL, et al. Clinical resting-state fMRI in the preoperative setting: are we ready for prime time? Top Magn Reson Imaging 2016;25(1):11–8.

16. Sair HI, Yahyavi-Firouz-Abadi N, Calhoun VD, et al. Presurgical brain mapping of the language network in patients with brain tumors using resting-state fMRI: comparison with task fMRI. Hum Brain Mapp 2016;37(3):913–23.

17. Smith SM, Fox PT, Miller KL, et al. Correspondence of the brain's functional architecture during activation and rest. Proc Natl Acad Sci U S A 2009; 106(31):13040–5.

18. Cordes D, Haughton VM, Arfanakis K, et al. Mapping functionally related regions of brain with functional connectivity MR imaging. AJNR Am J Neuroradiol 2000;21(9):1636–44.

19. Yeo BT, Krienen FM, Eickhoff SB, et al. Functional specialization and flexibility in human association cortex. Cereb Cortex 2015;25(10):3654–72.

20. Larson-Prior LJ, Zempel JM, Nolan TS, et al. Cortical network functional connectivity in the descent to sleep. Proc Natl Acad Sci U S A 2009;106(11): 4489–94.

21. Picchioni D, Pixa ML, Fukunaga M, et al. Decreased connectivity between the thalamus and the neocortex during human nonrapid eye movement sleep. Sleep 2014;37(2):387–97.

22. Samann PG, Wehrle R, Hoehn D, et al. Development of the brain's default mode network from wakefulness to slow wave sleep. Cereb Cortex 2011;21(9): 2082–93.

23. Tagliazucchi E, von Wegner F, Morzelewski A, et al. Automatic sleep staging using fMRI functional connectivity data. Neuroimage 2012;63(1):63–72.

24. Mhuircheartaigh RN, Rosenorn-Lanng D, Wise R, et al. Cortical and subcortical connectivity changes during decreasing levels of consciousness in humans: a functional magnetic resonance imaging study using propofol. J Neurosci 2010;30(27): 9095–102.

25. Mannfolk P, Nilsson M, Hansson H, et al. Can resting-state functional MRI serve as a complement to task-based mapping of sensorimotor function? A test-retest reliability study in healthy volunteers. J Magn Reson Imaging 2011;34(3):511–7.

26. Kristo G, Rutten GJ, Raemaekers M, et al. Task and task-free FMRI reproducibility comparison for motor network identification. Hum Brain Mapp 2014;35(1): 340–52.

27. Rosazza C, Aquino D, D'Incerti L, et al. Preoperative mapping of the sensorimotor cortex: comparative assessment of task-based and resting-state FMRI. PLoS One 2014;9(6):e98860.

28. Hou BL, Bhatia S, Carpenter JS. Quantitative comparisons on hand motor functional areas determined by resting state and task BOLD fMRI and anatomical MRI for pre-surgical planning of patients with brain tumors. Neuroimage Clin 2016;11:378–87.

29. Brier MR, Thomas JB, Snyder AZ, et al. Loss of intra-network and internetwork resting state functional connections with Alzheimer's disease progression. J Neurosci 2012;32(26):8890–9.

30. Power JD, Mitra A, Laumann TO, et al. Methods to detect, characterize, and remove motion artifact in resting state fMRI. Neuroimage 2014;84:320–41.

31. Fox MD, Zhang D, Snyder AZ, et al. The global signal and observed anticorrelated resting state brain networks. J Neurophysiol 2009;101(6): 3270–83.

32. Power JD, Plitt M, Laumann TO, et al. Sources and implications of whole-brain fMRI signals in humans. Neuroimage 2017;146:609–25.

33. Smyser CD, Inder TE, Shimony JS, et al. Longitudinal analysis of neural network development in preterm infants. Cereb Cortex 2010;20(12): 2852–62.

34. Hacker CD, Laumann TO, Szrama NP, et al. Resting state network estimation in individual subjects. Neuroimage 2013;82:616–33.

35. Corbetta M, Kincade JM, Ollinger JM, et al. Voluntary orienting is dissociated from target detection in human posterior parietal cortex. Nat Neurosci 2000;3(3):292–7.

36. Dale AM, Fischl B, Sereno MI. Cortical surface-based analysis. I. Segmentation and surface reconstruction. Neuroimage 1999;9(2):179–94.

37. Desikan RS, Segonne F, Fischl B, et al. An automated labeling system for subdividing the human

cerebral cortex on MRI scans into gyral based regions of interest. Neuroimage 2006;31(3):968–80.

38. Van Essen DC. A population-average, landmark- and surface-based (PALS) atlas of human cerebral cortex. Neuroimage 2005;28(3):635–62.

39. Marcus DS, Harwell J, Olsen T, et al. Informatics and data mining tools and strategies for the human connectome project. Front Neuroinform 2011;5:4.

40. Van Essen DC, Smith SM, Barch DM, et al. The WU-Minn Human Connectome Project: an overview. Neuroimage 2013;80:62–79.

41. Jaccard P. The distribution of the flora in the alpine zone. New Phytol 1912;11:37–50.

42. Batra P, Bandt SK, Leuthardt EC. Resting state functional connectivity magnetic resonance imaging integrated with intraoperative neuronavigation for functional mapping after aborted awake craniotomy. Surg Neurol Int 2016;7:13.

43. Roland JL, Hacker CD, Breshears JD, et al. Brain mapping in a patient with congenital blindness - a case for multimodal approaches. Front Hum Neurosci 2013;7:431.

44. Laumann TO, Snyder AZ, Mitra A, et al. On the stability of BOLD fMRI correlations. Cereb Cortex 2016. [Epub ahead of print].

45. Mitra A, Snyder AZ, Hacker CD, et al. Human cortical-hippocampal dialogue in wake and slow-wave sleep. Proc Natl Acad Sci U S A 2016; 113(44):E6868–76.

46. Burton H, Sinclair RJ, Wingert JR, et al. Multiple parietal operculum subdivisions in humans: tactile activation maps. Somatosens Mot Res 2008;25(3): 149–62.

47. Agarwal S, Sair HI, Yahyavi-Firouz-Abadi N, et al. Neurovascular uncoupling in resting state fMRI demonstrated in patients with primary brain gliomas. J Magn Reson Imaging 2016;43(3):620–6.

48. Zaca D, Jovicich J, Nadar SR, et al. Cerebrovascular reactivity mapping in patients with low grade gliomas undergoing presurgical sensorimotor mapping with BOLD fMRI. J Magn Reson Imaging 2014;40(2):383–90.

49. Mallela AN, Peck KK, Petrovich-Brennan NM, et al. Altered resting-state functional connectivity in the hand motor network in glioma patients. Brain Connect 2016. [Epub ahead of print].

50. Mitchell TJ, Hacker CD, Breshears JD, et al. A novel data-driven approach to preoperative mapping of functional cortex using resting-state functional magnetic resonance imaging. Neurosurgery 2013;73(6): 969–82 [discussion: 982–3].

Application of Resting State Functional MR Imaging to Presurgical Mapping: Language Mapping

Haris I. Sair, MD*, Shruti Agarwal, PhD, Jay J. Pillai, MD

KEYWORDS

- Presurgical brain mapping • Functional connectivity • Resting-state fMR imaging • Language

KEY POINTS

- Characterization of intrinsic language networks is feasible using resting state functional MR imaging (rs-fMR imaging) in healthy subjects, patients with epilepsy, and patients with brain lesions.
- In larger studies, interindividual variability in reliability of rs-fMR imaging language region localization is demonstrated.
- Language lateralization may be more effectively assessed compared with language center localization using rs-fMR imaging.

BACKGROUND

Blood-oxygen level–dependent (BOLD) functional MR imaging (fMR imaging) is widely used as a clinical tool for presurgical brain mapping. For lesions close to eloquent brain regions, the use of brain mapping with task-fMR imaging can result in reduced operative time and increased lesion resection; information from task-fMR imaging has also been shown to alter management by allowing the neurosurgeon to proceed with surgery when surgery was previously deemed too risky.[1]

Although task-fMR imaging is successfully used in routine clinical care for operative management, there are certain limitations to the technique. The nontrivial cost of implementation and maintenance of task-fMR imaging systems, including knowledgeable MR technologists to administer the test, raise the barrier of use in smaller institutions. For each brain function of interest to be interrogated, a sensitive and specific task paradigm must be designed while simultaneously attempting to diminish contributions from secondarily related brain regions. For language mapping, this means that several paradigms must be used to ensure adequate representation of the language network.

Patient-specific considerations also exist. Many of the patients who present for preoperative brain mapping may be neurologically debilitated because of the presence of large brain lesions and may be unable to comply with a given task. Although paradigms in various languages are available, nevertheless, occasionally one encounters patients for whom a paradigm in their native language is not available. In the pediatric population, selection of language paradigms may be limited because of varying visual and auditory language abilities and comprehension by age.

Resting state fMR imaging (rs-fMR imaging) has been investigated as an attractive alternative to task-fMR imaging. As no explicit task is given in rs-fMR imaging, the issue of patient compliance

Disclosure Statement: The authors have no relevant disclosures.
The Russell H. Morgan Department of Radiology and Radiological Science, Johns Hopkins University School of Medicine, 600 North Wolfe Street Phipps B100, Baltimore, MD 21287, USA
* Corresponding author.
E-mail address: hsair1@jhmi.edu

is significantly diminished, only necessitating basic instructions similar to routine MR imaging (primarily, to keep as motionless as possible). Although multiple task paradigms are usually necessary to interrogate a limited and specific brain function, rs-fMR imaging allows for simultaneous characterization of multiple brain networks within a reasonable acquisition time period of approximately 10 minutes. In this article, the authors review the major highlights of rs-fMR imaging language mapping for preoperative planning. Technical, methodological, developmental, and neurologic considerations that may affect reliable language mapping are described.

CONSIDERATIONS DURING RESTING STATE FUNCTIONAL MR IMAGING ACQUISITION

During rs-fMR imaging acquisition, visual status may have implications on reliability of intrinsic network characterization.[2] rs-fMR imaging can be acquired with eyes closed or eyes open, the latter either freely wandering or fixated to a graphical object. For the language network specifically, high reliability is seen in all visual conditions[3]; therefore, the method of most simple implementations may be optimal to ensure compliance across all subjects. At the authors' institution, they have used an eyes closed paradigm for rs-fMR imaging acquisition in brain tumor and epilepsy patients. One must also ensure that no cognitively directed instructions are given, as cognitive process may be altered depending on the specific instruction given. A common instruction is "keep your eyes closed, try to keep as still as possible without falling asleep, and don't think of anything in particular."

The effect of obtaining rs-fMR imaging following task-fMR imaging needs to be considered when interpreting studies of concordance and reliability. In many cases due to necessity, the rs-fMR imaging acquisition is added after routine clinical task-fMR imaging in order to ensure that critical clinically relevant image acquisition is not compromised due to factors such as patient fatigue. Rs-fMR imaging however is influenced by prior cognitive tasks; increases in connectivity between left and right middle frontal gyri and between posterior cingulate cortex and medial prefrontal cortex are found in rs-fMR imaging when a recent language-task fMR imaging has been performed.[4]

IMAGE PROCESSING

Variations in processing may affect connectivity metrics in rs-fMR imaging. The influence of head motion on connectivity is well known, with micro-movements causing loss of long-range connectivity within networks.[5] Physiologic nuisance from cardiopulmonary effects also alter connectivity. Motion correction using a 6-parameter affine transformation is commonly performed for task-fMR imaging as well as rs-fMR imaging. Following motion correction, the realignment parameters are included as nuisance regressors. Additional motion-related regressors may be included using derivatives of the original motion regressors as well as time shifts. For large shifts in sporadic motion during scanning, volume censoring based on relative spatial displacement (framewise displacement) or relative signal variances (derivative of root-mean-square variance over voxels) may be used, commonly known as "scrubbing."[5,6] Volume censoring should not be used in analysis of rs-fMR imaging in the frequency domain.

Physiologic nuisance regression may be performed using a wide variety of techniques, either prospectively (ideally) or retrospectively. A common method of nuisance regression is to estimate white matter and cerebrospinal fluid signal changes that are then regressed out of the fMR imaging dataset, such as in the CompCor method.[7] Caballero-Gaudes and Reynold[8] provide a comprehensive review of various methods to diminish influence of nonneural signals in BOLD fMR imaging datasets.

Global signal regression (GSR) has been used variably as a processing step in rs-fMR imaging analysis. Here, the mean BOLD signal across the entire set of voxels in a single acquisition volume is removed.[8] There is some controversy in the use of GSR in rs-fMR imaging.[9] As described later, specifically for language mapping using rs-fMR imaging, GSR may be disadvantageous because of some evidence that broad information about language systems may be present in the global signal.

CONNECTIVITY ANALYSIS

There are 2 major methods used for characterizing intrinsic language networks using rs-fMR imaging: seed-based analysis (SBA) and independent component analysis (ICA). SBA in general necessitates a priori knowledge of presumed language regions of the brain. Having selected a region of interest (ROI) as the seed, whole brain correlations of rs-fMR imaging BOLD time courses can be computed, generating spatial maps of the network of interest. There are several challenges in using SBA for language network characterization. First, the precise anatomic localization of language regions of the brain may be difficult to determine, because language function is more distributed across individuals compared with other systems such as the motor network.[10] SBA is less problematic when using productive language regions (Broca) as the seed, because there is relative constraint of anatomic distribution in the inferior frontal gyrus (IFG), although there certainly are gyral-level variations. For example, a seed ROI placed in the pars opercularis of the IFG may yield attention-related intrinsic networks in the dorsal aspect of the gyrus, compared with language-related regions in the ventral aspect. Attempting to seed primary receptive language areas (Wernicke) is more challenging because of the wider variation of functional localization in relation to anatomic landmarks. Further complicating the issue of high intersubject functional network variability is the presence of normal anatomic variations across individuals, which may be relatively high in the IFG (Fig. 1).[11] Even when limiting SBA in anatomically normal individuals, the selection of seed placement may result in multiple normal patterns of language networks. Broca region comprises Brodmann regions 44

and 45[12]; these regions demonstrate different connectivity patterns to the inferior parietal lobule (specifically the supramarginal gyrus, connected to area 44) and along the posterior superior temporal sulcus (connected to area 45).[13] Using this knowledge, Jakobsen and colleagues[14] were able to parcellate these subsegments of Broca region at the individual level. Thus, in SBA the expected topology of the language network may be different, but both correct depending on whether area 44 or 45 was used as the seed ROI.

Second, although in most cases language function is lateralized to the left hemisphere in right-handed individuals, for those whose language function may be bilaterally distributed or even completely on the contralateral right side, seeding only the left hemisphere may yield incorrect results. An option here is to generate seeds from bilateral hemispheres; however, without a known target spatial map of language function for a particular subject, it may be difficult to determine which side is the correct intrinsic language network (or the relative contribution of each side). Last, in clinical populations,

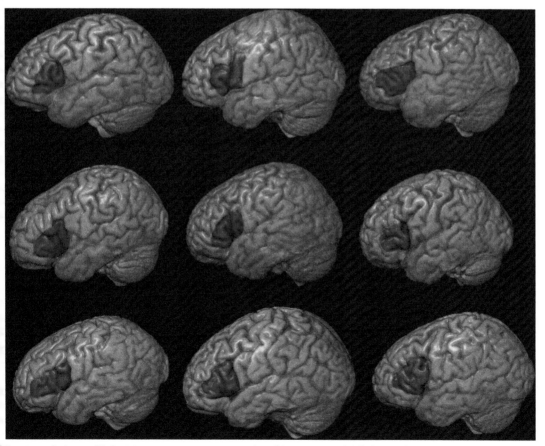

Fig. 1. Variations of left IFG anatomy across 9 sample subjects. Areas shaded in red are presumed to represent left IFG.

accurate placement of seed ROIs may be precluded for various reasons. Significant brain shifts in those with mass lesions may obscure known anatomic landmarks. Tumors may directly infiltrate language-related brain regions. Reorganization of brain function may also occur with slow-growing lesions or in patients with epilepsy.

ICA is a data-driven method that overcomes some of the limitations of SBA described above. ICA generates a maximally independent set of linear representations of multivariate signals, with the assumption that the signals are statistically independent of each other.[15] It has been shown to be a robust and efficient method to generate intrinsic brain networks. ICA is typically simpler at the onset for language network characterization because no decision on ROI placement is necessary. However, there is a different set of challenges in using ICA in rs-fMR imaging. There are many methods of estimating the optimum number of components (ie, ICA orders); however, it is not clear that a single method has emerged that can be accurately used across all settings for fMR imaging data.[16] Using low ICA orders, networks of interest may not be completely separated from other networks of no interest. On the opposite end of the spectrum, high ICA orders may cause fragmentation of the network of interest into subnetworks. Selecting the language network out of multiple components may also be difficult, compounded by the potential problem described above of subnetworks being split across components. Many of the studies to date use task-fMR imaging as the "gold standard" when selecting the correct rs-fMR imaging language map; however, in the authors' experience, when expert fMR imagers are asked to blindly select potential language maps from only rs-fMR imaging data, the accuracy is not high; this limits the utility of rs-fMR imaging as an independent tool for language network characterization when task-fMR imaging is not performed. A potential alternative is to use a population-based language template to narrow the candidate components, although issues of nonstandard (ie, right-hemisphere or mixed) language dominance, and changes in language network spatial distribution due to brain shifts or network reorganization, would limit this approach as in the SBA method.

RELIABILITY OF RESTING STATE FUNCTIONAL MR IMAGING METRICS

Accurate assessment of the reliability of rs-fMR imaging must be made if it is to be considered a viable clinical tool. Although reproducibility of rs-fMR imaging has been shown to be high in initial reports,[17] more recent studies highlight the individual variability of functional connectivity across subjects.[18,19] There seems to be converging evidence that although there is variability in the pattern of connectivity across individuals, the reproducibility of connectivity within a single subject is high. This pattern of reproducibility has introduced the concept of rs-fMR imaging "fingerprinting," the identification of a single subject based on functional connectivity, which necessitates a combination of a certain degree of intersubject variance while maintaining high intrasubject reproducibility.[18,19] Given a set of unlabeled test-retest rs-fMR imaging data, the authors' group showed that a blinded algorithm was accurately able to determine the correct pairs of test-retest rs-fMR imaging scans for a set of subjects.[18] Furthermore, they demonstrated that higher-order association cortices represented the brain regions that most contributed to the ability of the algorithm to identify unique subjects, including regions implicated in language function such as the inferior frontal gyri and the posterior temporal lobe. The implication of this is that at the state of rest, subject-level variability in the organization of brain networks may impede characterization of a specific network of interest. For example, in a subject whose language network might be strongly associated with the default mode network, it may be difficult to dissociate components of each.

Depending on the exact metric used for connectivity analysis, varying levels of intrasubject and intersubject reliability may be found. A dataset of 300 rs-fMR imaging scans from 30 healthy participants over 1 month (on average one scan every 3 days) showed relatively high intrasubject variability and low intersubject variability of graph theoretic metrics of language-related brain areas.[20]

RELIABILITY OF RESTING STATE FUNCTIONAL MR IMAGING LANGUAGE NETWORK IN HEALTHY SUBJECTS

In a large number of healthy subjects (970), Tomasi and Volkow[21] showed high reproducibility of language networks derived from rs-fMR imaging across multiple institutions with variable acquisition methods.

High-field scanning may improve sensitivity and specificity of rs-fMR imaging language networks by taking advantage of increased signal-to-noise ratio. In healthy controls, there is high intrasession and intersession (1 week separation between scans) reliability of language networks at 7 T, similar to or exceeding test-retest metrics of task-fMR imaging reliability.[22]

RESTING STATE FUNCTIONAL MR IMAGING IN PREOPERATIVE PLANNING: LANGUAGE LOCALIZATION

Most studies examining the clinical utility of rs-fMR imaging in preoperative planning have concentrated on motor mapping, which yields promising findings. For localization of hand motor brain regions, some reports indicate rs-fMR imaging to be comparable to direct cortical stimulation (DCS), with accuracy possibly even surpassing task-fMR imaging.[23,24]

For language mapping using rs-fMR imaging, fewer detailed studies exist. A caveat in comparing rs-fMR imaging language networks with task-fMR imaging language activation is alterations in network connectivity and recruitment of additional functional regions during a task compared with rest. Commonly, in addition to primary language regions of Broca (IFG) and Wernicke (superior temporal gyrus [STG]), additional sites of activation during task-fMR imaging language studies include the dorsolateral prefrontal cortex, ventral motor and premotor cortex, and the presupplementary motor area. Other networks not classically belonging to the language system may also demonstrate connectivity changes during a task; graph theoretic analysis of a semantic decision task demonstrated emergence of language-related modules during the task that were separate from modules detected at rest, and reduction in connectivity of hub region of the default mode network was noted.[25] Few studies directly compare rs-fMR imaging language networks to DCS, because of the difficulty of obtaining such data in a systematic fashion. Within this limitation however, there are several encouraging studies demonstrating the utility of rs-fMR imaging as a viable tool for preoperative language mapping.

In one of the earliest investigations of the utility of rs-fMR imaging language mapping patients with brain lesions, Tie and colleagues[26] demonstrate the feasibility of extracting language networks from rs-fMR imaging in individual subjects using ICA with template matching to select the language specific ICA component. Branco and colleagues[27] demonstrate fair concordance between rs-fMR imaging language maps derived from ICA and noun-verb language task fMR imaging in 15 subjects with brain lesions. In this study, using a template-matching procedure to identify rs-fMR imaging language networks, the degree of concordance between the ICA components

and the template were ranked from highest to lowest. The first ranked component correctly corresponded to the language network in 12 subjects (80%), and for the remaining 3, the second ranked component.

Studies directly comparing rs-fMR imaging language networks with DCS are limited. One of the first studies in a limited number of subjects used a novel machine-learning algorithm comprising a neural network to label each brain voxel by classifying the spatial pattern of its whole brain correlation. The language network derived from this scheme demonstrated respectable overlap with DCS, with area under the curve of 0.76, even in patients with lesion-related brain shifts in expected language regions.[28]

Cochereau and colleagues[29] recently published the largest dataset comparing rs-fMR imaging derived motor and language networks and DCS in patients with low-grade gliomas (DCS). SBA demonstrated high temporal correlations between regions of known language regions confirmed by DCS. ICA was successful in identifying language networks in 75% of the patients and was in general able to label eloquent language brain regions (greater than 90% concordance at 10 mm of error margin, and 70% at 5 mm of error margin between rs-fMR imaging and DCS). However, overall high interindividual variability of mapping accuracy was found, consistent with results of the authors' study comparing rs-fMR imaging versus task-fMR imaging language mapping.[30]

The authors' study comprised to date the largest dataset (49 subjects) comparing rs-fMR imaging language networks (using ICA) with a consistent set of language task-fMR imaging paradigms designed to activate the global language network, namely the Silent Word Generation, Sentence Completion, and Rhyming tasks. When conjunction analysis is performed, using these 3 paradigms reliability elicits language-specific brain regions while minimizing contributions from concurrent activation of nonlanguage regions. The authors found overall moderate concordance between rs-fMR imaging and task-fMR imaging at a group level, however with a concerning wide range of concordance across subjects (Fig. 2). Given the findings of some patients with excellent concordance, theoretically rs-fMR imaging has the potential to provide highly accurate language maps at the individual level; however, further studies are needed to improve reliability across all subjects. There is the possibility that there is a certain limit of obtaining reliable rs-fMR imaging language maps in an individual; however, in this case, a robust metric to determine the inherent reliability or accuracy of the rs-fMR imaging

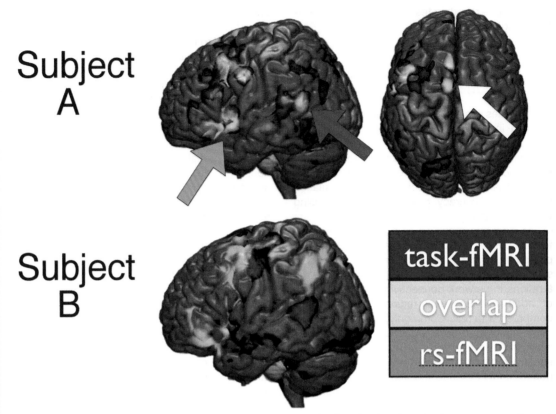

Fig. 2. Composite language task-fMR imaging activation maps (*red*) and rs-fMR imaging language maps (*green*) overlaid on MNI-152 brain template. Maps from 2 representative subjects are shown. Subject A (*top row*) demonstrates high overlap between task-fMR imaging and rs-fMR imaging (*regions of overlap indicated in yellow*) in both primary productive (*blue arrow*) and receptive (*purple arrow*) language regions. High overlap is also seen in the left-lateralized presupplemental motor area (pre-SMA; *white arrow*). Subject B (*bottom row*) however does not demonstrate any significant overlap.

language map, without a gold standard, must be detailed for this technique to be used as a clinical tool in lieu of task-fMR imaging.

For this reason, language network localization using only rs-fMR imaging should be used with caution at the current time, because no convincing metric is known to determine the intrinsic reliability of rs-fMR imaging language maps without a known target such as task-fMR imaging or DCS. A potential use of rs-fMR imaging at this time is as an adjunctive tool with task-fMR imaging in cases of limited activations, which nevertheless demonstrates a convergent focus of activation that then may be used as the seed to determine the global language network using rs-fMR imaging, although further studies are necessary to see whether targeted rs-fMR imaging analysis in this fashion improves accuracy compared with DCS.

Perhaps one explanation of the subject-level variability in language network detection success is the nature of the cognitive state during rs-fMR imaging acquisition. Although broadly classified as "rest," more accurately, this state encompasses a range of undirected cognitive functioning. Dynamic connectivity analysis of rs-fMR imaging demonstrates a consistent set of "states" during rest, with wide variation of functional network attribution for a particular anatomic region.[31] Decreased correlations between network modules are associated with self-reported measures of time spent in visual mental imagery and/ or inner language.[32] Thus, as expected, intrinsic rs-fMR imaging network correlations are likely related to the specific pattern of cognitive processes occurring during image acquisition. Intrinsic language maps may thus be characterized best in those with a higher frequency of time spent in language-related cognitive mind-wandering. To limit random mind-wandering and to constrain cognitive processes to improve network detection, "pseudo" rs-fMR imaging acquisitions using movie watching during scanning have also been used.[33]

Beyond rs-fMR imaging, very high concordance of intrinsic language network localization at rest versus task has also been shown using near-infrared spectroscopy in adults and children, indicating that highly reliable language-related signals exist in the brain at rest.[34]

RESTING STATE FUNCTIONAL MR IMAGING IN PREOPERATIVE PLANNING: LANGUAGE LATERALIZATION

A direct comparison of rs-fMR imaging and intra-carotid amobarbital procedure (IAP, commonly known as the "Wada" test) in 23 patients with intractable focal epilepsy showed 96% accuracy of rs-fMR imaging in language lateralization using CA with IAP as the gold standard.[35] Only in one patient was the result discordant; IAP demonstrated left language function, whereas rs-fMR imaging indicated probable bilateral language function. The relative simplicity of rs-fMR imaging analysis in this study is attractive in attempting to use rs-fMR imaging as a clinically viable tool; 20 CA components were estimated for all subjects using ICA (eliminating decision making about optimal number of target components for each subject), and a *bilateral* language network template comprising bilateral IFG, inferior parietal lobules, and superior temporal gyri was used to select the most probable language ICA component. Supporting the use of templates with bilateral language ROIs is an rs-fMR imaging SBA study demonstrating the role of the right hemisphere in language.[36] In healthy volunteers, the hemispheric global rs-fMR imaging signal also shows leftward asymmetry correlating with frontal and temporal brain regions related to semantic processing, suggesting that this rather crude measurement may be potentially used for language lateralization.[37] Caution must be exercised however because global functional connectivity may be impaired in patients with epilepsy, correlated with longer duration of epilepsy.[38] Furthermore, there is an increased likelihood of language reorganization in epilepsy patients.[39–41] In patients with rolandic epilepsy, specific altered connectivity is demonstrated between the motor network and the left inferior frontal gyrus (ie, Broca region).[42] In addition, discordant lateralization between expressive and receptive language regions can also occur.

SBA has also been used to determine language laterality with findings corroborating the above. Interestingly, in another study using SBA to determine language lateralization from rs-fMR imaging data in patients with temporal lobe epilepsy, seeding of the *contralateral* IFG appeared to be the most predictive of laterality index correlated with

that obtained using a verb generation task when spatially constraining analyses to sites of potential primarily language areas only (bilateral IFG, middle temporal gyrus [MTG], and STG).[43] In a large set of 44 patients referred for presurgical brain mapping with heterogeneous lesions from gliomas to cavernous malformations, assessment of connectivity between language regions and the frontal pole, superior frontal gyrus, and the supramarginal gyrus significantly correlated with task-fMR imaging lateralization.[44]

NEUROVASCULAR UNCOUPLING

A critical assumption in utilization of BOLD fMR imaging in assessing underlying neural function is the integrity of the normal neurovascular response associated with neural activity. Indeed, there are instances whereby this relationship is broken, termed neurovascular uncoupling (NVU).[45] NVU can occur in the vicinity of brain tumors. Recently, Agarwal and colleagues[46] showed the presence of NVU in rs-fMR imaging in a cohort of 7 patients with brain tumors. Furthermore, NVU was also shown in rs-fMR imaging at 7 T.[47]

MULTILINGUAL SUBJECTS

The organization of the multilingual brain is different than the organization of brains that are monolingual.[48,49] Altered RS functional connectivity of language control systems is shown in bilingual individuals.[50] Furthermore, there are differences in functional connectivity in bilinguals who learn 2 languages simultaneously versus those that learn them sequentially.[51] For multilingual patients then, a data-driven approach to characterizing rs-fMR imaging language networks may be preferable to account for these variabilities. On one hand, ICA may be able to separate distinct connectivity profiles for different languages within a subject. On the other hand, variable degrees of involvement of a comprehensive language network or possibly separate but overlapping networks for languages may result in a single combined ICA component for more than one language.

LANGUAGE PREDICTION

Intrinsic connectivity patterns may also be useful for prediction. The pattern of connectivity between 2 language-related brain regions is shown to be correlated with lexical retrieval and reading speed of a second learned language.[52] Connectivity between the left visual word form area and the left mid superior temporal gyrus correlates with reading speed and connectivity between the left anterior insula/frontal operculum, and the dorsal anterior cingulate cortex correlates with lexical retrieval of a second language, indicating innate baseline characteristics that can be used to predict an individual's ability to learn a second language. In another study, regional amplitude of low-frequency fluctuations (ALFF) in the left superior temporal gyrus was shown to correlate with learning of pitch patterns in a foreign language; additional non-language-related networks also demonstrated correlations with this learning, such as the default mode network where ALFF was negatively correlated.[53] The complex interplay between language-specific networks and nonlanguage networks may further yield insight into the functional organization of the intrinsic language network.

Rs-fMR imaging may also be used to determine neurocognitive outcome following neurologic intervention; graph theory measures of the left IFG correlate with language function following anterior temporal lobectomy in patients with temporal lobe epilepsy.[54]

CHILDREN

Rs-fMR imaging is perhaps most attractive as a preoperative mapping tool in the pediatric population, where compliance with task-fMR imaging may be significantly limited. Vadivelu and colleagues[55] present a small series of pediatric cases using rs-fMR imaging language mapping in patients undergoing epilepsy surgery using ICA. Although rs-fMR imaging may be most applicable in this group, unique challenges exist in the pediatric population. Changes in functional connectivity are seen during development,[56] and changes in functional connectivity patterns during development therefore must be fully characterized to ensure connectivity patterns for patients presenting at any age. During infancy, both the IFG and the STG show increasing interhemispheric symmetry of connectivity, which steadily decrease in both regions starting at approximately 11 to 12 months of age, indicating initiation of hemispheric functional specialization around that time.[57] In this longitudinal study of 71 infants, behavioral language scores were also shown to correlate with both early peaking of IFG interhemispheric symmetry (and therefore early initiation of hemispheric lateralization) and the magnitude of symmetry at peak.

SUMMARY

Rs-fMR imaging remains a promising tool for preoperative language mapping. Early reports with small numbers of patients with brain lesions indicated high concordance of language region localization between rs-fMR imaging and task-fMR imaging or DCS. More recent larger studies highlight the subject-level variability in concordance. Further large-scale studies are necessary to validate rs-fMR imaging as a clinically viable tool for preoperative language localization. Assessment of language lateralization with rs-fMR imaging appears to be higher in accuracy however, again large-scale studies for validation are necessary.

REFERENCES

1. Petrella JR, Shah LM, Harris KM, et al. Preoperative functional MR imaging localization of language and motor areas: effect on therapeutic decision making in patients with potentially resectable brain tumors Radiology 2006;240(3):793–802.
2. Patriat R, Molloy EK, Meier TB, et al. The effect of resting condition on resting-state fMRI reliability and consistency: a comparison between resting with eyes open, closed, and fixated. Neuroimage 2013;78:463–73.
3. Kollndorfer K, Fischmeister FPhS, Kasprian G, et al. A systematic investigation of the invariance of resting-state network patterns: is resting-state fMR ready for pre-surgical planning? Front Hum Neurosc 2013;7:95.
4. Waites AB, Stanislavsky A, Abbott DF, et al. Effect of prior cognitive state on resting state networks measured with functional connectivity. Hum Brain Mapp 2005;24(1):59–68.
5. Power JD, Barnes KA, Snyder AZ, et al. Spurious but systematic correlations in functional connectivity MRI networks arise from subject motion. Neuro image 2012;59(3):2142–54.
6. Power JD, Mitra A, Laumann TO, et al. Methods to detect, characterize, and remove motion artifact in resting state fMRI. Neuroimage 2014;84:320–41.
7. Behzadi Y, Restom K, Liau J, et al. A component based noise correction method (CompCor) for BOLD and perfusion based fMRI. Neuroimage 2007;37(1):90–101.
8. Caballero-Gaudes C, Reynolds RC. Methods for cleaning the BOLD fMRI signal. Neuroimage 2017 154:128–49.
9. Liu TT, Nalci A, Falahpour M. The global signal in fMRI: nuisance or information? Neuroimage 2017 150:213–29.
10. Sanai N, Mirzadeh Z, Berger MS. Functional outcome after language mapping for glioma resection. N Engl J Med 2008;358(1):18–27.
11. Keller SS, Highley JR, Garcia-Finana M, et al. Sulca variability, stereological measurement and asymmetry

of Broca's area on MR images. J Anat 2007;211(4): 534–55.

12. Amunts K, Schleicher A, Bürgel U, et al. Broca's region revisited: cytoarchitecture and intersubject variability. J Comp Neurol 1999;412(2):319–41.

13. Margulies DS, Petrides M. Distinct parietal and temporal connectivity profiles of ventrolateral frontal areas involved in language production. J Neurosci 2013;33(42):16846–52.

14. Jakobsen E, Liem F, Klados MA, et al. Automated individual-level parcellation of Broca's region based on functional connectivity. Neuroimage 2016. http:// dx.doi.org/10.1016/j.neuroimage.2016.09.069.

15. Calhoun VD, Potluru VK, Phlypo R, et al. Independent component analysis for brain fMRI does indeed select for maximal independence. PLos One 2013; 8(8):e73309.

16. Hui M, Li J, Wen X, et al. An empirical comparison of information-theoretic criteria in estimating the number of independent components of fMRI data. PLoS One 2011;6(12):e29274.

17. Damoiseaux JS, Rombouts SaRB, Barkhof F, et al. Consistent resting-state networks across healthy subjects. Proc Natl Acad Sci U S A 2006;103(37): 13848–53.

18. Airan RD, Vogelstein JT, Pillai JJ, et al. Factors affecting characterization and localization of interindividual differences in functional connectivity using MRI. Hum Brain Mapp 2016;37(5): 1986–97.

19. Finn ES, Shen X, Scheinost D, et al. Functional connectome fingerprinting: identifying individuals using patterns of brain connectivity. Nat Neurosci 2015; 18(11):1664–71.

20. Chen B, Xu T, Zhou C, et al. Individual variability and test-retest reliability revealed by ten repeated resting-state brain scans over one month. PLoS One 2015;10(12):e0144963.

21. Tomasi D, Volkow ND. Resting functional connectivity of language networks: characterization and reproducibility. Mol Psychiatry 2012;17(8):841–54.

22. Branco P, Seixas D, Castro SL. Temporal reliability of ultra-high field resting-state MRI for single-subject sensorimotor and language mapping. Neuroimage 2016. http://dx.doi.org/10.1016/j.neuroimage.2016. 11.029.

23. Zhang D, Johnston JM, Fox MD, et al. Preoperative sensorimotor mapping in brain tumor patients using spontaneous fluctuations in neuronal activity imaged with fMRI: initial experience. Neurosurgery 2009; 65(6 Suppl):226–36.

24. Qiu TM, Yan CG, Tang WJ, et al. Localizing hand motor area using resting-state fMRI: validated with direct cortical stimulation. Acta Neurochir (Wien) 2014;156(12):2295–302.

25. DeSalvo MN, Douw L, Takaya S, et al. Task-dependent reorganization of functional connectivity networks during visual semantic decision making. Brain Behav 2014;4(6):877–85.

26. Tie Y, Rigolo L, Norton IH, et al. Defining language networks from resting-state fMRI for surgical planning—a feasibility study. Hum Brain Mapp 2014; 35(3):1018–30.

27. Branco P, Seixas D, Deprez S, et al. Resting-state functional magnetic resonance imaging for language preoperative planning. Front Hum Neurosci 2016;10:11.

28. Mitchell TJ, Hacker CD, Breshears JD, et al. A novel data-driven approach to preoperative mapping of functional cortex using resting-state functional magnetic resonance imaging. Neurosurgery 2013;73(6): 969–82, 983.

29. Cochereau J, Deverdun J, Herbet G, et al. Comparison between resting state fMRI networks and responsive cortical stimulations in glioma patients. Hum Brain Mapp 2016;37(11):3721–32.

30. Sair HI, Yahyavi-Firouz-Abadi N, Calhoun VD, et al. Presurgical brain mapping of the language network in patients with brain tumors using resting-state fMRI: comparison with task fMRI. Hum Brain Mapp 2016;37(3):913–23.

31. Allen EA, Damaraju E, Plis SM, et al. Tracking whole-brain connectivity dynamics in the resting state. Cereb Cortex 2014;24(3):663–76.

32. Doucet G, Naveau M, Petit L, et al. Patterns of hemodynamic low-frequency oscillations in the brain are modulated by the nature of free thought during rest. Neuroimage 2012;59(4):3194–200.

33. Tie Y, Rigolo L, Ozdemir OA, et al. A new paradigm for individual subject language mapping: movie-watching fMRI. J Neuroimaging 2015;25(5):710–20.

34. Gallagher A, Tremblay J, Vannasing P. Language mapping in children using resting-state functional connectivity: comparison with a task-based approach. J Biomed Opt 2016;21(12):125006.

35. DeSalvo MN, Tanaka N, Douw L, et al. Resting-state functional MR imaging for determining language laterality in intractable epilepsy. Radiology 2016; 281(1):264–9.

36. Muller AM, Meyer M. Language in the brain at rest: new insights from resting state data and graph theoretical analysis. Front Hum Neurosci 2014;8:228.

37. McAvoy M, Mitra A, Coalson RS, et al. Unmasking language lateralization in human brain intrinsic activity. Cereb Cortex 2016;26(4):1733–46.

38. Englot DJ, Hinkley LB, Kort NS, et al. Global and regional functional connectivity maps of neural oscillations in focal epilepsy. Brain 2015;138(Pt 8): 2249–62.

39. Hamberger MJ, Cole J. Language organization and reorganization in epilepsy. Neuropsychol Rev 2011; 21(3):240.

40. Pravatà E, Sestieri C, Mantini D, et al. Functional connectivity MR imaging of the language network

in patients with drug-resistant epilepsy. AJNR Am J Neuroradiol 2011;32(3):532–40.

41. Waites AB, Briellmann RS, Saling MM, et al. Functional connectivity networks are disrupted in left temporal lobe epilepsy. Ann Neurol 2006;59(2):335–43.

42. Besseling RMH, Jansen JFA, Overvliet GM, et al. Reduced functional integration of the sensorimotor and language network in rolandic epilepsy. Neuroimage Clin 2013;2:239–46.

43. Doucet GE, Pustina D, Skidmore C, et al. Resting-state functional connectivity predicts the strength of hemispheric lateralization for language processing in temporal lobe epilepsy and normals. Hum Brain Mapp 2015;36(1):288–303.

44. Teghipco A, Hussain A, Tivarus ME. Disrupted functional connectivity affects resting state based language lateralization. Neuroimage Clin 2016;12:910–27.

45. Pillai JJ, Mikulis DJ. Cerebrovascular reactivity mapping: an evolving standard for clinical functional imaging. AJNR Am J Neuroradiol 2015;36(1):7–13.

46. Agarwal S, Sair HI, Yahyavi-Firouz-Abadi N, et al. Neurovascular uncoupling in resting state fMRI demonstrated in patients with primary brain gliomas. J Magn Reson Imaging 2016;43(3):620–6.

47. Agarwal S, Sair HI, Airan R, et al. Demonstration of brain tumor-induced neurovascular uncoupling in resting-state fMRI at ultrahigh field. Brain Connect 2016;6(4):267–72.

48. Berken JA, Gracco VL, Klein D. Early bilingualism, language attainment, and brain development. Neuropsychologia 2016;2017(98):220–7.

49. Wong B, Yin B, O'Brien B. Neurolinguistics: structure, function, and connectivity in the bilingual brain. Biomed Res Int 2016;2016:7069274.

50. Li L, Abutalebi J, Zou L, et al. Bilingualism alters brain functional connectivity between "control" regions and "language" regions: evidence from bimodal bilinguals. Neuropsychologia 2015;71:236–47.

51. Berken JA, Chai X, Chen JK, et al. Effects of early and late bilingualism on resting-state functional connectivity. J Neurosci 2016;36(4):1165–72.

52. Chai XJ, Berken JA, Barbeau EB, et al. Intrinsic functional connectivity in the adult brain and success in second-language learning. J Neurosci 2016;36(3):755–61.

53. Deng Z, Chandrasekaran B, Wang S, et al. Resting-state low-frequency fluctuations reflect individual differences in spoken language learning. Cortex 2016;76:63–78.

54. Doucet GE, Rider R, Taylor N, et al. Presurgery resting-state local graph-theory measures predict neurocognitive outcomes after brain surgery in temporal lobe epilepsy. Epilepsia 2015;56(4):517–26.

55. Vadivelu S, Wolf VL, Bollo RJ, et al. Resting-state functional MRI in pediatric epilepsy surgery. Pediatr Neurosurg 2014;49(5):261–73.

56. Xiao Y, Friederici AD, Margulies DS, et al. Longitudinal changes in resting-state fMRI from age 5 to age 6 years covary with language development. Neuroimage 2016;128:116–24.

57. Emerson RW, Gao W, Lin W. Longitudinal study of the emerging functional connectivity asymmetry of primary language regions during infancy. J Neurosci 2016;36(42):10883–92.

Limitations of Resting-State Functional MR Imaging in the Setting of Focal Brain Lesions

 CrossMark

Shruti Agarwal, PhD, Haris I. Sair, MD, Jay J. Pillai, MD*

KEYWORDS

• Resting-state fMR imaging • Motor activation • Neurovascular uncoupling • Presurgical mapping

KEY POINTS

The purpose of this article is to review the feasibility of blood oxygen level dependent (BOLD) resting-state functional MR imaging (rsfMR imaging) in the setting of focal brain lesions. We describe how assessment of resting-state functional connectivity can be adversely affected by the presence of various lesion-related confounds.

- Discussion of general confounds that adversely affect rsfMR imaging analysis.
- Challenges in processing/analysis of rsfMR imaging data in the setting of neurovascular uncoupling (NVU) and susceptibility artifact.
- Assessment of NVU related to focal brain lesions and its effect on visualization of different functional networks in lesions involving motor and language cortical areas with the use of various rsfMR imaging metrics.

INTRODUCTION

In 1995, Biswal and colleagues[1] discovered that, even during rest, in the absence of any explicit task, the blood oxygen level dependent (BOLD) signal within the brain's sensorimotor network fluctuated synchronously. Contrary to unstructured neuronal activity at rest as expected, a correlation has been found among brain regions that were known to function together within a single network. Later, in a series of experiments, Raichle and colleagues[2] showed that the brain is constantly active even when the person is not engaged in a specific task (ie, the resting state), and the brain's energy consumption is increased by less than 5% of its baseline energy consumption while performing a focused task. The findings suggested that networks of brain regions that activate or deactivate together during tasks maintain signatures of their connectivity even at rest.[3] "Resting-state functional connectivity"[4–6] is a promising approach to study the functional organization of both the healthy and abnormal brain, particularly in subjects who cannot complete challenging cognitive tasks. Unlike task-based functional MR imaging (tbfMR imaging), which typically highlights a single brain network associated with any given task, resting-state functional MR imaging (rsfMR imaging) allows one to observe many networks at once with a single imaging acquisition. The simplicity of the procedure and its relatively short duration are other advantages of rsfMR imaging. Further,

Disclosure Statement: No competing financial interests exist. This work was partially supported by National Institutes of Health grant R42 CA173976-02 (National Cancer Institute) (Principal Investigator: J.J. Pillai).
Division of Neuroradiology, The Russell H. Morgan Department of Radiology and Radiological Science, Johns Hopkins University School of Medicine, Phipps B-100, 1800 Orleans Street, Baltimore, MD 21287, USA
* Corresponding author.
E-mail address: jpillai1@jhmi.edu

synchronized resting-state networks (RSNs) have been found even during sleep and under anesthesia.[7,8] Scientists hope to use resting-state functional connectivity to help improve treatments for many different neurologic and neuropsychiatric conditions.[9–11]

Clinical applications of resting-state functional connectivity have continued to increase over the past decade. In recent years, there has been an increase in interest in the application of rsfMR imaging for presurgical planning in patients with brain tumors and other focal brain lesions, such as brain neoplasms, arteriovenous malformations, and other vascular malformations, cortical dysplasias, and other epileptogenic lesions. Presurgical mapping with tbfMR imaging has already been established as standard of care at many academic centers around the world, but rsfMR imaging has not yet been widely accepted for this purpose.

The purpose of this article was to review the feasibility of rsfMR imaging in the settings of focal brain lesions. Therefore, the remainder of the article will focus on various problems associated with performance and analysis of rsfMR imaging in the setting of focal brain lesions. This includes susceptibility artifacts and neurovascular uncoupling (NVU), which predominantly affect rsfMR imaging analysis in cases of structural brain lesions, as well as more generic problems, such as bulk head motion, which can result in similar image degradation.

SUSCEPTIBILITY EFFECTS

Susceptibility effects are often an issue at 3T and higher field strength. Susceptibility reflects the extent of magnetization of a substance in the presence of external magnetic field.[12] Diamagnetic substances, such as calcium in cortical bone, strongly disperse the external magnetic field, whereas tissues such as muscles, fat, and water are weakly diamagnetic. The largest susceptibilities, field distortions and MR artifacts are prominent around metal objects and implants.[13] These objects contain ferromagnetic materials such as Fe/Co/Ni, which strongly concentrate the external magnetic field. Susceptibility distortions are also seen at natural interfaces, such as at the skull base.[14] Susceptibility-induced signal loss from $T2^*$-dephasing results in "geometric distortion" with regions of signal void and "piling up" with regions of very bright signal resulting from accumulating signals assigned to the wrong areas. Susceptibility artifacts are worse at high fields and can be minimized by using shorter echo time (TE) values (less time for dephasing) and by using fast spin-echo instead of gradient-echo sequences.[15] Imaging at 7T is restricted by increased susceptibility artifacts near the frontal sinuses and skull base, resulting in spatial distortion and signal drop out, increased dielectric artifacts due to signal inhomogeneity, and shimming. "Z-shimming" results in a longer repetition time (TR), which means that portions of the original image not suffering from susceptibility-induced signal loss can be dephased by the z-shimming gradients and become worse. Such loss of fMR imaging signal due to dephasing cannot be restored by distortion correction techniques, such as field mapping, unwarping, and z-shimming, which are used to reassign recorded signals to the proper points in space from which they arose. Other ways to reduce susceptibility artifacts include increasing gradient strength, use of thinner slices, and use of parallel imaging techniques.[16,17]

HEAD MOTION AND PHYSIOLOGIC NOISE

Head motion[18] and physiologic noise from the respiratory and cardiac cycles[19] are unavoidable sources of variance that adversely affect rsfMR imaging signal. Although these problems are inherent in all applications of rsfMR imaging, these tend to be especially problematic in patients with focal brain lesions, because many of these patients are neurologically or cognitively impaired and thus may be less able to cooperate for satisfactory data collection. Because respiratory fluctuations produce aliased signals in the range of 0.1 to 0.3 Hz and cardiac pulsations produce signals in the range of 0.8 to 1.3 Hz, physiologic noise is a much greater problem for rsfMR imaging wherein low-frequency (0.01–0.1 Hz) BOLD fluctuations show strong correlations at rest even in distant gray matter regions. Physiologic noise becomes more prominent than thermal noise at higher fields, and, therefore, may reduce the effects of signal-to-noise ratio (SNR) improvement at 7T and higher fields. False-positive BOLD signals due to eye motion, random noise, partial volume effects, and physiologic pulsations along with postprocessing statistical issues, such as thresholding, clustering, and improper estimation of F values, may adversely impact the reliability of fMR imaging studies.

Head restraints or navigator echoes are used to reduce the effects of head motion.[20] Motion-detection parameters from a navigator echo can be used for motion correction during postprocessing. Similarly, signals representing physiologic cardiac and respiratory cycles can be obtained through the use of a respiratory belt. Besides these parameters obtained during image acquisition, there are retrospective motion and physiologic noise-correction methods available.[21–24] These include motion correction considering head as a rigid body with 3 directions of translation (displacement) and 3 axes of rotation, removal of low-frequency drifts (known as "detrending"), correction for the non-neural noise from white matter and cerebrospinal fluid (known as "nuisance regression"[25,26]), and removal of volumes with excessive motion, which is known as "scrubbing."[27] Fig. 1, shows surgical hardware–related susceptibility artifacts at 3T.

Fig. 2 shows 3T rsfMR imaging and 7T rsfMR imaging comparison indicating geometric distortion at ultrahigh field.

NEUROVASCULAR UNCOUPLING

Impaired BOLD fMR imaging activation in the eloquent cortex in the vicinity of brain tumors or other focal brain lesions can lead to inaccurate presurgical planning, which can result in inadvertent eloquent cortical resection. These false-negative or abnormally decreased BOLD responses in the vicinity of focal brain lesions often occur due to the disruption of coupling between neuronal activity and adjacent microvasculature, known as NVU.[28,29] Such NVU also may adversely affect other applications of task and rsfMR imaging in the setting of focal brain lesions that may alter regional hemodynamics or otherwise disrupt local networks. The mechanisms underlying brain tumor–induced neurovascular uncoupling are not yet completely understood, but preclinical studies have suggested that tumors induce a variety of physiologic changes in the microenvironment that may contribute to this phenomenon.[30] Previous studies[31–39] have demonstrated prevalence of NVU in high-grade gliomas as well as with low-grade gliomas. NVU in high-grade gliomas is due to tumor angiogenesis that compromises cerebral autoregulatory capacity in the tumoral and peritumoral regions.[34,38] The mechanism underlying NVU in low-grade gliomas differs from that of high-grade gliomas because glial tumors are infiltrating lesions that disrupt the neuronal contacts with surrounding microvasculature and astrocytes,[40–42] also known as "gliovascular uncoupling,"[43] and that in turn results in reduced cerebrovascular reactivity (CVR).

NVU is a critical limitation of clinical fMR imaging and has been widely studied in task-based BOLD fMR imaging (tbfMR imaging).[31,33,34,37,38] NVU is characterized by the presence of abnormally decreased tbfMR imaging activation in the ipsilesional hemisphere when the patient neither exhibits substantial neurologic deficit that would be indicative of tumor-related destruction of eloquent cortex, nor displays inability to adequately perform the required tasks.[31] NVU may not necessarily be an all-or-none (ie, binary) phenomenon, but rather may be present to variable degrees, resulting in variable degrees of reduction of expected ipsilesional BOLD activation in eloquent cortical regions and complete absence of detectable activation only in some cases.

Evaluating CVR is often useful for identifying cortical regions affected by NVU.[43] CVR is defined as the change in cerebral blood flow (CBF) per change in a vasoactive stimulus. Mostly either breath-hold (BH) or exogenous gas administration methods are used for CVR mapping.[43] The BH method has been used to induce hypercapnia and thus produce an increase in the arterial partial pressure of CO_2 with time, which consequently raises CBF through a vasodilatory mechanism. In most patients, the BH technique is easier to implement and produces similarly useful BOLD CVR maps as those achieved by using gas-inhalation techniques.[44,45] BOLD BH CVR maps display the change in the BOLD-MR imaging signal in response to the BH hypercapnia challenge relative to a normocapnic baseline condition. BH CVR maps have been compared with T2* dynamic susceptibility contrast (DSC) MR perfusion imaging to demonstrate the increased effectiveness of BH CVR over DSC perfusion imaging in the detection of NVU in patients with brain tumors of varying grades.[35] In another study, BH CVR maps were compared with tbfMR imaging and were shown as an effective method for assessment of NVU in patients with low-grade perirolandic tumors.[31]

Biswal and colleagues[46] showed that in rsfMR imaging only very low frequency amplitude (0.01, 0.03, and 0.04 Hz) correlated with BH-related activity. Studies also have been performed to represent resting-state fluctuation of amplitude (RSFA) as an alternative approach to represent CVR.[47–50] These studies examined the correlation between end-tidal CO_2 fluctuations and low-frequency BOLD fluctuations available from rsfMR imaging and established RSFA as a strong CVR correlate.[47,48] A recent study proposed a different resting-state CVR map that exploits the natural variation in respiration to map CVR using resting-state BOLD data.[51] Because of its easy implementation and less stringent requirements for patient compliance, rsfMR imaging has been attracting wide attention for use as a preoperative mapping

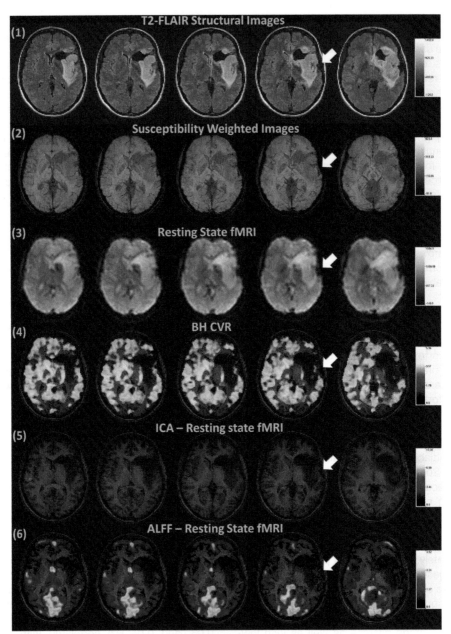

Fig. 1. Surgical hardware–related susceptibility artifacts at 3T. Susceptibility artifact related to a left craniotomy in a patient with World Health Organization (WHO) grade II diffuse astrocytoma. White arrow pointing to the surgical hardware–related susceptibility artifact in T2-FLAIR structural images (*row 1*), susceptibility-weighted images (*row 2*), and resting-state BOLD fMR images (rsfMR images) (*row 3*). Note that the degree of susceptibility-related anatomic distortion is greater on the EPI images (*row 3*) than on the anatomic images (*row 1*). Row 4 shows BH CVR map (z score >2.5) overlaid on T1-weighted images. Notice that the BH CVR map shows ipsilesional apparent loss of regional vascular reactivity (*white arrow*), but this is partially caused by surgical hardware–related susceptibility artifact rather than NVU. Row 5 displays the auditory RSN from ICA of rsfMR imaging (z score >4.0) overlaid on T1-weighted images. Row 6 shows map of frequency-domain metrics ALFF (ALFF >0.6) overlaid on T1-weighted images. Notice ipsilesional absent (*white arrow*) resting-state BOLD signal within the auditory RSN component along the tumor, as well as decreased tumor ALFF.

tool.[52,53] However, rsfMR imaging also suffers from similar important clinical limitations of false-negative BOLD signals due to brain-tumor–related NVU[54–56]; thus, to use rsfMR imaging as a reliable presurgical tool, it becomes all the more important to study NVU in cases of focal resectable brain lesions, such as tumors, to evaluate its effects on rsfMR imaging.

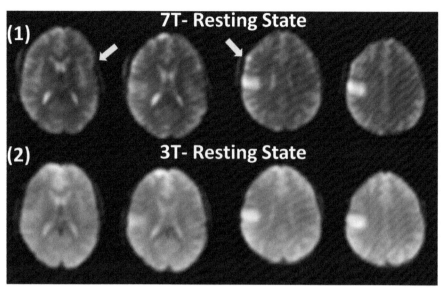

Fig. 2. Comparison of 3T and 7T rsfMR imaging (geometric distortion at ultrahigh field). Top row shows "geometric distortion" (*yellow arrow*) in multiple 2D fast echo planar imaging T2*-weighted BOLD sequences for rsfMR imaging at ultrahigh (7T) field (TR/TE 2500/22 ms, acceleration factor = 3) acquired in a patient with grade II oligoastrocytoma referred for fMR imaging presurgical mapping at our institution. Bottom row displays the corresponding slices of rsfMR images acquired at 3T using multiple 2D GE-EPI T2*-weighted BOLD sequence (TR/TE 2000/30 ms). Notice that geometric distortions were much less prominent at 3T.

EXAMPLES OF EACH OF THE PREVIOUSLY MENTIONED LIMITATIONS IN THE SETTING OF FOCAL BRAIN PATHOLOGY

In the remainder of this article, various examples of the previously described limitations of resting-state functional connectivity related to focal brain lesions is provided. All of the presented data were acquired and processed using the following protocol at our institution:

3T scanning was performed using our standard clinical sequences for fMR imaging studies on a 3.0-T S Trio MRI system (Siemens Medical Solutions, Erlangen, Germany) equipped with a 12-channel head matrix coil. Imaging protocol included a 3-dimensional (3D) T1 magnetization prepared rapid acquisition gradient echo (MPRAGE) (TR = 2300 ms, inversion time [TI] = 900 ms, TE = 3.5 ms, 9° flip angle, 24-cm field of view [FOV], 256 × 256 × 176 matrix, slice thickness 1 mm) as well as an axial 2-dimensional (2D) T2 fluid-attenuated inversion recovery (FLAIR) imaging sequence (TR = 9000 ms, TI = 2500 ms, TE = 116 ms, flip angle = 1418, FOV = 17.2 cm × 23 cm, acquisition matrix = 240 × 320 × 53, slice thickness = 3 mm with 3-mm gap between slices) for structural imaging and multiple 2D gradient-echo–echo planar imaging (GE-EPI) T2*-weighted BOLD sequences for both task and resting functional imaging (TR = 2000 ms, TE = 30 ms, flip angle = 90°,

FOV = 24 cm, acquisition matrix = 64 × 64 × 33, slice thickness = 4 mm with 1-mm gap between slices, interleaved acquisition).

7T scanning was performed using research sequences on a 7.0-T Philips MR imaging system equipped with a 32-channel head matrix coil. Imaging protocol included a 3D T1 3D MPRAGE imaging sequence (TR = 4.023 ms, TE = 1.81 ms, flip angle = 7, FOV = 22 cm, acquisition matrix = 224 × 224 × 180, slice thickness = 1 mm) for structural imaging and multiple 2D fast echo planar imaging T2*-weighted BOLD sequences for functional imaging (TR = 2500 ms, TE = 22 ms, flip angle = 80, FOV = 19.2 cm, acquisition matrix = 128 × 128 × 31, slice thickness = 3 mm). The BOLD parallel imaging acceleration (SENSE) factor = 3.

For *rsfMR imaging*, subjects were instructed to remain still with eyes closed without falling asleep during the scanning period of 6 minutes.[55–57] For *motor-task fMR imaging*, bilateral simultaneous sequential finger tapping (FingM) task to map hand representation area and vertical tongue movement task to map face representation area of primary motor cortex (PMC) were used.[31] Both paradigms were block design with alternating active and control blocks lasting 30 seconds each for a total of 3 minutes. For *language-task fMR imaging*, sentence completion task to map both expressive and receptive language areas was used. This paradigm was block design with alternating active and control blocks lasting 20 seconds each for a total of 4 minutes.[58] A *BH* task includes normal breathing period of 40 seconds followed by a 4-second block of inspiration that immediately preceded a 16-second BH period.[31] This cycle was repeated 4 times, and at the end of the last BH period, an additional normal breathing period of 20 seconds was added.

Instructions for all tasks were visually cued. A comprehensive prescan training session outside the MR imaging scanner ensured full patient understanding of task instructions and confirmed the patient's ability to adequately perform the tasks. Patient task performance was monitored during the scan via use of a respiratory belt for the BH task and use of both an liquid-crystal display monitor in the scan suite and real-time fMR imaging for patient observation and assessment of activation, respectively.

SPM12 (Wellcome Trust Center for Neuroimaging, London, UK) software implemented in Matlab R2014b (The Mathworks, Natick, MA) was used for preprocessing of BH, tbfMR imaging, and rsfMR imaging data (slice timing correction, realignment, normalization to Montreal Neurological Institute (MNI) space at 2-mm voxel resolution, and spatially smoothing using a 6-mm full-width half-maximum Gaussian kernel). For the motor and BH tasks, z-score maps were obtained using general linear model analysis using SPM software (reflecting motor activation vs rest and hypercapnia vs baseline, respectively).

On the preprocessed rsfMR imaging data, detrending for removal of systematic linear trend and low-frequency (0.01–0.08 Hz) bandpass filtering was performed using the REST (version 1.8)[59] toolkit. An Automated Anatomic Labeling template[60,61] was used to obtain a seed region circumscribing the combination of precentral gyri and postcentral gyri in contralesional (CL) hemisphere (ie, contralateral to tumor). Pearson linear correlation was calculated using the REST toolkit between the seed region in CL to ipsilesional precentral gyri and postcentral gyri (ie, ipsilateral to tumor) to obtain the functional connectivity map (seed correlation analysis [SCA] map) of the sensorimotor network.[55] Subsequently, ALFF (amplitude of low-frequency fluctuation[62]) and ReHo (regional homogeneity[63,64]) maps were calculated. fALFF (fractional ALFF[65]) maps were calculated from detrended rsfMR imaging data. For ReHo maps, smoothing was done after ReHo map calculation, not during preprocessing of rsfMR imaging data. Two additional preprocessing steps, "scrubbing" and "nuisance regression," were performed on rsfMR imaging data before

independent component analysis (ICA)[66–69] computation. Outlier volumes (ie, volumes with excessive variation in volume-to-volume global signal and motion) identified with the ART repair toolbox[70] were removed to generate "scrubbed" rsfMR imaging data. White matter and cerebrospinal fluid masks were used to regress physiologic noise (ie, "nuisance regression") from the fMR imaging time series.[71] GIFT toolbox[72] was used to perform ICA with 30 target components. The single best candidate ICA component for the rsfMR imaging sensorimotor network was selected.[55]

For the BH task, during clinical scanning, the real-time respiratory bellows on the MR imaging scanner console were observed for quality control purposes. On more rigorous quantitative post hoc evaluation of respiratory waveform plots, variations in the signals during the BH period were found within 10% of the corresponding median value, which indicates the stability of the baseline during the BH period and confirms patient compliance during performance of the BH task.

Fig. 3 shows an example of respiratory waveform and its quantitative evaluation for quality control purposes. The figure also displays BH CVR maps obtained at 3T and 7T with specific mention of motion and susceptibility artifact–related degradation of the CVR maps.

The following section describe critical evaluation of rsfMR imaging in the assessment of brain tumor–related NVU.

NEUROVASCULAR UNCOUPLING EFFECTS ON RESTING-STATE FUNCTIONAL CONNECTIVITY (SEED CORRELATION ANALYSIS AND INDEPENDENT COMPONENT ANALYSIS)

Standard methods for determining various rsfMR imaging networks (RSN) include SCA and ICA of voxel time series.[73] Such analysis methods focus on the similarities of interregional time series, and, therefore, investigate temporal synchronization of low-frequency fluctuations (<0.1 Hz); that is, functional connectivity.[74] Agarwal and colleagues[55] demonstrated NVU on rsfMR imaging using ICA and SCA analysis approaches in patients with perirolandic tumors. In another study, they further assessed brain tumor–related NVU in rsfMR imaging at ultrahigh field (7T) and demonstrated that the higher SNR at 7T does not fully mitigate the effects of such NVU.[56] Mallela and colleagues[54] examined the correlation of rsfMR imaging data with tumor characteristics and clinical information to characterize functional reorganization of RSNs and the limitations of rsfMR imaging in high-grade gliomas due to NVU.

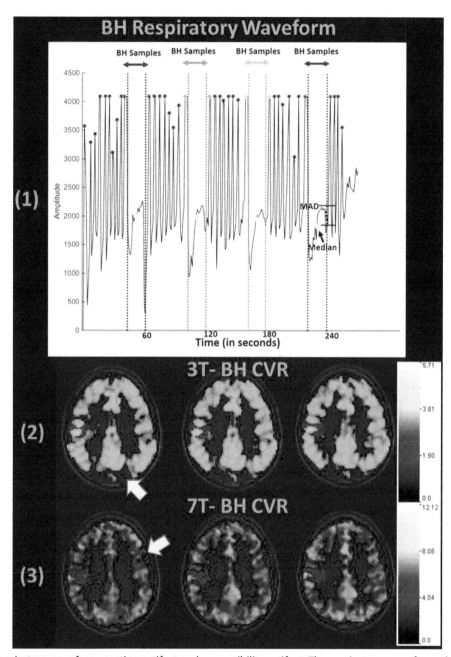

Fig. 3. Respiratory waveform, motion artifact and susceptibility artifact. The respiratory wave form plot (*row 1*) for the 4-minute 20-second (ie, 260 seconds)-long BH paradigm. Red, green, cyan, and magenta blocks indicate the BH periods, which are each 16 seconds long. Yellow dot in each BH block represents the median value of all samples within the respective block. In each BH block, median absolute deviation, which represents the median deviation of the absolute values of the differences of amplitude between each individual sample and the median of all samples within each BH block, was less than 10% of the median value of all samples within each respective BH block, indicating the overall stability of the baseline within each BH block, which in turn confirms the patient compliance during BH. Row 2 displays BH CVR map (z score >3.0) obtained at 3T. Note the artifact (*white arrow*) in image because of head motion that is not adequately corrected even when the respiratory waveform provides adequate quality control numbers. Row 3 displays BH CVR map (z score >4.0) obtained at 7T. Note the artifact created because of susceptibility (*white arrow*). Irrespective of artifact, 7T images shows high SNR and better resolution relative to 3T.

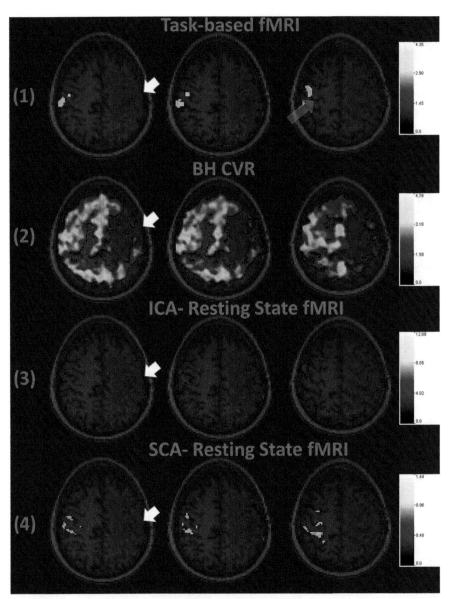

Fig. 4. Patient with left hemispheric glioblastoma demonstrating severe NVU: task, BH, SCA, and ICA maps overlaid on precontrast T1-weighted anatomic images. Patient with a left hemispheric WHO grade IV glioblastoma. Top row shows the BOLD sensorimotor activation map obtained from a bilateral simultaneous sequential finger tapping task overlaid on T1-weighted structural images. Suprathreshold voxels (z score >3.5) in the expected hand representation area of the PMC are highlighted in yellow-white. Blue arrow points to the central sulcus. Note that there is absence of ipsilesional activation (*white arrow*) during task performance in the left PMC. Second row shows BOLD BH CVR maps overlaid on T1-weighted anatomic images of the same patient displaying decreased regional CVR in the ipsilesional hemisphere (z score >1.5). Third and fourth rows show the BOLD resting-state sensorimotor network maps of the same patient displaying the functional connectivity maps derived from SCA (*yellow-orange suprathreshold voxels; z* score >1.0) and ICA (z score >3.0) overlaid on structural T1-weighted images. Note that absent activation during task performance and decreased ipsilesional CVR in the expected hand, representation area of the left PMC (precentral gyrus) corresponds to absence of BOLD signal in the resting-state sensorimotor network within the same cortical region on the functional connectivity SCA and ICA maps. Ipsilesional reduction in BOLD signal on all maps compared with the contralesional PMC in the setting of preserved motor function and bilateral robust finger movement is indicative of lesion-induced NVU. Color bar indicates z score in all panels.

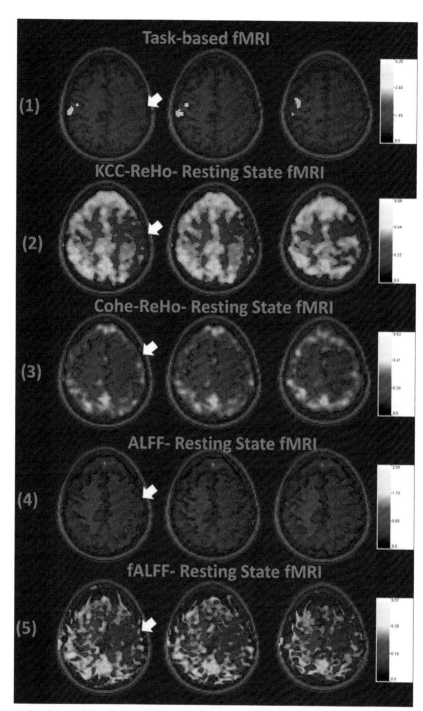

Fig. 5. Patient with left hemispheric glioblastoma demonstrating severe NVU: task, ReHo, ALFF. Patient with a left hemispheric WHO grade IV glioblastoma. Top row shows the BOLD sensorimotor activation map obtained from a bilateral simultaneous sequential finger tapping task overlaid on T1-weighted structural images. Suprathreshold voxels (z score >3.5) in the expected hand representation area of the primary motor cortex are highlighted in yellow-white. Second and third rows show ReHo maps, KCC-ReHo and Cohe-ReHo, respectively (KCC >0.35 and Cohe >0.26), from rsfMR imaging. Fourth and fifth rows show maps of frequency-domain metrics ALFF and fALFF (ALFF >0.4 and fALFF >0.25) from rsfMR images. Note that absent activation during task performance corresponds to absence/decrease of BOLD signal within the same cortical region on KCC-ReHo, Cohe-ReHo, ALFF, and fALFF rsfMRI maps. The abnormally reduced ipsilesional task-based activation in the absence of corresponding neurologic deficits or impaired task performance is direct evidence of NVU, whereas the findings on the other maps are resting-state correlates of such NVU. This is a case of clinically significant NVU, because the NVU affects regions in which critical motor activation is expected. White arrow in each map points to the ipsilesional decreased/absent BOLD signal.

Fig. 4 displays a case of left hemispheric glioblastoma demonstrating severe NVU affecting the sensorimotor network. NVU is demonstrated on task fMR imaging, BH CVR, and functional connectivity maps obtained from SCA and ICA.

NEUROVASCULAR UNCOUPLING EFFECTS ON REGIONAL HOMOGENEITY (KENDALL COEFFICIENT OF CONCORDANCE AND COHERENCE TO EVALUATE)

Zang and colleagues[63] proposed ReHo metrics of rsfMR imaging signals as a voxel-based measure of brain activity that evaluates the synchronization between the time series of a given voxel and its nearest neighbors. This measure was based on the hypothesis that intrinsic brain activity is manifested by clusters of voxels rather than single voxels. They used the Kendall coefficient of concordance (KCC)[75] as an index to evaluate the similarity of the time series within a cluster of a given voxel and its nearest neighbor voxels (KCC-ReHo). Values of KCC range from 0 to 1, with higher values indicating greater similarity between the BOLD signal of a given voxel and that of its neighbors. Later, Liu and colleagues[64] applied coherence to evaluate ReHo (Cohe-ReHo) in healthy participants as well as in patients with attention-deficit/hyperactivity disorder (ADHD). ReHo has been widely used to evaluate resting-state cortical activity.[75–80] ReHo does not require a priori definition of regions of interest and can provide information about the local/regional activity of regions throughout the brain. Liu and colleagues[64] showed that the 2 measurements, KCC-ReHo and Cohe-ReHo, differed mainly in some brain regions in which physiologic noise is dominant. We have shown previously that ReHo is sensitive to NVU in the sensorimotor network as well.[81] ReHo findings may possibly complement findings on tbfMR imaging used for presurgical planning.

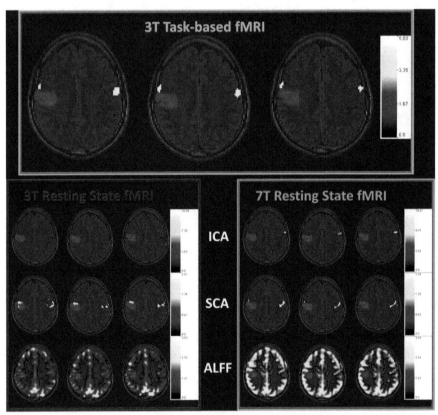

Fig. 6. Mild NVU depicted via task fMRI, ALFF, SCA, and ICA: patient with a right perirolandic tumor of grade II oligoastrocytoma. Motor-task–based activation at 3T (*green box*) and sensorimotor network resting-state functional connectivity (SCA and ICA) maps along with frequency-domain metrics ALFF at 3T (*purple box*) as well as 7T (*blue box*) are displayed. This is a case of mild NVU. Notice ipsilesional decreased activation and ipsilesional decreased resting-state BOLD signal within the sensorimotor network (as assessed with both SCA and ICA) along the tumor as well as mildly decreased tumor ALFF. This case illustrates that SNR advantages for rsfMR imaging provided by ultrahigh field strength (7T) may not fully mitigate the effects of brain tumor–related NVU on rsfMR imaging.

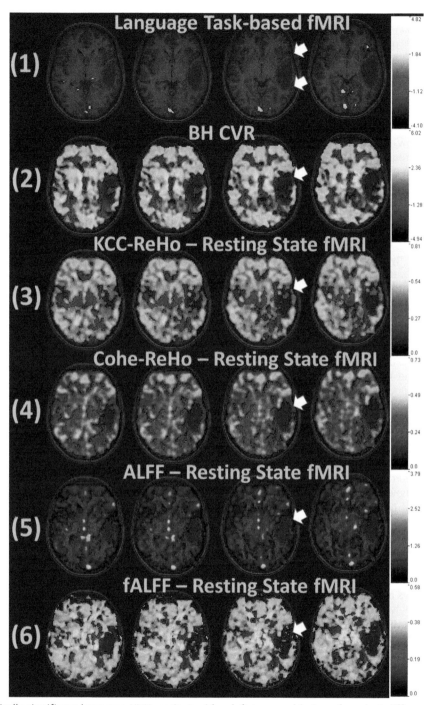

Fig. 7. Clinically significant language NVU: patient with a left temporal lesion of grade II diffuse astrocytoma/ grade III anaplastic astrocytoma. Top row shows language activation map (tbfMR imaging) for a sentence comple- tion task (z score >3.8) overlaid on T1-weighted structural images. Note that absent activation (*white arrow*) dur- ing task performance both in the Broca and Wernicke language areas. Second row shows BOLD BH CVR maps overlaid on T1-weighted anatomic images of the same patient displaying decreased regional CVR in the ipsile- sional hemisphere (z score >2.5). Third and fourth rows show KCC-ReHo and Cohe-ReHo maps (KCC >0.42 and Cohe >0.3) from rsfMR images. Fifth and sixth rows show maps of frequency-domain metrics ALFF and fALFF (ALFF >0.35 and fALFF >0.32) from rsfMR images. Note that absent activation during task performance and decreased ipsilesional CVR in the expected Broca and Wernicke areas of the left temporal lobe corresponds to absence/decrease of BOLD signal within the same cortical region on KCC-ReHo, Cohe-ReHo, ALFF, and fALFF

NEUROVASCULAR UNCOUPLING EFFECTS ON FREQUENCY-DOMAIN METRICS (AMPLITUDE OF LOW-FREQUENCY FLUCTUATIONS AND FRACTIONAL AMPLITUDE OF LOW-FREQUENCY FLUCTUATIONS)

rsfMR imaging focuses on spontaneous low-frequency fluctuations (<0.1 Hz) in the BOLD signal. Studies have found that the relative magnitude of these low-frequency fluctuations can differ between brain regions and between subjects, and thus may act as a marker of individual differences or dysfunction. Biswal and colleagues[1] found that amplitude of low-frequency fluctuations was higher in gray matter than in white matter. Subsequently, as a measure of amplitude of regional activity (unlike SCA and ICA, which measure functional connectivity), frequency-domain rsfMR imaging metrics were developed, such as ALFF,[62] defined as the total power within the frequency range between 0.01 and 0.08 Hz indexing the strength or intensity of low-frequency fluctuations, and fALFF,[65] which is defined as the ratio of the power spectrum of the low-frequency (0.01–0.08 Hz) range to that of the entire frequency range representing the relative contribution of specific low-frequency fluctuation to the whole frequency range. Their usefulness in characterizing rsfMR imaging properties in healthy[82–85] and diseased populations[86–88] has been studied. Studies[89] have also been performed using ALFF to reduce the distortions in task-based activation due to regional variance in neurovascular coupling. Our group has recently shown that ALFF may be sensitive for detection of NVU in brain tumors that affect the sensorimotor network.[90] Reliability of ALFF in gray matter regions tends to be higher than for fALFF. **Fig. 5** displays a case of a left hemispheric glioblastoma with severe NVU, as assessed on motor-task fMR imaging, ReHo, and ALFF.

Fig. 6 displays a case of mild NVU affecting the sensorimotor network, as depicted via task fMR imaging and rsfMR imaging, including ALFF, ICA, and SCA approaches.

NEUROVASCULAR UNCOUPLING EFFECTS ON MAPPING OF THE LANGUAGE NETWORK

In case of the relatively nonlateralized primary sensorimotor network, contralesional values can serve as an internal reference standard with which the NVU-affected ipsilesional side can be studied at a single subject level in cases of unilateral lesion-induced NVU. In the preceding sections, regional alterations in ReHo and the frequency-domain rsfMR imaging metrics ALFF and fALFF were shown to correspond to similar ipsilesional abnormal activation reductions on tbfMR imaging and decreased BOLD signal in BH CVR maps in the setting of lesion-induced NVU involving sensorimotor cortical areas. The abnormally reduced ipsilesional task-based activation in the absence of corresponding neurologic deficits or impaired task performance is direct evidence of NVU, whereas the findings on the other maps are resting-state correlates of such NVU. Although some of the asymmetry observed may be due to differences in handedness, this degree of asymmetry is greater than what would be expected based on differences in handedness alone.[31,91,92] rsfMR imaging–based frequency-domain and regional homogeneity metrics are not restricted by network specificity and provide information about the local/regional activity of regions throughout the brain. Therefore, they can be advantageous in the assessment of brain-tumor–related NVU in more lateralized networks,[93] like language. Although this remains to be determined in the future, we present here 2 cases with lesions involving language areas representing clinically significant and insignificant NVU, respectively.

Fig. 7 illustrates a case of clinically significant language NVU, because the NVU affects regions in which critical language activation is expected.

Fig. 8 illustrates a case of clinically insignificant language NVU, because the ipsilesional expected critical language activation in the Broca area and Wernicke area is still detectable despite the NVU.

NEUROVASCULAR UNCOUPLING IN THE CONTEXT OF NETWORK/GRAPH THEORETIC ANALYSIS

Graph theory is increasingly being used to describe functional and anatomic connectivity in the brain. For network analysis, nodes (or vertices) at the voxel level, gyral level, or at much larger anatomic levels are defined via cortical parcellation. Nodes that have correlated activity or direct

---

rsfMR imaging maps. The abnormally reduced ipsilesional task-based activation in the absence of corresponding neurologic deficits or impaired task performance is direct evidence of NVU, whereas the findings on the other maps are resting-state correlates of such NVU. This is a case of clinically significant NVU, because the NVU affects regions in which critical language activation is expected. White arrow in each map points to the ipsilesional decreased/absent BOLD signal.

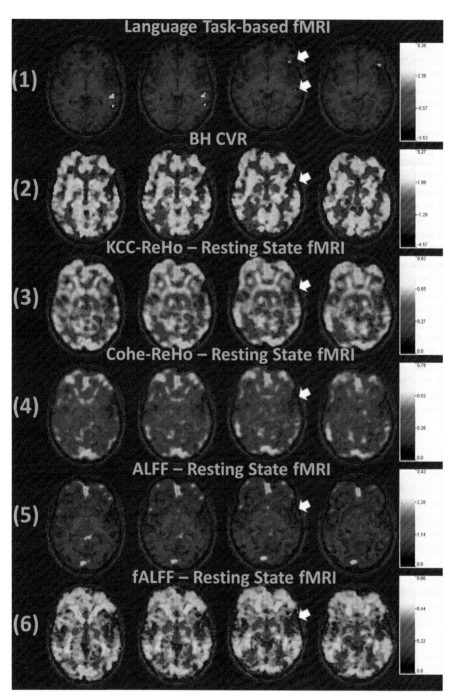

Fig. 8. Clinically insignificant language NVU: patient with a left temporal lobe grade II diffuse astrocytoma. Top row shows language activation map (tbfMR imaging) for a sentence completion task (*z* score >3.7) overlaid on T1-weighted structural images. Note the decreased activation (*white arrow*) during task performance in both Broca and Wernicke areas. Second row shows BOLD BH CVR maps overlaid on T1-weighted anatomic images of the same patient displaying decreased regional CVR in the ipsilesional hemisphere (*z* score >2.2). Third and fourth rows show KCC-ReHo and Cohe-ReHo maps (KCC >0.39 and Cohe >0.27) from rsfMR images. Fifth and sixth rows show frequency-domain metrics ALFF and fALFF maps (ALFF >0.5 and fALFF >0.34) from rsfMR images. Note that decreased activation during task performance and decreased ipsilesional CVR in the expected Broca and Wernicke areas of the left temporal lobe correspond to decreased BOLD signal within the same cortical region on KCC-ReHo, Cohe-ReHo, ALFF, and fALFF rsfMR imaging maps. In this case, the reduced ipsilesional task-based activation in the absence of corresponding neurologic deficits or impaired task performance is direct evidence of NVU, whereas the findings on the other maps are resting-state correlates of such NVU. However, because the ipsilesional expected critical language activation in Broca and Wernicke areas is still detectable despite the NVU, this is a case of clinically insignificant NVU. White arrow in each map points to the ipsilesional decreased BOLD signal.

physical connections are linked by "edges." A network with nodes and links is represented either graphically or as a numerical array (also known as "adjacency matrix"). Various different graph theoretic metrics can then be defined in terms of various parameters, such as path length and number of connections to individual nodes within the whole brain network. Such metrics include degree centrality, small worldness, global and local efficiency, among many others. Graph theory has been used to study many neurologic disorders, such as Alzheimer disease, autism spectrum disorder, and schizophrenia. A full discussion of these methods is beyond the scope of this article, and instead are addressed more fully in other articles in this *Neuroimaging Clinics* issue. However, it is worth mentioning that such graph theoretic metrics represent another method of analysis of rsfMR imaging data that also may be adversely affected by the effects of NVU in the setting of focal brain lesions such as tumors. In fact, several studies have shown that the effects of brain gliomas may not just be limited to local network disruption, but also may affect global networks with distant disruptions as well as local ones.[94–97]

SUMMARY

In this review, limitations affecting the results of presurgical mapping with rsfMR imaging are discussed. Methods of image acquisition, monitoring, and analysis are still evolving, and there is a need to standardize these to ensure reliability of rsfMR imaging results in clinical scenarios. In the near future, with the wide range of ongoing research in rsfMR imaging, these issues likely will be overcome and will open new windows into brain functional connectivity that will enhance both research and clinical applications of rsfMR imaging.

REFERENCES

1. Biswal B, Yetkin FZ, Haughton VM, et al. Functional connectivity in the motor cortex of resting human brain using echo-planar MRI. Magn Reson Med 1995;34(4):537–41.
2. Raichle ME, MacLeod AM, Snyder AZ, et al. A default mode of brain function. Proc Natl Acad Sci U S A 2001;98(2):676–82.
3. Greicius MD, Krasnow B, Reiss AL, et al. Functional connectivity in the resting brain: a network analysis of the default mode hypothesis. Proc Natl Acad Sci U S A 2003;100(1):253–8.
4. Barkhof F, Haller S, Rombout SARB. Resting-state functional MR imaging: a new window to the brain. Radiology 2014;272:29–49.
5. Power JD, Schlaggar BL, Petersen SE. Studying brain organization via spontaneous fMRI signal. Neuron 2014;84:681–96.
6. Van Dijk KR, Hedden T, Venkataraman A, et al. Intrinsic functional connectivity as a tool for human connectomics: theory, properties, and optimization. J Neurophysiol 2010;103:297–321.
7. Vincent JL, Patel GH, Fox MD, et al. Intrinsic functional architecture in the anaesthetized monkey brain. Nature 2007;447(7140):83–6.
8. Sämann PG, Wehrle R, Hoehn D, et al. Development of the brain's default mode network from wakefulness to slow wave sleep. Cereb Cortex 2011;21(9):2082–93.
9. Zhang D, Raichle ME. Disease and the brain's dark energy. Nat Rev Neurol 2010;6(1):15–28.
10. Uddin LQ, Supekar K, Menon V. Reconceptualizing functional brain connectivity in autism from a developmental perspective. Front Hum Neurosci 2013;7:458.
11. Fox MD, Buckner RL, Liu H, et al. Resting-state networks link invasive and noninvasive brain stimulation across diverse psychiatric and neurological diseases. Proc Natl Acad Sci U S A 2014;111(41):E4367–75.
12. Schenck JF. The role of magnetic susceptibility in magnetic resonance imaging: MRI magnetic compatibility of the first and second kinds. Med Phys 1996;23:815–50.
13. Liu H, Martin AJ, Truwit C. Interventional MRI at high field (1.5T): needle artifacts. J Magn Reson Imaging 1998;8:214–9.
14. Elster AD. Sellar susceptibility artifacts: theory and implications. AJNR Am J Neuroradiol 1993;14:129–36.
15. Port JD, Pomper MG. Quantification and minimization of magnetic susceptibility artifacts on GRE images. J Comput Assist Tomogr 2000;24:958–64.
16. Glover GH. 3D z-shim method for reduction of susceptibility effects in BOLD fMRI. Magn Reson Med 1999;42:290–9.
17. Weiskopf N, Hutton C, Josephs O, et al. Optimal EPI parameters for reduction of susceptibility-induced BOLD senstivity losses: a whole-brain analysis at 3 T and 1.5 T. Neuroimage 2006;33:493–504.
18. Maclaren J, Herbst M, Speck O, et al. Prospective motion correction in brain imaging: a review. Magn Reson Med 2013;69:621–36.
19. Triantafyllou C, Hoge RD, Krueger G, et al. Comparison of physiological noise at 1.5 T, 3 T and 7 T and optimization of fMRI acquisition parameters. Neuroimage 2005;26:243–50.
20. Friedman L, Glover GH. Report on a multicenter fMRI quality assurance protocol. J Magn Reson Imaging 2006;23:827–39.
21. Bright MG, Murphy K. Removing motion and physiological artifacts from intrinsic BOLD fluctuations using short echo data. Neuroimage 2013;64:526–37.

22. Mikl M, Maraček R, Hluštík P, et al. Effects of spatial smoothing on fMRI group inferences. Magn Reson Imaging 2008;26:490–503.

23. Sladky R, Friston KJ, Tröstl J, et al. Slice-timing effects and their correction in functional MRI. Neuroimage 2011;58:588–94.

24. Tanabe J, Miller D, Tregellas J, et al. Comparison of detrending methods for optimal fMRI preprocessing. Neuroimage 2002;15:902–7.

25. Dagli MS, Ingeholm JE, Haxby JV. Localization of cardiac-induced signal change in fMRI. Neuroimage 1999;9:407–15.

26. Windischberger C, Langenberger H, Sycha T, et al. On the origin of respiratory artifacts in BOLD-EPI of the human brain. Magn Reson Imaging 2002;20: 575–82.

27. Power JD, Barnes KA, Snyder AZ, et al. Spurious but systematic correlations in functional connectivity MRI networks arise from subject motion. Neuroimage 2011;59:2142–54.

28. Attwell D, Buchan AM, Charpak S, et al. Glial and neuronal control of brain blood flow. Nature 2010; 468(7321):232–43.

29. Villringer A, Dirnagl U. Coupling of brain activity and cerebral blood flow: basis of functional neuroimaging. Cerebrovasc Brain Metab Rev 1995;7(3):240–76.

30. Lee J, Lund-Smith C, Borboa A, et al. Glioma-induced remodeling of the neurovascular unit. Brain Res 2009;1288:125–34.

31. Zacà D, Jovicich J, Nadar SR, et al. Cerebrovascular reactivity mapping in patients with low grade gliomas undergoing presurgical sensorimotor mapping with BOLD fMRI. J Magn Reson Imaging 2014;40(2): 383–90.

32. DeYoe E, Ulmer JL. Method for measuring neurovascular uncoupling in fMRI. US Patent 7469159. 2008.

33. Holodny AI, Schulder M, Liu WC, et al. The effect of brain tumors on BOLD functional MR imaging activation in the adjacent motor cortex: implications for image-guided neurosurgery. AJNR Am J Neuroradiol 2000;21:1415–22.

34. Hou BL, Bradbury M, Peck KK, et al. Effect of brain tumor neovasculature defined by rCBV on BOLD fMRI activation volume in the primary motor cortex. Neuroimage 2006;32:489–97.

35. Pillai JJ, Zacà D. Comparison of BOLD cerebrovascular reactivity mapping and DSC MR perfusion imaging for prediction of neurovascular uncoupling potential in brain tumors. Technol Cancer Res Treat 2012;11(4):361–74.

36. Pillai JJ, Zacá D. Clinical utility of cerebrovascular reactivity mapping in patients with low grade gliomas. World J Clin Oncol 2011;2(12):397–403.

37. Ulmer JL, Krouwer HG, Mueller WM, et al. Pseudoreorganization of language cortical function at fMR imaging: a consequence of tumor-induced neurovascular uncoupling. AJNR Am J Neuroradiol 2003;24:213–7.

38. Jiang Z, Krainik A, David O, et al. Impaired fMRI activation in patients with primary brain tumors. Neuroimage 2010;52:538–48.

39. Zaca D, Hua J, Pillai JJ. Cerebrovascular reactivity mapping for brain tumor presurgical planning. World J Clin Oncol 2011;2(7):289–98.

40. Chaitanya GV, Minagar A, Alexander JS. Neuronal and astrocytic interactions modulate brain endothelial properties during metabolic stresses of in vitro cerebral ischemia. Cell Commun Signal 2014;12:7.

41. Pelligrino DA, Vetri F, Xu HL. Purinergic mechanisms in gliovascular coupling. Semin Cell Dev Biol 2011; 22:229–36.

42. Watkins S, Robel S, Kimbrough IF, et al. Disruption of astrocyte-vascular coupling and the blood-brain barrier by invading glioma cells. Nat Commun 2014;5:4196.

43. Pillai JJ, Mikulis DJ. Cerebrovascular reactivity mapping: an evolving standard for clinical functional imaging. AJNR Am J Neuroradiol 2015;36(1):7–13.

44. Kastrup A, Krüger G, Neumann-Haefelin T, et al. Assessment of cerebrovascular reactivity with functional magnetic resonance imaging: comparison of CO(2) and breath holding. Magn Reson Imaging 2001;19:13–20.

45. Magon S, Basso G, Farace P, et al. Reproducibility of BOLD signal change induced by breath holding. Neuroimage 2009;45:702–12.

46. Biswal BB, Kannurpatti SS, Rypma B. Hemodynamic scaling of fMRI-BOLD signal: validation of low frequency spectral amplitude as a scalability factor. Magn Reson Imaging 2007;25(10):1358–69.

47. Kannurpatti SS, Biswal BB. Detection and scaling of task-induced fMRI BOLD response using resting state fluctuations. Neuroimage 2008;40:1567–74.

48. Wise RG, Ide K, Poulin MJ, et al. Resting fluctuations in arterial carbon dioxide induce significant low frequency variations in BOLD signal. Neuroimage 2004;21:1652–64.

49. Kannurpatti SS, Motes MA, Rypma B, et al. Increasing measurement accuracy of age-related BOLD signal change: minimizing vascular contributions by resting-state-fluctuation-of-amplitude scaling. Hum Brain Mapp 2011;32:1125–40.

50. Kannurpatti SS, Motes MA, Biswal BB, et al. Assessment of unconstrained cerebrovascular reactivity marker for large age-range fMRI studies. PLoS One 2014;9(2):e88751.

51. Liu P, Li Y, Pinho M, et al. Cerebrovascular reactivity mapping without gas challenges. Neuroimage 2016; 146:320–6.

52. Shimony JS, Zhang D, Johnston JM, et al. Resting-state spontaneous fluctuations in brain activity: a new paradigm for presurgical planning using fMRI. Acad Radiol 2009;16:578–83.

53. Liu H, Buckner RL, Talukdar T, et al. Task-free presurgical mapping using functional magnetic

resonance imaging intrinsic activity. J Neurosurg 2009;111:746–54.

54. Mallela AN, Peck KK, Petrovich-Brennan NM, et al. Altered resting-state functional connectivity in the hand motor network in glioma patients. Brain Connect 2016;6(8):587–95.

55. Agarwal S, Sair HI, Yahyavi-Firouz-Abadi N, et al. Neurovascular uncoupling in resting state fMRI demonstrated in patients with primary brain gliomas. J Magn Reson Imaging 2016;43(3):620–6.

56. Agarwal S, Sair HI, Airan R, et al. Demonstration of brain tumor-induced neurovascular uncoupling in resting-state fMRI at ultrahigh field. Brain Connect 2016;6(4):267–72.

57. Patriat R, Molloy EK, Meier TB, et al. The effect of resting condition on resting-state fMRI reliability and consistency: a comparison between resting with eyes open, closed, and fixated. Neuroimage 2013;78:463–73.

58. Zacà D, Nickerson JP, Pillai JJ. Role of semantic paradigms for optimization of language mapping in clinical fMRI studies. AJNR Am J Neuroradiol 2013;34(10):1966–71.

59. Song XW, Dong ZY, Long XY, et al. REST: a toolkit for resting-state functional magnetic resonance imaging data processing. PLoS One 2011;6: e25031.

60. Smith SM. Fast robust automated brain extraction. Hum Brain Mapp 2002;17:143–55.

61. Tzourio-Mazoyer N, Landeau B, Papathanassiou D, et al. Automated anatomical labeling of activations in SPM using a macroscopic anatomical parcellation of the MNI MRI single-subject brain. Neuroimage 2002;15:273–89.

62. Zang YF, He Y, Zhu CZ, et al. Altered baseline brain activity in children with ADHD revealed by resting-state functional MRI. Brain Dev 2007;29:83–91.

63. Zang Y, Jiang T, Lu Y, et al. Regional homogeneity approach to fMRI data analysis. Neuroimage 2004; 22(1):394–400.

64. Liu D, Yan C, Ren J, et al. Using coherence to measure regional homogeneity of resting-state fMRI signal. Front Syst Neurosci 2010;4:24.

65. Zou QH, Zhu CZ, Yang Y, et al. An improved approach to detection of amplitude of low-frequency fluctuation (ALFF) for resting-state fMRI: fractional ALFF. J Neurosci Methods 2008;172:137–41.

66. McKeown MJ, Makeig S, Brown GG, et al. Analysis of fMRI data by blind separation into independent spatial components. Hum Brain Mapp 1998;6:160–88.

67. Beckman CF. Modelling with independent components. Neuroimage 2012;62:891–901.

68. Calhoun VD, Adali T, Hasen LK, et al. ICA of functional MRI data: an overview. 4th International Symposium on Independent Component Analysis and Blind Signal Separation. Nara, Japan, April 1–4, 2003. p. 281–8.

69. Hyvärinen A, Oja E. Independent component analysis: algorithms and applications. Neural Netw 2000;13:411–3.

70. Mazaika PK, Hoeft F, Glover GH, et al. Methods and software for fMRI analysis for clinical subjects. Neurolmage 2009;47(1):S39–41.

71. Behzadi Y, Restom K, Liau J, et al. A component based noise correction method (CompCor) for BOLD and perfusion based fMRI. Neuroimage 2007;37:90–101.

72. Correa N, Adali T, Li YO, et al. Comparison of blind source separation algorithms for fMRI using a new Matlab toolbox: GIFT. In: Proceedings of the ICASSP, Philadelphia, March 18–23, 2005.

73. Lee MH, Smyser CD, Shimony JS. Resting-state fMRI: a review of methods and clinical applications. AJNR Am J Neuroradiol 2013;34:1866–72.

74. Rosazza C, Minati L, Ghielmetti F, et al. Functional connectivity during resting-state functional MR imaging: study of the correspondence between independent component analysis and region-of-interest-based methods. AJNR Am J Neuroradiol 2012;33:180–7.

75. Kendall MG, Gibbons JD. Rank correlation methods. London: E. Arnold; 1990.

76. Tian L, Ren J, Zang Y. Regional homogeneity of resting state fMRI signals predicts stop signal task performance. Neuroimage 2012;60(1):539–44.

77. Wu T, Zang Y, Wang L, et al. Normal aging decreases regional homogeneity of the motor areas in the resting state. Neurosci Lett 2007;423(3):189–93.

78. Liu H, Liu Z, Liang M, et al. Decreased regional homogeneity in schizophrenia: a resting state functional magnetic resonance imaging study. Neuroreport 2006;17(1):19–22.

79. Liu Y, Wang K, Yu C, et al. Regional homogeneity, functional connectivity and imaging markers of Alzheimer's disease: a review of resting-state fMRI studies. Neuropsychologia 2008;46(6):1648–56.

80. Cao Q, Zang Y, Sun L, et al. Abnormal neural activity in children with attention deficit hyperactivity disorder: a resting-state functional magnetic resonance imaging study. Neuroreport 2006;17(10): 1033–6.

81. Agarwal S, Sair HI, Pillai JJ. Brain Connect 2017; 7(4):228–35.

82. Di X, Kim EH, Huang CC, et al. The influence of the amplitude of low-frequency fluctuations on resting-state functional connectivity. Front Hum Neurosci 2013;7:118.

83. Taylor PA, Gohel S, Di X, et al. Functional covariance networks: obtaining resting-state networks from inter-subject variability. Brain Connect 2012;2(4):203–17.

84. Yuan R, Di X, Kim EH, et al. Regional homogeneity of resting-state fMRI contributes to both neurovascular and task activation variations. Magn Reson Imaging 2013;31(9):1492–500.

85. Gohel S, Biswal BB. Functional integration between brain regions at rest occurs in multiple-frequency bands. Brain Connect 2015;5(1):23–34.

86. Yan C, Liu D, He Y, et al. Spontaneous brain activity in the default mode network is sensitive to different resting-state conditions with limited cognitive load. PLos One 2009;4(5):e5743.

87. Hu S, Chao HH, Zhang S, et al. Changes in cerebral morphometry and amplitude of low-frequency fluctuations of BOLD signals during healthy aging: correlation with inhibitory control. Brain Struct Funct 2014; 219(3):983–94.

88. Biswal BB, Mennes M, Zuo XN, et al. Toward discovery science of human brain function. Proc Natl Acad Sci U S A 2010;107(10):4734–9.

89. Di X, Kannurpatti SS, Rypma B, et al. Calibrating BOLD fMRI activations with neurovascular and anatomical constraints. Cereb Cortex 2013;23(2): 255–63.

90. Agarwal S, Lu H, Pillai JJ. Value of frequency domain resting state fMRI metrics ALFF & fALFF in the assessment of brain tumor-induced neurovascular uncoupling. Brain Connect 2017. [Epub ahead of print].

91. Solodkin A, Hlustik P, Noll DC, et al. Lateralization of motor circuits and handedness during finger movements. Eur J Neurol 2001;8:425–34.

92. Dassonville P, Zhu XH, Uurbil K, et al. Functional activation in motor cortex reflects the direction and the degree of handedness. Proc Natl Acad Sci U S A 1997;94:14015–8.

93. Zacà D, Nickerson JP, Deib G, et al. Effectiveness of four different clinical fMRI paradigms for preoperative regional determination of language lateralization in patients with brain tumors. Neuroradiology 2012; 54:1015–25.

94. Maesawa S, Bagarinao E, Fujii M, et al. Evaluation of resting state networks in patients with gliomas: connectivity changes in the unaffected side and its relation to cognitive function. PLoS One 2015;10(2): e0118072.

95. Esposito R, Mattei PA, Briganti C, et al. Modifications of default-mode network connectivity in patients with cerebral glioma. PLoS One 2012;7:e40231.

96. Harris RJ, Bookheimer SY, Cloughesy TF, et al. Altered functional connectivity of the default mode network in diffuse gliomas measured with pseudo-resting state fMRI. J Neurooncol 2014; 116(2):373–9.

97. Park JE, Kim HS, Kim SJ, et al. Alteration of long-distance functional connectivity and network topology in patients with supratentorial gliomas. Neuroradiology 2016;58(3):311–20.

Applications of Resting-State Functional Connectivity to Neurodegenerative Disease

Juan Zhou, PhD[a,b,*], Siwei Liu, PhD[a], Kwun Kei Ng, PhD[a],
Juan Wang, PhD[a]

KEYWORDS

- Resting-state fMR imaging • Functional connectivity • Alzheimer disease
- Frontotemporal dementia • Neurodegenerative disease • Mild cognitive impairment • Risk factors
- Amyloid beta

KEY POINTS

- Resting-state functional MR imaging–based functional connectivity method maps symptoms-associated functional network deterioration in vivo in neurodegenerative diseases.
- Distinct syndrome-specific network functional connectivity changes in clinical and prodromal Alzheimer disease (AD) and frontotemporal dementia (FTD) variants.
- Specific gene expressions moderate functional connectivity in clinical and asymptomatic AD and FTD.
- Amyloid beta accumulation is associated with atypical functional connectivity patterns in preclinical AD.
- Better cohort stratification and advanced computational and statistical techniques are essential for better prognosis and personalized treatment.

INTRODUCTION

Neurodegeneration, characterized by gradual and selective spreading of pathologic changes in a target brain network, leads to specific behavioral and cognitive dysfunctions. Alzheimer disease (AD) and frontotemporal dementia (FTD) are the 2 most common causes of neurodegenerative diseases among patients younger than 65 years,[1,2] whereas AD is more common among patients older than 65 years. AD usually begins with episodic memory loss with prominent medial temporal, posterior cingulate/precuneus, and lateral temporoparietal atrophy.[3,4] In contrast, 3 behavioral or language-related subtypes make up the clinical FTD spectrum: behavioral variant (bvFTD),[5] semantic variant primary progressive aphasia (svPPA), and nonfluent/agrammatic primary progressive aphasia (nfaPPA).[6] BvFTD features prominent social misconduct and emotional deficits with anterior cingulate, frontoinsular, striatal, and frontopolar degeneration. SvPPA results in loss

Disclosure Statement: The authors have nothing to disclose.
This work was supported by the Biomedical Research Council, Singapore (BMRC 04/1/36/372), the National Medical Research Council, Singapore (NMRC/CBRG/0088/2015 and NMRC/CIRG/1446/2016 and 1416/2015), Duke-NUS Medical School Signature Research Programme funded by Ministry of Health, Singapore (J. Zhou).
[a] Center for Cognitive Neuroscience, Neuroscience and Behavioral Disorders Programme, Duke-National University of Singapore Medical School, 8 College Road, #06-15, Singapore 169857, Singapore; [b] Agency for Science, Technology and Research-National University of Singapore (A*STAR-NUS), Clinical Imaging Research Centre, Centre for Translational Medicine (MD6), 14 Medical Drive, #B1-01, Singapore 117599, Singapore
* Corresponding author. Duke-National University of Singapore Medical School, 8 College Road, #06-15, Singapore 169857.
E-mail address: helen.zhou@duke-nus.edu.sg

of word and object meaning accompanied by left predominant temporal pole and subgenual cingulate involvement. nfaPPA presents with nonfluent, effortful, and agrammatic speech and is associated with left frontal operculum, dorsal anterior insula, and precentral gyrus atrophy. Moreover, presence of the apolipoprotein E (APOE) ε4 is the strongest genetic risk factor of sporadic AD.[7] FTD syndromes, in contrast, result from a group of distinct underlying molecular pathologic entities referred to collectively as frontotemporal lobar degeneration (FTLD). FTLD is further divided into 3 major molecular classes including tau (FTLD-tau), transactive response DNA-binding protein of 43 kDA (TDP-43, FTLD-TDP), and, least commonly, fused in sarcoma (FUS) protein (FTLD-FUS).[8] Although most patients have sporadic disease, several autosomal dominant culprit genes have been identified, with mutations in the genes encoding microtubule-associated protein tau (MAPT), progranulin (GRN), and C9orf72 accounting for most known genetic causes.[9]

A network-based neurodegeneration hypothesis was proposed 2 decades ago based on neuropathology studies[10] and transgenic animal models.[11] As effective, disease-specific, and personalized treatments are emerging for neurodegenerative diseases, an objective, noninvasive, biologically based network-sensitive neuroimaging assay is needed to predict risk, diagnose early, stage, and monitor the course and treatment of neurodegenerative diseases. Researchers have demonstrated that, unlike traditional region-based approaches, connectivity-based approaches can map large-scale networks in health and detect the network-level alterations in disease. This review focuses on the recent findings on resting-state functional MR imaging–based (rsfMR imaging) functional connectivity alterations in neurodegenerative diseases,[12–19] especially AD and FTD. as well as preclinical populations.[20] Specifically, we first introduce the rsfMR imaging–based functional connectivity methods and then highlight 3 major aspects: can resting-state functional connectivity analyses (1) reveal syndrome-specific network changes in neurodegenerative diseases, (2) uncover disease mechanism and the underlying neuropathology, and (3) detect early changes and track disease severity. Last we discuss the possible future directions.

MAPPING BRAIN CIRCUITS: RESTING-STATE FUNCTIONAL MAGNETIC RESONANCE IMAGING

Resting-state fMR imaging can be easily acquired in cognitively impaired populations and has offered valuable insights in the study of AD.[21] Instead of the changes evoked by specific stimuli, rsfMR imaging captures the macroscopic hemodynamic fluctuations at slow frequencies (<0.1 Hz). Regions showing synchronized spontaneous activities are functionally connected, as they also tend to coactivate or deactivate with similar spatial patterns during task,[22] and are often supporting highly relevant cognitive functions.[23,24] Therefore, functional connectivity derived from rsfMR imaging reveals network-based intrinsic functional connectivity.[25] These intrinsic connectivity networks (ICNs) change systematically at different vigilance and wakefulness conditions, developmental stages, and have homologues across species, suggesting their fundamental role in cognition.[21] Importantly, the interaction among networks is also critical to normal and aberrant cognitive performance and mental states,[26] and as such have offered valuable insights about the symptom manifestation and pathologic mechanisms of many neurodegenerative diseases.

Functional connectivity is often measured by temporal correlations between spatially distributed brain regions based on rsfMR imaging data. **Fig. 1** summarizes 4 primary methods for deriving functional connectivity from rsfMR imaging data. Seed-based analysis extracts ICNs by correlating the blood-oxygenation-level-dependent (BOLD) signals of a seed region to other target regions or with the rest of the brain (see **Fig. 1**A).[23] The representativeness and utility of the connectivity and network is therefore seed-dependent, as showcased by Seeley and colleagues,[27] who used 5 characteristic seeds of 5 distinctive neurodegenerative syndromes and showed the correspondence between unique syndrome and specific ICNs (**Fig. 2**).

Other approaches consider multiple brain regions simultaneously. In independent component analysis (ICA), spontaneous BOLD signals from all brain voxels are decomposed into spatially nonoverlapping and temporally coherent networks[28] (see **Fig. 1**B). Wu and colleagues[29] used ICA to extract ICNs associated with high-level cognition and reported that at-risk individuals, namely APOE ε4 carriers, had lower within-network functional connectivity that might precede cognitive decline. In analysis using parcellation-based connectivity matrices, the brain is segregated into predefined regions of interest (ROIs).[30] The functional connectivity between all pairs of regions are computed and arranged in matrix format (see **Fig. 1**C). Univariate or multivariate statistical analysis is then performed on the matrices to identify discernable differences between groups or conditions.[31]

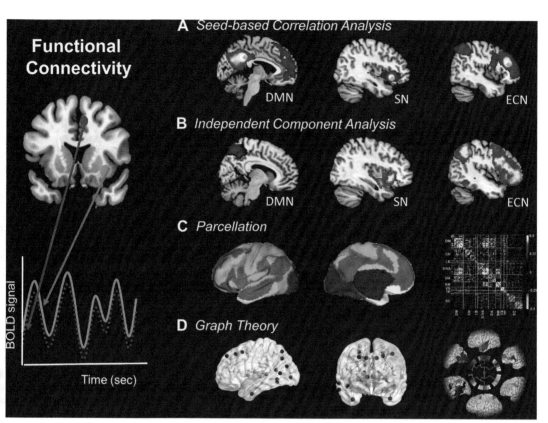

Fig. 1. Summary of common techniques to derive functional connectivity from rsfMR imaging data. Intrinsic functional connectivity describes the synchronized spontaneous low-frequency BOLD fluctuations (<0.1 Hz) between brain regions during task-free or resting-state condition (*left panel*). There are several analytical methods to derive functional connectivity from rsfMR imaging data. (*A*) In seed-based correlation analysis, large-scale functional connectivity networks are extracted with respect to a seed region (*green dots*). Three networks of primary interest in studies of neurodegenerative diseases are illustrated. (*B*) In ICA, multiple brain networks are identified by maximizing the spatial independence of the hemodynamic signals. A network comprises brain regions sharing the similar hemodynamic time course. Seed-based and ICA typically give very similar networks. (*C*) In parcellation-based connectivity matrix analysis, the connectivity patterns between a set of predefined brain regions (eg, functional parcellations[171]) are represented as a matrix and subject to statistical analysis. (*D*) In graph theoretic analysis, topological measures that describe different properties of the organization of the connectivity strength (edges) across multiple regions (nodes) or networks (nodes of the same color), that is, connectome, are examined. Abstraction of the brain as a graph also allows informative visualization, such as connectogram (modified from Nieto-Castanon[172] under the Creative Common License). BOLD, blood oxygenation level dependent; DMN, default mode network; ECN, executive control network; ICA, independent component analysis; SN, salience network.

Graph theoretic approach (see **Fig. 1**D) is highly useful in capturing and visualizing complex brain interactions embedded in these high dimensional matrices. In a brain graph, each ROI is a node and the functional connectivity between a pair of ROIs is an edge. Nodes and edges may be clustered and segregated such that nodes can belong to the same or different networks and edges can indicate within-network or between-network connectivity. Graph theoretic measures then capture these systematic organizations at nodal, network, and whole-brain levels.[32,33] By modeling connectivity as complex networks, graph theoretic analyses provide a new avenue to characterize

macroscopic brain topology and reveal disease mechanisms.[34–36] As detailed later in this article, Zhou and colleagues[37] derived functional connectivity matrices based on 1128 ROIs (635,628 ROI pairs) and used graph theoretic measures on such huge functional connectome matrices to derive topological parameters to examine the network-based neurodegenerative hypothesis.

With these methods, rsfMR imaging provides a novel network-sensitive, immediately repeatable, noninvasive tool to examine human functional connectome. Importantly, these methods are broadly applicable to both static and time-varying functional connectivity, the latter of which

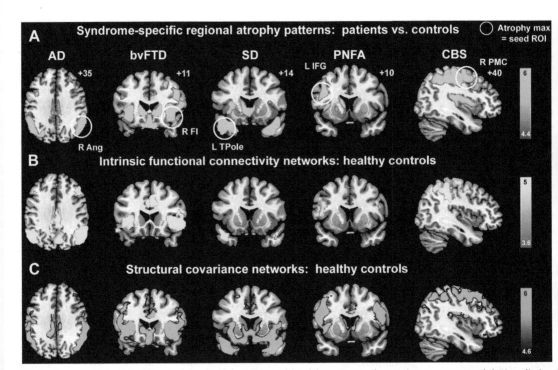

Fig. 2. Convergent syndromic atrophy, healthy ICN, and healthy structural covariance patterns. (*A*) Five distinct clinical syndromes showed dissociable atrophy patterns, whose cortical maxima (*circled*) provided seed ROIs for ICN and structural covariance analyses. (*B*) ICN mapping experiments identified 5 distinct networks anchored by the 5 syndromic atrophy seeds. (*C*) Healthy subjects further showed GM volume covariance patterns that recapitulated results shown in (*A*) and (*B*). Color bars indicate *t*-scores. In coronal and axial images, the left side of the image corresponds to the left side of the brain. ANG, angular gyrus; FI, frontoinsula; IFGoper, inferior frontal gyrus, pars opercularis; PMC, premotor cortex; TPole, temporal pole. (*Adapted from* Seeley WW, Crawford RK, Zhou J, et al. Neurodegenerative diseases target large-scale human brain networks. Neuron 2009;62(1):42–52.)

better captures neural dynamics at a finer time scale and is shown to be of clinical utility.[38]

CAN RESTING-STATE FUNCTIONAL MR IMAGING–BASED CONNECTIVITY ANALYSES REVEAL SYNDROME-SPECIFIC NETWORK CHANGES?

To date, rsfMR imaging has been widely used to chart normal human functional connectivity architecture[24,39,40] and predict individual differences in human behavior and cognition.[41–43] Such typical architecture provides important framework to understanding diseases. Seeley and colleagues[27] confirmed that spatial atrophy patterns in 5 distinct neurodegenerative syndromes, including AD and variants of FTD, mirror normal human ICNs derived from rsfMR imaging (see **Fig. 2**, rows 1 and 2). Specifically, AD causes atrophy within a posterior hippocampal-cingulo-temporal-parietal network, which resembles the "default mode network" (DMN) in health.[39,44,45] BvFTD, in contrast, features atrophy in anterior insula, anterior cingulate cortex (ACC), and subcortical and thalamic regions, mirroring the "Salience Network" (SN) in

health.[43,46,47] The SN is often activated in response to social-emotionally significant internal and external stimuli,[48,49] whereas elements of the DMN are usually involved in episodic memory and visuospatial imagery.[44,50,51] Notably, although the anterior SN degenerates in bvFTD, posterior cortical functions survive or even thrive, at times associated with emergent visual creativity.[52,53] AD, in contrast, maintains socioemotional functions and features episodic memory loss and visuospatial dysfunction.

Based on the inversely correlated relationship between the salience and DMNs in the healthy brain[54,55] and the opposing symptom-deficit profiles of AD and bvFTD, Seeley and colleagues[56] proposed a "reciprocal networks" model in which each network exerts an inhibitory influence on the other. This model has led to the hypothesis of divergent functional connectivity changes in AD and bvFTD. Zhou and colleagues[57] later tested this hypothesis by comparing AD and bvFTD to age-matched healthy controls using task-free fMR imaging ICN technique. As predicted, the SN connectivity was disrupted in bvFTD but enhanced in AD, whereas the DMN connectivity was disrupted in AD but enhanced in bvFTD (Fig. 3). The findings were largely consistent with previous studies on the DMN connectivity reductions in AD.[58–60] Several studies using other imaging modalities supported the divergent patterns in AD and bvFTD.[61,62] The reciprocal model is further supported by a fornix/hypothalamus deep brain stimulation (DBS) study on patients with AD.[63] All patients with AD after 1 month and 12 months of DBS showed consistent increased metabolism in the DMN regions along with improvements and/or slowing in the rate of cognitive decline; more interestingly, they also presented robust decreased metabolism in the SN regions (ACC and medial frontal cortex).

Graph theoretic analyses on functional connectivity revealed decreased clustering coefficient and characteristic path length closer to the theoretic values of random networks in patients with AD,[64] in parallel with findings using other imaging modalities.[59,62,65,66] Weakening of intermodular connectivity was outspoken and strongly related to cognitive impairment in AD.[64] This observation was in line with a global reduction of functional long-distance links between frontal and caudal brain regions.[65] Taken together, the randomization of the brain functional networks in AD suggested a loss of global information integration through degeneration in a distributed network. The opposite trend exhibited by bvFTD toward an overly

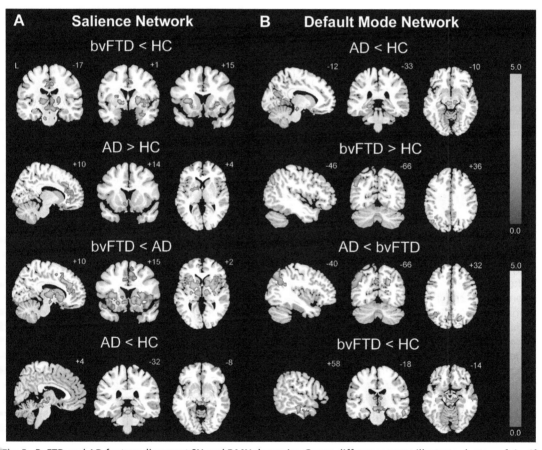

Fig. 3. BvFTD and AD feature divergent SN and DMN dynamics. Group difference maps illustrate clusters of significantly reduced or increased connectivity for each ICN. In the SN (A), patients with bvFTD showed distributed connectivity reductions compared with healthy controls (HCs) and patients with AD, whereas patients with AD showed increased connectivity in ACC and ventral striatum compared with healthy controls. In the DMN (B), patients with AD showed several connectivity impairments compared with HCs and patients with bvFTD, whereas patients with bvFTD showed increased left angular gyrus connectivity. Patients with bvFTD and AD further showed focal brainstem connectivity disruptions within their "released" network (DMN for bvFTD, SN for AD). Results are displayed at a joint height and extent probability threshold of P<.05, corrected at the whole-brain level. Color bars represent t-scores, and statistical maps are superimposed on the Montreal Neurologic Institute template brain. (*Adapted from* Zhou J, Greicius MD, Gennatas ED, et al. Divergent network connectivity changes in behavioral variant frontotemporal dementia and Alzheimer's disease. Brain 2010;133(5):1352–67.)

ordered topology in electroencephalogram (EEG) data might imply the divergent effect of the disease on distributed large-scale networks.[62]

A significant portion of patients with AD does exhibit nonmemory deficits in language, executive function, and higher visual functions.[67] These patients make up 3 major types of AD variants, namely the early-onset AD (EOAD), the logopenic variant of primary progressive aphasia (lvPPA), and the posterior cortical atrophy (PCA). Structural imaging studies found that these AD variants share common atrophy in the DMN, especially the posterior cingulate cortex.[68,69] PET studies examining glucose metabolism found hypometabolism in distinct brain regions that were associated with executive function, language, or visual functions corresponding well to the variant-specific deficits.[70] Recent rsfMR imaging study compared functional connectivity at the atrophy regions either common across and specific to AD variants and found common connectivity in posterior DMN and precuneus, suggesting DMN involvements were shared among AD variants.[70] For variant-specific atrophy region, intrinsic networks related to variant-specific cognitive deficits were identified. Atrophy specific to the lvPPA was seated in the language network,[70] which was similarly found in another study comparing lvPPA and amnesic patients with AD matched on amyloid deposition.[71] Anterior SN and right executive-control network were specific to the EOAD.[70,72] Atrophy regions specific to the PCA were linked with the higher visual network,[70] where disrupted functional connectivity was also reported in a later study examining dorsal and ventral visual networks separately in PCA[73] (Fig. 4). The topographic similarity between the variant-specific atrophy and the deficit-related functional networks support the network-based propagation of the neurodegenerative diseases, in which similar local pathologic changes and disease-related aggregate spread in different brain networks may underline the clinico-anatomical variations in AD.

Similarly, emerging studies used rsfMR imaging to assess distinct network disruptions in FTD variants. SvPPA was associated with extensive functional connectivity disruption between the anterior temporal lobe and multiple speech-processing areas.[74] To our knowledge, functional connectivity of nfaPPA has not yet been examined, but it might be related to the network anchored by the inferior frontal gyrus.[75] More importantly, a link between specific functional connectivity changes and behavioral impairment in FTD variants is established. Farb and colleagues[76] found that high level of behavioral dysfunction was associated with enhanced prefrontal connectivity in bvFTD, whereas low level of behavioral dysfunction was associated with reduced lateral prefrontal connectivity in svPPA. Recent studies using graph theoretic analyses on whole-brain functional connectome revealed distinct abnormal network topology in bvFTD and svPPA. Notably, patients with bvFTD featured loss of hubs in frontal lobes involving ACC, orbitofrontal cortex, and caudate nucleus, which were associated with executive dysfunction[77] (Fig. 5), whereas patients with svPPA had loss of hubs and reduced nodal degree in the inferior and ventral temporal regions and occipital cortices.[78] Additionally, the network centrality combined with social-executive behavioral measures had been applied to distinguish patients with bvFTD from healthy controls and fronto-insular stroke with a high classification rate.[79] Taken together, disruption of optimal brain connectome configurations were driven by specific symptom-associated networks, supporting the network breakdown mechanism in neurodegeneration.

CAN RESTING-STATE FUNCTIONAL MR IMAGING–BASED CONNECTIVITY ANALYSES UNCOVER DISEASE MECHANISM AND THE UNDERLYING NEUROPATHOLOGY?

That each neurodegenerative syndrome reflects a large-scale network breakdown has been established, as discussed previously, through a variety of convergent approaches. But what do we know about how disease progresses to create a network-related spatial pattern? At least 4 disease-general hypotheses have been put forth and can be summarized: (1) "nodal stress," in which regions subject to heavy network traffic (ie, "hubs") undergo activity-related "wear and tear" that gives rise to or worsens disease[80,81]; (2) "transneuronal spread," in which some toxic agent propagates along network connections, perhaps through "prionlike" templated conformational change[82–89]; (3) "trophic failure," in which network connectivity disruption undermines internodal trophic factor support, accelerating disease within nodes lacking collateral trophic sources[90–92]; and (4) "shared vulnerability," in which networked regions feature a common gene or protein expression signature[93] that confers disease-specific susceptibility, evenly distributed throughout the network. These non–mutually exclusive candidate network degeneration mechanisms make competing predictions about how healthy network architecture should influence disease-associated regional vulnerability. Notably, although "network degeneration" is often understood to mean "network-based spread," only the "transneuronal

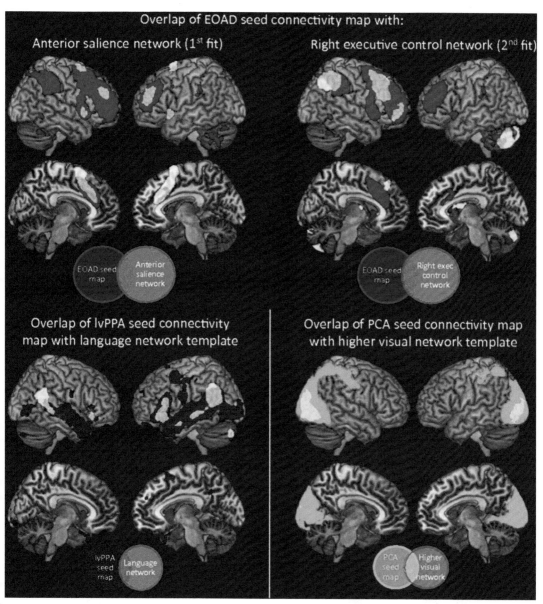

Fig. 4. Overlap of seed-based connectivity networks of specifically atrophied ROIs with best-fitting functional network templates. The EOAD seed connectivity map showed 2 strong fits: the anterior salience network showed the best fit with the left hemisphere connectivity map, and the right executive-control network showed the best fit with the right connectivity map. The lvPPA seed and PCA seed connectivity maps showed the best fit with the language and higher visual networks, respectively. (*Adapted from* Lehmann M, Ghosh PM, Madison C, et al. Diverging patterns of amyloid deposition and hypometabolism in clinical variants of probable Alzheimer's disease. Brain 2013;136(Pt 3):844–58.)

spread" model proposes that progression represents physical spreading of a pathologic process along axons connecting individual neurons.

The ideal approach for examining disease progression and predicting neurodegeneration from brain connectivity would be to follow individuals from health to disease, exploring connectivity-vulnerability interactions within single subjects.

Although this approach may prove challenging for the FTD syndromes, longitudinal analyses of this type are beginning to be pursued for AD-type dementia through large, ongoing, collaborative longitudinal studies. To date, efforts to investigate disease progression mechanisms have mainly relied on cross-sectional data. As discussed in relation to disease onset, for each of 5

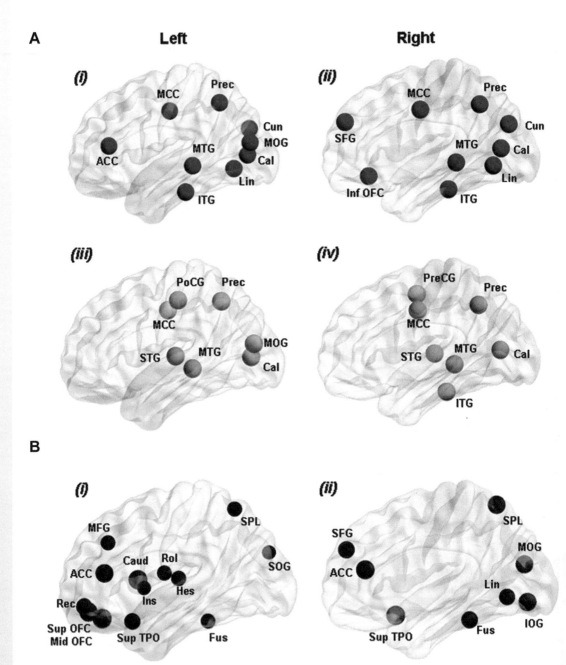

Fig. 5. Graph theoretic analysis reveal reduced nodal degree in bvFTD patients. (A) Cortical hubs of the functional networks of healthy controls (i, ii) and patients with the behavioral variant of frontotemporal dementia (bvFTD) (iii, iv). Hubs were identified as brain regions having either integrated nodal degree or betweenness centrality 1 SD greater than the network average. (B) Regions showing decreased integrated nodal degree (i, ii) in patients with bvFTD compared with healthy controls. Node size is proportional to the difference in the value of the integrated nodal parameters between the 2 groups. Cal, calcarine cortex; Caud, caudate nucleus; Cun, cuneus; Fus, fusiform gyrus; Hes, Heschl gyrus; Ins, insula; IOG, inferior occipital gyrus; ITG, inferior temporal gyrus; Lin, lingual gyrus; MCC, middle cingulate cortex; MFG, middle frontal gyrus; MOG, middle occipital gyrus; MTG, middle temporal gyrus; PoCG, postcentral gyrus; Prec, precuneus; PreCG, precentral gyrus; Rec, gyrus rectus; Rol, rolandic operculum; SFG, superior frontal gyrus; SOG, superior occipital gyrus; SPL, t superior parietal lobule; STG, superior temporal gyrus; TPO, temporal pole. (Adapted from Agosta F, Sala S, Valsasina P, et al. Brain network connectivity assessed using graph theory in frontotemporal dementia. Neurology 2013;81(2):134–43.)

syndromes Zhou and colleagues[37] identified critical network epicenters whose normal connectivity profiles most resembled the syndrome-associated atrophy patterns. Graph theoretic analyses in healthy subjects revealed that regions with higher total connectional flow and, more consistently, shorter functional paths to the epicenters, showed greater syndrome-associated vulnerability (Fig. 6). Across all 5 syndromes, network nodes subject to greater intranetwork total information flow were found to undergo greater atrophy. This observation raised the possibility that activity-dependent mechanisms, such as oxidative stress, local extracellular milieu fluctuations, or glia-dependent phenomena, influence regional vulnerability; this influence might be a key factor in determining sites of initial onset or secondary onset (ie, progression).

Second, nodes with shorter connectional paths to an epicenter showed greater vulnerability, suggesting that transneuronal spread represents one of the key factors driving early target network degeneration, most likely by physical transmission of toxic disease proteins or other agents along axons. In other words, epicenter infiltration by disease may provide privileged but graded access across the network that determines where the disease will arrive next. Although trophic factor insufficiency or a shared gene or protein expression profile may help to determine sites of onset, the findings of this study were difficult to reconcile with predictions made by these models regarding the graded vulnerability seen within the target networks. To extend the anatomic scope of the analyses, the investigators further examined

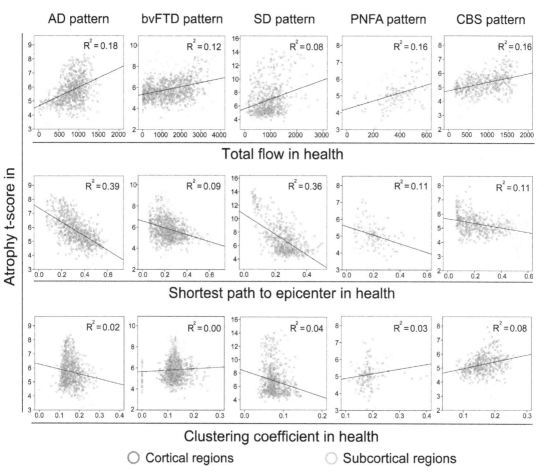

Fig. 6. Intranetwork graph theoretic connectivity measures in health predict atrophy severity in disease. Regions with high total connectional flow (row 1) and shorter functional paths to the epicenters (row 2) showed significantly greater disease vulnerability ($P<.05$ familywise error corrected for multiple comparisons in AD, bvFTD, SD, PNFA, and CBS), whereas inconsistent weaker or nonsignificant relationships were observed between clustering coefficient and atrophy (row 3). Cortical regions, blue circles; subcortical regions, orange circles. (*From* Zhou J, Gennatas ED, Kramer JH, et al. Predicting regional neurodegeneration from the healthy brain functional connectome. Neuron 2012;73(6):1216–27; with permission.)

connectivity-vulnerability relationships within the "off-target" networks to determine how nodal characteristics influence downstream vulnerability. Here, overwhelmingly, the evidence supported the transneuronal spread model. In summary, the findings best fit a model in which initial vulnerability may reflect a node's centrality (ie, "hubness") within the target network, whereas downstream vulnerability more closely related to a node's connectional proximity to the most vulnerable "epicenter" regions.

Maps of functional connectivity provide a means to understand why certain lesions and connectional abnormalities are particularly disruptive. One step further, it may predict the underlying AD or FTD pathology. Using task-free fMR imaging, Buckner and colleagues[80] showed that functional connectivity hubs in the healthy brain were mainly located in the DMN areas. More importantly, by mapping in vivo Aβ deposition with Pittsburg Compound B PET in patients with AD and controls, they found that the DMN cortical hubs in health resembled the high Aβ accumulation in AD compared with controls. This finding suggested that hubs, while acting as critical way stations for information processing, may also augment the underlying pathologic cascade in AD. Disruption of functional connectivity between the DMN regions may represent an early functional consequence of Aβ pathology before clinical AD. A recent study found significant disruptions of whole-brain connectivity in amyloid-positive patients with mild cognitive impairment in typical cortical hubs (posterior cingulate cortex/precuneus), strongly overlapping with regional hypometabolism.[94]

Intriguingly, subtle connectivity disruptions and hypometabolism were already present in amyloid-positive asymptomatic subjects and both connectivity and metabolism measures had positive correlation with each other and a negative correlation with amyloid burden (also see Brier and colleagues[95]). Two studies have indicated that the amount of Aβ deposits was negatively correlated with the DMN connectivity (ventral medial prefrontal cortex, angular gyrus, and medial posterior regions), and the lower connectivity was associated with poorer working memory performance in normal aging.[96,97] Gili and colleagues[98] found similar functional connectivity disruption of the DMN in AD and mild cognitive impairment (MCI), prodromal stage of AD, compared with controls. Interestingly, the posterior cingulate cortex showed reduced connectivity in patients with MCI in the absence of gray matter (GM) atrophy, which, in contrast, detectable at the stage of fully developed AD. This study indicated that

functional disconnection precedes GM atrophy during AD pathologic process.

More recent studies on early AD and cognitively healthy older adults point to a more complex picture regarding the association between amyloid and functional connectivity. On the one hand, a lack of association between Aβ and DMN functional connectivity was reported[99]; on the other hand, the relationship between the DMN and cerebrospinal fluid (CSF) Aβ biomarker was found in a subnetwork of the DMN with a hub in the right dorsal ACC; this subnetwork was distinct from another one that was more associated with the tau biomarker and had a hub in the right anterior entorhinal cortex.[100] Such divergent associations with the DMN functional connectivity between Aβ and tau markers are consistent with, and may help understand, the known discrepancies between the 2 pathologies (eg, locus of deposition, symptoms predictive power[95,101]).

Furthermore, the influence of Aβ deposition may extend beyond DMN into functional connectivity within the fronto-parietal network, within the attentional networks, and the "anticorrelation" between these networks.[102,103] Some of these correlations are surprisingly positive, which might reflect compensatory reorganization to combat neural and cognitive decline.[102,104] Koch and colleagues[105] examined the relationship among Aβ pathology, functional connectivity, and cognitive performance in patients with prodromal AD and healthy controls. They extracted brain networks from rsfMR imaging and task fMR imaging during a demanding visuo-motor dual task (Fig. 7). Consistent with other studies, Aβ accumulation was negatively correlated with DMN connectivity. Furthermore, although the resting-state functional connectivity in the posterior DMN was lower in patients than in controls, the task connectivity in the same region showed the reversed pattern, and such higher task connectivity was associated with poorer task performance. Importantly, similar results were also found for the posterior right attentional network (rATN). However, only the DMN but not rATN resting-state functional connectivity statistically moderated the association between Aβ pathology and task performance. These findings prompt a network-based neurodegeneration hypothesis to account for how these changes "outside" of the epicenters may arise (for instance, through between-network connections[37,95]), and whether or how they are differentially associated with symptoms.

Based on the divergent functional connectivity patterns among patients with dementia and healthy controls, researchers have begun to

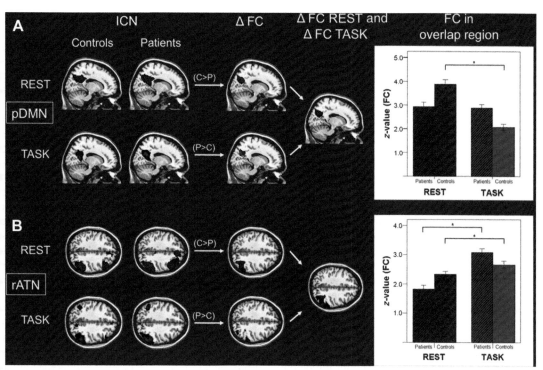

Fig. 7. Spatially consistent functional connectivity (FC) changes of posterior default mode network (pDMN) and right attentional network (rATN) across rest and task in patients. Columns 1 and 2: ICNs characterized by spatial patterns of FC during rest (*lines* 1 and 3) and task (*lines* 2 and 4) concerning the pDMN (*A*) and rATN (*B*). Columns 3 and 4: Results of the ICN group comparisons for FC maps between patients and controls (ΔFC) for rest and task condition as well as corresponding spatial overlaps of group differences (ΔFC Rest and ΔFC Task). Right side: Bar plots representing averaged FC values for overlapping group differences for each group, condition, and ICN. Paired *t* tests revealed FC differences across conditions (*P*<.05, * Significant result, pDMN T = 0.9 (patients)/7.7 (controls); rATN T = −7.8/−2.1). (*Adapted from* Koch K, Myers NE, Göttler J, et al. Disrupted intrinsic networks link amyloid-β pathology and impaired cognition in prodromal Alzheimer's disease. Cerebral Cortex 2015;25(12):4678–88.)

develop functional connectivity-based biomarkers to distinguish among dementia subtypes and controls. Using rsfMR imaging, Greicius and colleagues[58] calculated the goodness-of-fit score to the DMN at the individual level and achieved 85% of sensitivity and 75% of specificity differentiating AD from controls. The clustering coefficient derived from graph theoretic analyses of rsfMR imaging distinguished AD participants from the controls with a sensitivity of 72% and specificity of 78%.[59] A recent study computed whole-brain correlation-based connectivity among 116 ROIs and achieved 85% of sensitivity and 80% of specificity between the AD group and the non-AD group (MCI and controls).[106] Using graph theoretic measures, Khazaee and colleagues[107] were able to classify patients with AD or MCI and control individuals with 93.3% accuracy; furthermore, hub counting showed a progressive decrease from control to AD, suggesting that AD is characterized by aberrant network communication. Such

classification success and implication on hub disruption is consistent with the findings of Dai and colleagues,[108] which also demonstrated hub-oriented impairment, in addition to disrupted internetwork connectivity, in AD compared with controls. Based on the observations that bvFTD and AD feature divergent connectivity effects on the SN and DMN, Zhou and colleagues[57] illustrated that a summary score incorporating both networks might better differentiate bvFTD from AD and each patient group from healthy controls, achieving the sensitivity of 92% and specificity of 96% in 3-group classification and 100% differentiation between AD and bvFTD. This suggested that functional network–based patterns, sensitive to decreases and increases, and divergent among syndromes, might prove more specific to predict disease diagnoses and predict the underlying pathology. Published work on differential diagnoses using functional networks in the language variants of FTD remains scarce. Current connectivity approaches require replication in an independent clinical dataset and validation in pathologically verified clinical samples.

CAN RESTING-STATE FUNCTIONAL MR IMAGING–BASED CONNECTIVITY ANALYSES DETECT EARLY CHANGES AND TRACK DISEASE SEVERITY?

As neurodegeneration spreads from its initial target to the entire network accompanied by multi-domain cognitive deficits, network-based break-down measured by connectivity analyses could be a potential sensitive marker to detect onset and track disease severity at the individual level. By examining the functional connectivity cross-sectionally in healthy elderly controls and patients with mild, moderate, or severe AD by rsfMR imaging, Zhang's group[60] found that all patients with AD consistently disrupted the functional connectivity between posterior cingulate cortex and the DMN regions, including medial prefrontal cortex, precuneus, and hippocampus, which intensified as the stage of AD progression increased. However, this study did not take into account the global atrophy volume and regional atrophy at posterior cingulate cortex. Similar to AD, specific regions of connectivity disruption within the SN can track disease severity of FTD. BvFTD clinical severity (CDR-SB) correlated with loss of right frontoinsular SN connectivity and with biparietal DMN connectivity enhancement, demonstrating that not only connectivity reduction but also enhancement have potential to track disease progression.[57]

Characterizing the earliest stages of cognitive impairment is receiving increasing attention in the field of aging and dementia research. MCI is a transitional state between healthy elderly individuals and mild AD, which is at high risk for developing AD. Emerging evidence on MCI showed a similar AD pattern of reduced DMN connectivity, including posterior cingulate cortex, medial prefrontal cortex, precuneus, and hippocampus.[4,98,109–112] Functional connectivity strength also was correlated with cognitive performance and can discriminate MCI from healthy controls.[113] In a recent longitudinal study, the DMN connectivity score (derived from task fMR imaging) distinguished patients with MCI who underwent cognitive decline and conversion to AD from those who remained stable over a 2-year to 3-year follow-up period, independent of global atrophy and demographics.[114] Looking at resting-state instead of task functional connectivity, another longitudinal study came to similar conclusions. In particular, functional connectivity of precuneus at baseline showed high sensitivity and specificity

in classifying amnesic MCI converting to AD against those nonconvertors.[115]

In parallel with consistent neuroimaging findings on symptomatic FTD and patients with AD, researchers recently became excited about studying the functional architecture changes in the high-risk population, aiming to develop disease-prevention strategies.[116,117] Genetic studies show unequivocally that the apolipoprotein ε4 (APOE ε4) allele is associated with an increased risk of EOAD and late-onset AD.[118,119] Functional connectivity studies on asymptomatic carriers of the APOE ε4 allele observed both decreased and increased connectivity at the DMN regions previously defined as having abnormal connectivity in AD[120–122] (see review by Seeley[123]). The connectivity changes in the DMN were observed before any manifestations of cognitive changes and in the absence of Aβ deposition[124] and white matter degradation.[125] Chen and colleagues[126] applied graph theoretic measures and found that ε4 carriers had lower nodal efficiency in bilateral hippocampus, right para-hippocampal gyrus, bilateral amygdala, and right Heschl gyrus (Fig. 8). To note, although these regions are generally implicated in memory-related processes, in this study it was their structural connectivity but not functional connectivity that was statistically associated with memory impairment, suggesting the usefulness of multimodal imaging. A recent task-free fMR imaging study revealed decreased connectivity between posterior cingulate cortex and regions of the posterior DMN while increased connectivity between ACC and the SN regions in the APOE ε4 carriers relative to noncarriers.[127] This finding was amazingly consistent with the reciprocal model between the SN and DMN. Results as such may therefore point to a genetic moderation of the network-based neurodegeneration.

What complicates the implication of the APOE-functional connectivity relationship is that compensatory reorganization[128] of brain networks may be prevalent in ε4 carriers to maintain cognitive performance. Functional connectivity that is higher in carriers compared with noncarriers is often interpreted as such. For instance, Matura and colleagues[129] reported higher functional connectivity between left posterior cingulate cortex (PCC) and left middle temporal gyrus in ε4 carriers compared with noncarriers. Using eigenvalue centrality (EC) a voxelwise measure computed as the sum of centralities of all neighbors connected to a given voxel, Luo and colleagues[130] found lower EC in left media temporal lobe and left lingual gyrus and increased EC in left middle frontal gyrus for the ε4 carriers. Although the lower functional connectivity in the medial temporal regions was consistent with

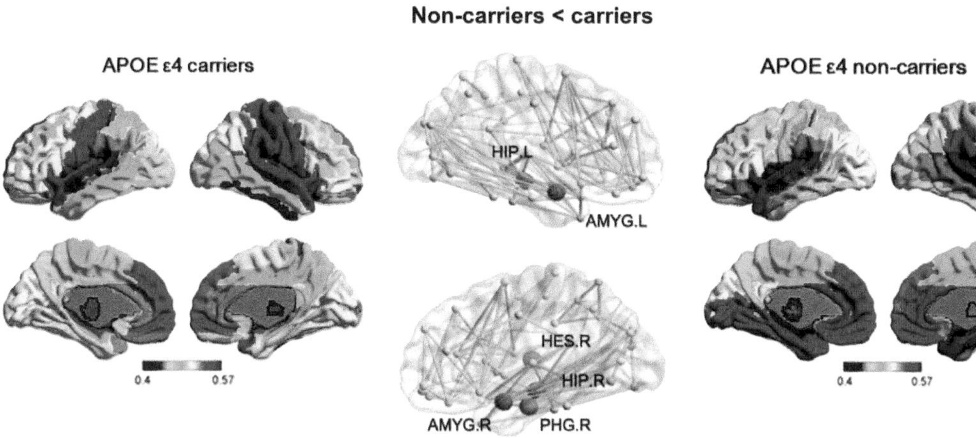

Fig. 8. Cognitively normal elderly APOE ε4 carriers showed lower nodal efficiency in the medial temporal lobe areas (middle panel). This lower nodal efficiency was consistent between functional and structural connectivity at the right parahippocampal gyrus (PHG.R; orange node). Age, gender, and education were considered as covariates in the analysis. Left and right panels show the topological distribution of mean nodal efficiency of ε4 carriers and noncarriers, respectively. AMYG, amygdala; HES, Heschl gyrus; HIP, hippocampus; L, Left; PHG, parahippocampal gyrus; R, Right. (*Adapted from* Chen Y, Chen K, Zhang J, et al. Disrupted functional and structural networks in cognitively normal elderly subjects with the APOE e4 allele. Neuropsychopharmacology 2015;40(5):1181–91. Figure 1b and Figure 2.)

impaired episodic memory, the higher connectivity in the middle temporal gyrus was speculated to reflect compensation. Consistent with these observations, McKenna and colleagues[131] found lower functional connectivity in early mild cognitive impairment (EMCI) patients than healthy controls but these changes were not evident in carriers compared with noncarriers. One possibility would be that compensatory reorganization of brain networks have protected some ε4 carriers from advancing into EMCI. Finally, using a longitudinal dataset, Ye and colleagues[132] observed a genotype-by-diagnosis interaction of the longitudinal changes in functional connectivity between hippocampus and right frontal regions in preclinical control individuals and patients with MCI. Specifically, cognitively normal ε4 carriers showed an increased connectivity across time, whereas MCI ε4 carriers showed a decrease. The investigators postulated this reversed trend to reflect a compensatory reorganization of the brain dynamics that is exhausted eventually, leading to the onset of clinical conditions. Future research needs to establish what compensatory mechanisms may be in play, whether they also follow a network trajectory, and how ε4 genotype can influence such mechanisms, for instance by replenishing reduced temporal dynamics complexity between brain regions through altering hemodynamic synchrony.[133]

Despite its robustness in risk elevation, presence of the ε4 allele does not guarantee a fate to dementia. Studies also suggest that the influence of APOE genotype on brain network organization may not necessarily be pathologic per se.[134,135] Therefore, it is plausible that the APOE genotype interacts with other risk factors and demographic characteristics during the lifespan to make its host more vulnerable to late-onset dementia.[136–138] For instance, female ε4 carriers have long been shown to suffer higher risk of AD.[119] Using hippocampal seeds, Heise and colleagues[139] reported lower hippocampus-precuneus/PCC connectivity in female ε4 carriers compared with male carriers and female noncarriers; it was also the only group to show a cross-sectional association between age and hippocampal functional connectivity. Besides gender, APOE genotype may also interact with Aβ pathology to elevate susceptibility to pathologic neurodegeneration.[136,140,141]

Similarly, recent rsfMR imaging work moves toward characterizing the early functional connectivity changes in subjects with genetic risk for FTD. The SN functional connectivity abnormalities were found in presymptomatic C90rf72, GRN, and MAPT carriers,[142,143] which was consistently involved in bvFTD, demonstrating that the network changes exist decades before disease onset.[144] However, no agreement on the pattern of changes has been made yet.[142,143,145] To date, researchers have started to investigate the issue by considering technical factors,[146] the possible influence of different pathology,[147] and distinct temporal and spatial profiles.[146] Such validation is essential for validating rsfMR imaging functional connectivity as a biomarker of the prodromal changes.

Last, work on intervention has begun to use rsfMR imaging functional connectivity to evaluate intervention efficacy. For instance, Goveas and colleagues[148] applied such analysis to identify the neural correlates of cognitive improvement in subjects with mild AD after 12 weeks of donepezil treatment. After donepezil treatment, neural correlates of cognitive improvement measured by Mini-Mental State Examination scores were identified in the hippocampal connectivity with left parahippocampus, dorsolateral prefrontal cortex, and inferior frontal gyrus. Stronger recovery in the network connectivity was associated with cognitive improvement. This finding suggested that rsfMR imaging connectivity approach may be further developed to monitor and predict AD treatment response in clinical pharmacologic trials.

SUMMARY AND FUTURE DIRECTIONS

Characterizing brain networks, such as rsfMR imaging–based functional connectivity changes, can explain how an endophenotype of molecular pathologic changes, such as cortical amyloid and tau accumulation, has built up in an individual brain leading to symptoms. The hub characteristics of a brain region and the degree of their functional connectivity and structural integration explain why certain brain networks are more vulnerable than others to brain diseases such as AD. Network-based principles have begun to shed light on group-level changes across a host of neurodegenerative disease syndromes.[149] To aid in the search for treatments, however, these methods will need to be developed for use in tracking single subjects over time. We summarize the possible future directions in the following.

First, differential diagnosis is required to tease apart variance in neurodegenerative disease associated with individual differences in clinico-anatomical variations and treatment responses.[70,76,142,143] The clinical utility of rsfMR imaging–based functional connectivity, as well as other modalities, will certainly benefit from better appreciation of disease heterogeneity through, for instance, more refined population stratification based on genetic, demographic, and environmental factors.[150,151] Rapidly increasing access to large and shared databases across multiple sites[152] can help overcome drawbacks of small-sample studies on disease variants and improve the stability and reproducibility of rsfMR imaging data analysis.[153]

Second, the strength of rsfMR imaging to discover covert neural changes in asymptomatic population opens up the opportunities of early detection and intervention, where outcomes can be substantial.[117,139,149,151,154,155] A combination of rsfMR imaging functional connectivity, and multimodal data, such as structural MR imaging, diffusion MR imaging,[156,157] other noninvasive detection techniques,[158] and better understanding of disease heterogeneity will greatly improve the sensitivity and specificity of existing methods.[115,157]

Third, many of these advancements will be attributable to breakthroughs in computational and statistical techniques. Methodological improvement, such as deriving functional connectivity with higher tempo-spatial fidelity (eg, Bayesian network modeling,[159] dynamic functional connectivity[160,161]; multi-atlas approach[162]), and machine learning[107,108,163] on whole-brain functional connectome (static or dynamic) or nonlinear statistical methods, will allow us to discover more robust and valid features of the diseases, and thus promise higher accuracy and generalizability in the detection at the preclinical stage, predictions on disease onset, progression, and treatment response.

Finally, longitudinal design is essential for moving from group predictions of disease progression toward individual prospective. More longitudinal data could help validate or clarify the rich knowledge gained from cross-sectional studies, such as the critical role of increased functional connectivity in the precuneus in MCI conversion,[115] the different longitudinal patterns relating to the left and right frontoparietal networks between patients with bvFTD and patients with AD,[164] the differential manifestation of APOE ε4 effect on DMN connectivity between MCI converters and nonconverters,[165] and the change of rate of functional connectivity alternations at early and late stages of MCI,[166] to name but a few. There is a need to further develop the rsfMR imaging method to better map cognitive dysfunctions with neural changes.[167–170]

In summary, rsfMR imaging–based functional connectivity offers a flexible and powerful way to describe the interrelationship of the neural signals among various brain regions. Research in the healthy population has revealed the hierarchical and topological organizations of these connectivities as intrinsic networks supporting cognitive functions. Disruptions of typical organization and interactions within and between functional networks implicate abnormal cognition and behavior. This raised the plausibility of the same principle underlying neurodegenerative diseases, assaulting the brain in a systematic, network-oriented fashion. To date, network-sensitive neuroimaging work (using rsfMR imaging) supports this network-based neurodegeneration hypothesis

This can serve as a significant first step toward predicting disease onset, variant manifestation, and progression. Future studies will continue to improve the working model to incorporate moderating factors, elucidate exception cases, and capitalize on translational opportunities.

REFERENCES

1. Ratnavalli E, Brayne C, Dawson K, et al. The prevalence of frontotemporal dementia. Neurology 2002;58(11):1615–21.

2. Ikeda M, Ishikawa T, Tanabe H. Epidemiology of frontotemporal lobar degeneration. Dement Geriatr Cogn 2004;17(4):265–8.

3. Hyman BT, Damasio AR, Van Hoesen GW, et al. Alzheimer's disease: cell-specific pathology isolates the hippocampal formation. Science 1984; 298:83–95.

4. Mitchell TW, Mufson EJ, Schneider JA, et al. Para-hippocampal tau pathology in healthy aging, mild cognitive impairment, and early Alzheimer's disease. Ann Neurol 2002;51(2):182–9.

5. Seeley WW, Zhou J, Kim EJ. Frontotemporal dementia: what can the behavioral variant teach us about human brain organization? Neuroscientist 2011;18(4):373–85.

6. Gorno-Tempini ML, Hillis AE, Weintraub S, et al. Classification of primary progressive aphasia and its variants. Neurology 2011;76(11):1006–14.

7. Dubois B, Feldman HH, Jacova C, et al. Research criteria for the diagnosis of Alzheimer's disease: revising the NINCDS-ADRDA criteria. Lancet Neurol 2007;6(8):734–46.

8. Mackenzie IR, Neumann M, Bigio EH, et al. Nomenclature and nosology for neuropathologic subtypes of frontotemporal lobar degeneration: an update. Acta Neuropathol 2010; 119(1):1–4.

9. Whitwell JL, Weigand SD, Boeve BF, et al. Neuroimaging signatures of frontotemporal dementia genetics: C9ORF72, tau, progranulin and sporadics. Brain 2012;135(Pt 3):794–806.

10. Braak H, Braak E. Neuropathological staging of Alzheimer-related changes. Acta Neuropathol 1991;82(4):239–59.

11. Palop JJ, Chin J, Roberson ED, et al. Aberrant excitatory neuronal activity and compensatory remodeling of inhibitory hippocampal circuits in mouse models of Alzheimer's disease. Neuron 2007;55(5):697–711.

12. Bokde AL, Ewers M, Hampel H. Assessing neuronal networks: understanding Alzheimer's disease. Prog Neurobiol 2009;89(2):125–33.

13. Pievani M, de Haan W, Wu T, et al. Functional network disruption in the degenerative dementias. Lancet Neurol 2011;10(9):829–43.

14. Sperling RA, Dickerson BC, Pihlajamaki M, et al. Functional alterations in memory networks in early Alzheimer's disease. Neuromolecular Med 2010; 12(1):27–43.

15. Sorg C, Riedl V, Perneczky R, et al. Impact of Alzheimer's disease on the functional connectivity of spontaneous brain activity. Curr Alzheimer Res 2009;6(6):541–53.

16. Dickerson BC, Sperling RA. Large-scale functional brain network abnormalities in Alzheimer's disease: insights from functional neuroimaging. Behav Neurol 2009;21(1):63–75.

17. Guye M, Bettus G, Bartolomei F, et al. Graph theoretical analysis of structural and functional connectivity MRI in normal and pathological brain networks. MAGMA 2010;23(5–6):409–21.

18. Di Biasio F, Vanacore N, Fasano A, et al. Neuropsychology, neuroimaging or motor phenotype in diagnosis of Parkinson's disease-dementia: which matters most? J Neural Transm (Vienna) 2012; 119(5):597–604.

19. Firbank MJ, Allan LM, Burton EJ, et al. Neuroimaging predictors of death and dementia in a cohort of older stroke survivors. J Neurol Neurosurg Psychiatr 2012;83(3):263–7.

20. Zhou J, Seeley WW. Network dysfunction in Alzheimer's disease and frontotemporal dementia: implications for psychiatry. Biol Psychiatry 2014; 75(7):565–73.

21. Teipel S, Grothe MJ, Zhou J, et al. Measuring cortical connectivity in Alzheimer's disease as a brain neural network pathology: toward clinical applications. J Int Neuropsychol Soc 2016;22:138–63.

22. Smith SM, Fox PT, Miller KL, et al. Correspondence of the brain's functional architecture during activation and rest. Proc Natl Acad Sci 2009;106(31): 13040–5.

23. Biswal B, Yetkin FZ, Haughton VM, et al. Functional connectivity in the motor cortex of resting human brain using echo-planar MRI. Magn Reson Med 1995;34:537–41.

24. Biswal BB, Mennes M, Zuo XN, et al. Toward discovery science of human brain function. Proc Natl Acad Sci U S A 2010;107(10):4734–9.

25. Menon V. Large-scale brain networks and psychopathology: a unifying triple network model. Trends Cogn Sci 2011;15:483–506.

26. Cole MW, Repovš G, Anticevic A. The frontoparietal control system: a central role in mental health. Neuroscientist 2014;20:652–64.

27. Seeley WW, Crawford RK, Zhou J, et al. Neurodegenerative diseases target large-scale human brain networks. Neuron 2009;62(1):42–52.

28. McKeown MJ, Hansen LK, Sejnowski TJ. Independent component analysis of functional MRI: what is signal and what is noise? Curr Opin Neurobiol 2003;13:620–9.

29. Wu X, Li Q, Yu X, et al. A triple network connectivity study of large-scale brain systems in cognitively normal APOE4 carriers. Front Aging Neurosci 2016;8:231.

30. Wig GS, Laumann TO, Petersen SE. An approach for parcellating human cortical areas using resting-state correlations. Neuroimage 2014;93(Pt 2):276–91.

31. Zhou B, Yao H, Wang P, et al. Aberrant functional connectivity architecture in Alzheimer's disease and mild cognitive impairment: a whole-brain, data-driven analysis. Biomed Res Int 2015;2015: e495375.

32. Sporns O. Network attributes for segregation and integration in the human brain. Curr Opin Neurobiol 2013;23:162–71.

33. Fornito A, Zalesky A, Breakspear M. Graph analysis of the human connectome: promise, progress, and pitfalls. Neuroimage 2013;80:426–44.

34. Bullmore E, Sporns O. Complex brain networks: graph theoretical analysis of structural and functional systems. Nat Rev Neurosci 2009;10(3): 186–98.

35. He Y, Evans A. Graph theoretical modeling of brain connectivity. Curr Opin Neurol 2010;23(4): 341–50.

36. Bassett DS, Bullmore ET. Human brain networks in health and disease. Curr Opin Neurol 2009;22(4): 340–7.

37. Zhou J, Gennatas ED, Kramer JH, et al. Predicting regional neurodegeneration from the healthy brain functional connectome. Neuron 2012; 73(6):1216–27.

38. Braun U, Schäfer A, Bassett DS, et al. Dynamic brain network reconfiguration as a potential schizophrenia genetic risk mechanism modulated by NMDA receptor function. Proc Natl Acad Sci U S A 2016;113:12568–73.

39. Greicius MD, Krasnow B, Reiss AL, et al. Functional connectivity in the resting brain: a network analysis of the default mode hypothesis. Proc Natl Acad Sci U S A 2003;100(1):253–8.

40. Damoiseaux JS, Rombouts SARB, Barkhof F, et al. Consistent resting-state networks across healthy subjects. Proc Natl Acad Sci 2006;103(37): 13848–53.

41. Di Martino A, Shehzad Z, Kelly C, et al. Relationship between cingulo-insular functional connectivity and autistic traits in neurotypical adults. Am J Psychiatry 2009;166(8):891–9.

42. Hampson M, Driesen NR, Skudlarski P, et al. Brain connectivity related to working memory performance. J Neurosci 2006;26(51):13338–43.

43. Seeley WW, Menon V, Schatzberg AF, et al. Dissociable intrinsic connectivity networks for salience processing and executive control. J Neurosci 2007;27(9):2349–56.

44. Buckner RL, Snyder AZ, Shannon BJ, et al. Molecular, structural, and functional characterization of Alzheimer's disease: evidence for a relationship between default activity, amyloid, and memory. J Neurosci 2005;25(34):7709–17.

45. Toussaint PJ, Maiz S, Coynel D, et al. Characteristics of the default mode functional connectivity in normal ageing and Alzheimer's disease using resting state fMRI with a combined approach of entropy-based and graph theoretical measurements. Neuroimage 2014;101:778–86.

46. Boccardi M, Sabattoli F, Laakso MP, et al. Frontotemporal dementia as a neural system disease. Neurobiol Aging 2005;26(1):37–44.

47. Seeley WW, Crawford R, Rascovsky K, et al. Frontal paralimbic network atrophy in very mild behavioral variant frontotemporal dementia. Arch Neurol 2008; 65(2):249–55.

48. Craig AD. How do you feel–now? The anterior insula and human awareness. Nat Rev Neurosc 2009;10(1):59–70.

49. Chong JS, Ng GJ, Lee SC, et al. Salience network connectivity in the insula is associated with individual differences in interoceptive accuracy. Brain Struct Funct 2017;222(4):1635–44.

50. Zysset S, Huber O, Samson A, et al. Functional specialization within the anterior medial prefrontal cortex: a functional magnetic resonance imaging study with human subjects. Neurosci Lett 2003; 335(3):183–6.

51. Cavanna AE, Trimble MR. The precuneus: a review of its functional anatomy and behavioural correlates. Brain 2006;129(3):564–83.

52. Miller BL, Cummings J, Mishkin F, et al. Emergence of artistic talent in frontotemporal dementia. Neurology 1998;51(4):978–82.

53. Seeley WW, Matthews BR, Crawford RK, et al. Unravelling bolero: progressive aphasia, transmodal creativity and the right posterior neocortex. Brain 2008;131(Pt 1):39–49.

54. Greicius MD, Menon V. Default-mode activity during a passive sensory task: uncoupled from deactivation but impacting activation. J Cogn Neurosc 2004;16(9):1484–92.

55. Fox MD, Snyder AZ, Vincent JL, et al. The human brain is intrinsically organized into dynamic, anticorrelated functional networks. Proc Natl Acad Sci U S A 2005;102(27):9673–8.

56. Seeley WW, Allman JM, Carlin DA, et al. Divergent social functioning in behavioral variant frontotemporal dementia and Alzheimer disease: reciprocal networks and neuronal evolution. Alzheimer Dis Assoc Disord 2007;21(4):S50–7.

57. Zhou J, Greicius MD, Gennatas ED, et al. Divergent network connectivity changes in behavioral variant frontotemporal dementia and Alzheimer's disease. Brain 2010;133(5):1352–67.

58. Greicius MD, Srivastava G, Reiss AL, et al. Default-mode network activity distinguishes Alzheimer's disease from healthy aging: evidence from functional MRI. Proc Natl Acad Sci U S A 2004; 101(13):4637–42.

59. Supekar K, Menon V, Rubin D, et al. Network analysis of intrinsic functional brain connectivity in Alzheimer's disease. PLoS Comput Biol 2008;4(6): e1000100.

60. Zhang HY, Wang SJ, Liu B, et al. Resting brain connectivity: changes during the progress of Alzheimer disease. Radiology 2010;256(2): 598–606.

61. Hu W, Wang Z, Lee V, et al. Distinct cerebral perfusion patterns in FTLD and AD. Neurology 2010; 75(10):881–8.

62. de Haan W, Pijnenburg Y, Strijers R, et al. Functional neural network analysis in frontotemporal dementia and Alzheimer's disease using EEG and graph theory. BMC Neurosci 2009;10(1):101.

63. Laxton AW, Tang-Wai DF, McAndrews MP, et al. A phase I trial of deep brain stimulation of memory circuits in Alzheimer's disease. Ann Neurol 2010; 68(4):521–34.

64. de Haan W, van der Flier WM, Koene T, et al. Disrupted modular brain dynamics reflect cognitive dysfunction in Alzheimer's disease. Neuroimage 2012;59(4):3085–93.

65. Sanz-Arigita EJ, Schoonheim MM, Damoiseaux JS, et al. Loss of 'small-world' networks in Alzheimer's disease: graph analysis of FMRI resting-state functional connectivity. PLoS One 2010;5(11):e13788.

66. Stam CJ, de Haan W, Daffertshofer A, et al. Graph theoretical analysis of magnetoencephalographic functional connectivity in Alzheimer's disease. Brain 2009;132(Pt 1):213–24.

67. Snowden JS, Stopford CL, Julien CL, et al. Cognitive phenotypes in Alzheimer's disease and genetic risk. Cortex 2007;43(7):835–45.

68. Lehmann M, Rohrer JD, Clarkson MJ, et al. Reduced cortical thickness in the posterior cingulate gyrus is characteristic of both typical and atypical Alzheimer's disease. J Alzheimers Dis 2010; 20(2):587–98.

69. Migliaccio R, Agosta F, Rascovsky K, et al. Clinical syndromes associated with posterior atrophy: early age at onset AD spectrum. Neurology 2009;73(19): 1571–8.

70. Lehmann M, Ghosh PM, Madison C, et al. Diverging patterns of amyloid deposition and hypometabolism in clinical variants of probable Alzheimer's disease. Brain 2013;136(Pt 3):844–58.

71. Whitwell JL, Jones DT, Duffy JR, et al. Working memory and language network dysfunctions in logopenic aphasia: a task-free fMRI comparison with Alzheimer's dementia. Neurobiol Aging 2015; 36(3):1245–52.

72. Gour N, Felician O, Didic M, et al. Functional connectivity changes differ in early and late-onset Alzheimer's disease. Hum Brain Mapp 2014;35(7): 2978–94.

73. Migliaccio R, Gallea C, Kas A, et al. Functional connectivity of ventral and dorsal visual streams in posterior cortical atrophy. J Alzheimers Dis 2016; 51(4):1119–30.

74. Guo CC, Gorno-Tempini ML, Gesierich B, et al. Anterior temporal lobe degeneration produces widespread network-driven dysfunction. Brain 2013;136(Pt 10):2979–91.

75. Wilson SM, Galantucci S, Tartaglia MC, et al. The neural basis of syntactic deficits in primary progressive aphasia. Brain Lang 2012;122(3):190–8.

76. Farb NA, Grady CL, Strother S, et al. Abnormal network connectivity in frontotemporal dementia: evidence for prefrontal isolation. Cortex 2013; 49(7):1856–73.

77. Agosta F, Sala S, Valsasina P, et al. Brain network connectivity assessed using graph theory in frontotemporal dementia. Neurology 2013;81(2):134–43.

78. Agosta F, Galantucci S, Valsasina P, et al. Disrupted brain connectome in semantic variant of primary progressive aphasia. Neurobiol Aging 2014; 35(11):2646–55.

79. Sedeno L, Couto B, Garcia-Cordero I, et al. Brain network organization and social executive performance in frontotemporal dementia. J Int Neuropsychol Soc 2016;22(2):250–62.

80. Buckner RL, Sepulcre J, Talukdar T, et al. Cortical hubs revealed by intrinsic functional connectivity: mapping, assessment of stability, and relation to Alzheimer's disease. J Neurosci 2009;29(6): 1860–73.

81. Saxena S, Caroni P. Selective neuronal vulnerability in neurodegenerative diseases: from stressor thresholds to degeneration. Neuron 2011;71(1): 35–48.

82. Baker HF, Ridley RM, Duchen LW, et al. Induction of beta (A4)-amyloid in primates by injection of Alzheimer's disease brain homogenate. Comparison with transmission of spongiform encephalopathy. Mol Neurobiol 1994;8(1):25–39.

83. Frost B, Diamond MI. Prion-like mechanisms in neurodegenerative diseases. Nat Rev Neurosci 2010;11(3):155–9.

84. Frost B, Ollesch J, Wille H, et al. Conformational diversity of wild-type Tau fibrils specified by templated conformation change. J Biol Chem 2009; 284(6):3546–51.

85. Jucker M, Walker LC. Pathogenic protein seeding in Alzheimer disease and other neurodegenerative disorders. Ann Neurol 2011;70(4):532–40.

86. Lee JK, Jin HK, Endo S, et al. Intracerebral transplantation of bone marrow-derived mesenchymal stem cells reduces amyloid-beta deposition and

rescues memory deficits in Alzheimer's disease mice by modulation of immune responses. Stem Cells 2010;28(2):329–43.

87. Ridley RM, Baker HF, Windle CP, et al. Very long term studies of the seeding of beta-amyloidosis in primates. J Neural Transm 2006;113(9):1243–51.

88. Walker LC, Levine H 3rd, Mattson MP, et al. Inducible proteopathies. Trends Neurosci 2006;29(8):438–43.

89. Prusiner SB. Some speculations about prions, amyloid, and Alzheimer's disease. N Engl J Med 1984; 310(10):661–3.

90. Salehi A, Delcroix JD, Belichenko PV, et al. Increased app expression in a mouse model of Down's syndrome disrupts NGF transport and causes cholinergic neuron degeneration. Neuron 2006;51(1):29–42.

91. Appel SH. A unifying hypothesis for the cause of amyotrophic lateral sclerosis, parkinsonism, and Alzheimer disease. Ann Neurol 1981;10(6):499–505.

92. Klupp E, Grimmer T, Tahmasian M, et al. Prefrontal hypometabolism in Alzheimer disease is related to longitudinal amyloid accumulation in remote brain regions. J Nucl Med 2015;56(3):399–404.

93. Richiardi J, Altmann A, Milazzo AC, et al. BRAIN NETWORKS. Correlated gene expression supports synchronous activity in brain networks. Science 2015;348(6240):1241–4.

94. Drzezga A, Becker JA, Van Dijk KR, et al. Neuronal dysfunction and disconnection of cortical hubs in non-demented subjects with elevated amyloid burden. Brain 2011;134(Pt 6):1635–46.

95. Brier MR, Thomas JB, Ances BM. Network dysfunction in Alzheimer's disease: refining the disconnection hypothesis. Brain Connect 2014; 4(5):299–311.

96. Kikuchi M, Hirosawa T, Yokokura M, et al. Effects of brain amyloid deposition and reduced glucose metabolism on the default mode of brain function in normal aging. J Neurosci 2011;31(31):11193–9.

97. Mormino EC, Smiljic A, Hayenga AO, et al. Relationships between beta-amyloid and functional connectivity in different components of the default mode network in aging. Cereb Cortex 2011; 21(10):2399–407.

98. Gili T, Cercignani M, Serra L, et al. Regional brain atrophy and functional disconnection across Alzheimer's disease evolution. J Neurol Neurosurg Psychiatr 2011;82(1):58–66.

99. Adriaanse SM, Sanz-Arigita EJ, Binnewijzend MAA, et al. Amyloid and its association with default network integrity in Alzheimer's disease. Hum Brain Mapp 2014;35(3):779–91.

100. Malpas CB, Saling MM, Velakoulis D, et al. Differential functional connectivity correlates of cerebrospinal fluid biomarkers in dementia of the Alzheimer's type. Neurodegener Dis 2015;16: 147–51.

101. Song Z, Insel PS, Buckley S, et al. Brain amyloid-β burden is associated with disruption of intrinsic functional connectivity within the medial temporal lobe in cognitively normal elderly. J Neurosci 2015;35(7):3240–7.

102. Elman JA, Madison CM, Baker SL, et al. Effects of beta-amyloid on resting state functional connectivity within and between networks reflect known patterns of regional vulnerability. Cereb Cortex 2016; 26(2):695–707.

103. Myers N, Pasquini L, Göttler J, et al. Within-patient correspondence of amyloid-β and intrinsic network connectivity in Alzheimer's disease. Brain 2014; 137(Pt 7):2052–64.

104. Lim HK, Nebes R, Snitz B, et al. Regional amyloid burden and intrinsic connectivity networks in cognitively normal elderly subjects. Brain 2014; 137(12):3327–38.

105. Koch K, Myers NE, Göttler J, et al. Disrupted intrinsic networks link amyloid-β pathology and impaired cognition in prodromal Alzheimer's disease. Cereb Cortex 2015;25(12):4678–88.

106. Chen G, Ward BD, Xie C, et al. Classification of Alzheimer disease, mild cognitive impairment, and normal cognitive status with large-scale network analysis based on resting-state functional MR imaging. Radiology 2011;259(1):213–21.

107. Khazaee A, Ebrahimzadeh A, Babajani-Feremi A, Alzheimer's Disease Neuroimaging Initiative. Classification of patients with MCI and AD from healthy controls using directed graph measures of resting-state fMRI. Behav Brain Res 2017; 322(Pt B):339–50.

108. Dai Z, Yan C, Li K, et al. Identifying and mapping connectivity patterns of brain network hubs in Alzheimer's disease. Cereb Cortex 2015;25(10): 3723–42.

109. Sorg C, Riedl V, Muhlau M, et al. Selective changes of resting-state networks in individuals at risk for Alzheimer's disease. Proc Natl Acad Sci 2007; 104(47):18760–5.

110. Han Y, Wang J, Zhao Z, et al. Frequency-dependent changes in the amplitude of low-frequency fluctuations in amnestic mild cognitive impairment: a resting-state fMRI study. Neuroimage 2011;55(1): 287–95.

111. Qi Z, Wu X, Wang Z, et al. Impairment and compensation coexist in amnestic MCI default mode network. Neuroimage 2010;50(1):48–55.

112. Rombouts SA, Barkhof F, Goekoop R, et al. Altered resting state networks in mild cognitive impairment and mild Alzheimer's disease: an fMRI study. Hum Brain Mapp 2005;26(4):231–9.

113. Wang J, Zuo X, Dai Z, et al. Disrupted functional brain connectome in individuals at risk for Alzheimer's disease. Biol Psychiatry 2013;73(5): 472–81.

114. Petrella JR, Sheldon FC, Prince SE, et al. Default mode network connectivity in stable vs progressive mild cognitive impairment. Neurology 2011;76(6): 511–7.

115. Serra L, Cercignani M, Mastropasqua C, et al. Longitudinal changes in functional brain connectivity predicts conversion to Alzheimer's disease. J Alzheimers Dis 2016;51(2):377–89.

116. Papenberg G, Salami A, Persson J, et al. Genetics and functional imaging: effects of APOE, BDNF, COMT, and KIBRA in aging. Neuropsychol Rev 2015;25(1):47–62.

117. Sperling R, Mormino E, Johnson K. The evolution of preclinical Alzheimer's disease: implications for prevention trials. Neuron 2014;84(3): 608–22.

118. Strittmatter WJ, Saunders AM, Schmechel D, et al. Apolipoprotein E: high-avidity binding to beta-amyloid and increased frequency of type 4 allele in late-onset familial Alzheimer disease. Proc Natl Acad Sci U S A 1993;90(5):1977–81.

119. Riedel BC, Thompson PM, Brinton RD. Age, APOE and sex: triad of risk of Alzheimer's disease. J Steroid Biochem Mol Biol 2016;160:134–47.

120. Fleisher AS, Sherzai A, Taylor C, et al. Resting-state BOLD networks versus task-associated functional MRI for distinguishing Alzheimer's disease risk groups. Neuroimage 2009;47(4):1678–90.

121. Filippini N, MacIntosh BJ, Hough MG, et al. Distinct patterns of brain activity in young carriers of the APOE-epsilon4 allele. Proc Natl Acad Sci U S A 2009;106(17):7209–14.

122. Damoiseaux JS, Seeley WW, Zhou J, et al. Gender modulates the APOE ε4 effect in healthy older adults: convergent evidence from functional brain connectivity and spinal fluid tau levels. J Neurosci 2012;32(24):8254–62.

123. Seeley WW. Divergent network connectivity changes in healthy APOE epsilon4 carriers: disinhibition or compensation? Arch Neurol 2011;68(9): 1107–8.

124. Sheline YI, Morris JC, Snyder AZ, et al. APOE4 allele disrupts resting state fMRI connectivity in the absence of amyloid plaques or decreased CSF Abeta42. J Neurosci 2010;30(50):17035–40.

125. Patel KT, Stevens MC, Pearlson GD, et al. Default mode network activity and white matter integrity in healthy middle-aged ApoE4 carriers. Brain Imaging Behav 2013;7(1):60–7.

126. Chen Y, Chen K, Zhang J, et al. Disrupted functional and structural networks in cognitively normal elderly subjects with the APOE e4 allele. Neuropsychopharmacology 2015;40(5):1181–91.

127. Machulda MM, Jones DT, Vemuri P, et al. Effect of APOE epsilon4 status on intrinsic network connectivity in cognitively normal elderly subjects. Arch Neurol 2011;68(9):1131–6.

128. Damoiseaux JS. Resting-state fMRI as a biomarker for Alzheimer's disease? Alzheimers Res Ther 2012;4(2):8.

129. Matura S, Prvulovic D, Butz M, et al. Recognition memory is associated with altered resting-state functional connectivity in people at genetic risk for Alzheimer's disease. Eur J Neurosci 2014; 40(7):3128–35.

130. Luo X, Qiu T, Jia Y, et al. Intrinsic functional connectivity alterations in cognitively intact elderly APOE ε4 carriers measured by eigenvector centrality mapping are related to cognition and CSF biomarkers: a preliminary study. Brain Imaging Behav 2016;1–12. Available at: https://link.springer. com/article/10.1007/s11682-016-9600-z.

131. McKenna F, Koo B-B, Killiany R, Alzheimer's Disease Neuroimaging Initiative. Comparison of ApoE-related brain connectivity differences in early MCI and normal aging populations: an fMRI study. Brain Imaging Behav 2016;10(4): 970–83.

132. Ye Q, Su F, Shu H, et al. The apolipoprotein E gene affects the three-year trajectories of compensatory neural processes in the left-lateralized hippocampal network. Brain Imaging Behav 2016;1–13. Available at: https://link.springer.com/article/10. 1007/s11682-016-9623-5.

133. Yang AC, Huang C-C, Liu M-E, et al. The APOE ε4 allele affects complexity and functional connectivity of resting brain activity in healthy adults. Hum Brain Mapp 2014;35(7):3238–48.

134. Trachtenberg AJ, Filippini N, Ebmeier KP, et al. The effects of APOE on the functional architecture of the resting brain. Neuroimage 2012; 59(1):565–72.

135. Shu H, Shi Y, Chen G, et al. Opposite neural trajectories of Apolipoprotein E ε4 and ε2 alleles with aging associated with different risks of Alzheimer's Disease. Cereb Cortex 2014;26(4): bhu237.

136. Reinvang I, Espeseth T, Westlye LT. APOE-related biomarker profiles in non-pathological aging and early phases of Alzheimer's disease. Neurosci Biobehav Rev 2013;37(8):1322–35.

137. Sheline YI, Raichle ME, Snyder AZ, et al. Amyloid plaques disrupt resting state default mode network connectivity in cognitively normal elderly. Biol Psychiatry 2010;67(6):584–7.

138. Dennis EL, Thompson PM. Functional brain connectivity using fMRI in aging and Alzheimer's disease. Neuropsychol Rev 2014;24(1):49–62.

139. Heise V, Filippini N, Trachtenberg AJ, et al. Apolipoprotein E genotype, gender and age modulate connectivity of the hippocampus in healthy adults. Neuroimage 2014;98:23–30.

140. Liu Y, Tan L, Wang H-F, et al. Multiple effect of APOE genotype on clinical and neuroimaging

biomarkers across Alzheimer's disease spectrum. Mol Neurobiol 2016;53(7):4539–47.

141. Lim YY, Villemagne VL, Laws SM, et al. APOE and BDNF polymorphisms moderate amyloid β-related cognitive decline in preclinical Alzheimer's disease. Mol Psychiatry 2014;20(11): 1322–8.

142. Dopper EG, Rombouts SA, Jiskoot LC, et al. Structural and functional brain connectivity in presymptomatic familial frontotemporal dementia. Neurology 2014;83(2):e19–26.

143. Borroni B, Alberici A, Cercignani M, et al. Granulin mutation drives brain damage and reorganization from preclinical to symptomatic FTLD. Neurobiol Aging 2012;33(10):2506–20.

144. Premi E, Cauda F, Gasparotti R, et al. Multimodal fMRI resting-state functional connectivity in granulin mutations: the case of fronto-parietal dementia. PLoS One 2014;9(9):e106500.

145. Pievani M, Paternicò D, Benussi L, et al. Pattern of structural and functional brain abnormalities in asymptomatic granulin mutation carriers. Alzheimers Dement 2014;10(5):354–63.e1.

146. Gordon E, Rohrer JD, Fox NC. Advances in neuroimaging in frontotemporal dementia. J Neurochem 2016;138(S1):193–210.

147. Ahmed RM, Devenney EM, Irish M, et al. Neuronal network disintegration: common pathways linking neurodegenerative diseases. J Neurol Neurosurg Psychiatr 2016;87(11):1234–41.

148. Goveas JS, Xie C, Ward BD, et al. Recovery of hippocampal network connectivity correlates with cognitive improvement in mild Alzheimer's disease patients treated with donepezil assessed by resting-state fMRI. J Magn Reson Imaging 2011; 34(4):764–73.

149. Greicius MD, Kimmel DL. Neuroimaging insights into network-based neurodegeneration. Curr Opin Neurol 2012;25(6):727–34.

150. Hampel H, O'Bryant SE, Castrillo JI, et al. Precision medicine: the golden gate for detection, treatment and prevention of Alzheimer's disease. J Prev Alzheimers Dis 2016;3:243–59.

151. Pievani M, Filippini N, van den Heuvel MP, et al. Brain connectivity in neurodegenerative diseases–from phenotype to proteinopathy. Nat Rev Neurol 2014;10(11):620–33.

152. Cui J, Zufferey V, Kherif F. In-vivo brain neuroimaging provides a gateway for integrating biological and clinical biomarkers of Alzheimer's disease. Curr Opin Neurol 2015;28(4):351–7.

153. Teipel SJ, Wohlert A, Metzger C, et al. Multicenter stability of resting state fMRI in the detection of Alzheimer's disease and amnestic MCI. Neuroimage Clin 2017;14:183–94.

154. Reiman EM, Langbaum JB, Tariot PN, et al. CAP–advancing the evaluation of preclinical Alzheimer disease treatments. Nat Rev Neurol 2016;12:56–61.

155. Shi L, Zhao L, Wong A, et al. Mapping the relationship of contributing factors for preclinical Alzheimer's disease. Sci Rep 2015;5:11259.

156. Qiu Y, Liu S, Hilal S, et al. Inter-hemispheric functional dysconnectivity mediates the association of corpus callosum degeneration with memory impairment in AD and amnestic MCI. Sci Rep 2016;6: 32573.

157. Schouten TM, Koini M, de Vos F, et al. Combining anatomical, diffusion, and resting state functional magnetic resonance imaging for individual classification of mild and moderate Alzheimer's disease. Neuroimage Clin 2016;11:46–51.

158. Liu S, Ong YT, Hilal S, et al. The association between retinal neuronal layer and brain structure is disrupted in patients with cognitive impairment and Alzheimer's disease. J Alzheimers Dis 2016; 54(2):585–95.

159. Rajapakse JC, Wang Y, Zheng X, et al. Probabilistic framework for brain connectivity from functional MR images. IEEE Trans Med Imaging 2008;27(6):825–33.

160. Cordova-Palomera A, Kaufmann T, Persson K, et al. Disrupted global metastability and static and dynamic brain connectivity across individuals in the Alzheimer's disease continuum. Sci Rep 2017;7:40268.

161. Wang C, Ong JL, Patanaik A, et al. Spontaneous eyelid closures link vigilance fluctuation with fMRI dynamic connectivity states. Proc Natl Acad Sci U S A 2016;113(34):9653–8.

162. Liu M, Zhang D, Shen D, Alzheimer's Disease Neuroimaging Initiative. View-centralized multi-atlas classification for Alzheimer's disease diagnosis. Hum Brain Mapp 2015;36:1847–65.

163. Dyrba M, Grothe M, Kirste T, et al. Multimodal analysis of functional and structural disconnection in Alzheimer's disease using multiple kernel SVM. Hum Brain Mapp 2015;36:2118–31.

164. Hafkemeijer A, Möller C, Dopper EGP, et al. A longitudinal study on resting state functional connectivity in behavioral variant frontotemporal dementia and Alzheimer's disease. J Alzheimers Dis 2017;55:521–37.

165. Su F, Shu H, Ye Q, et al. Integration of multilocus genetic risk into the default mode network longitudinal trajectory during the Alzheimer's disease process. J Alzheimers Dis 2016;56(2):491–507.

166. Zhang Y, Simon-Vermot L, Araque Caballero MÁ, et al. Enhanced resting-state functional connectivity between core memory-task activation peaks is associated with memory impairment in MCI. Neurobiol Aging 2016;45:43–9.

167. Chapman SB, Aslan S, Spence JS, et al. Neural mechanisms of brain plasticity with complex

cognitive training in healthy seniors. Cereb Cortex 2015;25:396–405.

168. Hill NTM, Mowszowski L, Naismith SL, et al. Computerized cognitive training in older adults with mild cognitive impairment or dementia: a systematic review and meta-analysis. Am J Psychiatry 2017;174(4):329–40.

169. Suo C, Singh MF, Gates N, et al. Therapeutically relevant structural and functional mechanisms triggered by physical and cognitive exercise. Mol Psychiatry 2016;21(11):1633–42.

170. Ng KK, Lo JC, Lim JK, et al. Reduced functional segregation between the default mode network and the executive control network in healthy older adults: a longitudinal study. Neuroimage 2016; 133:321–30.

171. Yeo BT, Krienen FM, Sepulcre J, et al. The organization of the human cerebral cortex estimated by intrinsic functional connectivity. J Neurophysiol 2011;106(3):1125–65.

172. Nieto-Castanon A. CONN toolbox representation of positive and negative (anti-) correlations in fcMRI. Available at: http://www.neurobureau.org/wp-content/uploads/2014/06/36e695feb0f6a36ab7cf0 8f3ab8ecebe6ed9046b5a65bb9c8f18597153ffa55 4a553fa4990edd8dfeae7e17a9cbfff50a6e327d6 4822693fcc27046ea88174a2.png. 2014. Accessed January 25, 2017.

Applications of Resting State Functional MR Imaging to Traumatic Brain Injury

Thomas J. O'Neill, MD, Elizabeth M. Davenport, PhD,
Gowtham Murugesan, MS, Albert Montillo, PhD,
Joseph A. Maldjian, MD*

KEYWORDS

• Resting state • BOLD • fMR imaging • TBI • Graph theory • Machine learning
• Magnetoencephalography

KEY POINTS

- Resting state functional MR imaging (rs-fMR imaging) is typically not applicable to the individual in a clinical setting.
- Graph theory and machine learning methods are beginning to identify traumatic brain injury–specific features in rs-fMR imaging for group studies and starting to show promise as assistive tools for individual diagnoses.
- Resting state magnetoencephalography has a higher temporal resolution and may be able to supplement rs-fMR imaging findings.
- Moving rs-fMR imaging into the clinic should be approached with cautious optimism.

INTRODUCTION

A traumatic brain injury (TBI) can be caused by a bump, blow, or jolt to the head. TBIs can also be caused by penetrating, or open, head injuries. In the United States, approximately 1.7 million TBIs occur each year. More than 1.3 million result in an emergency department visit, 275,000 result in hospitalizations, and 52,000 result in deaths. On average, the most common cause of TBI is falls, and the rates are highest among very young children and adults older than the age of 75.[1] Most TBI cases are closed-head injuries, but some are open-head injuries, which occur when the skull is fractured or penetrated.

TBI encompasses a spectrum of brain abnormality with many variables affecting the type and severity of injury. Mechanism of injury plays a prominent role; however, the distribution of local forces sustained by the brain parenchyma during injury, and patient factors, including individual anatomic differences, age, gender, medications/substance use, and medical history, can also dramatically affect the severity of injury and subsequent patient outcome.[2–4] Multiple factors are used to classify the severity of the TBI. The most common include the Glasgow Coma Scale and the Abbreviated Injury Scale–Head.[5] The severity of the injury is often classified from mild to severe. The effects of mild TBI (mTBI) are often not visible on conventional imaging, whereas severe TBI can manifest as an obvious finding, such as an open-head injury or hematoma.

Disclosure Statement: The authors have nothing to disclose.
Radiology, University of Texas Southwestern, 5323 Harry Hines Boulevard, Dallas, TX 75390, USA
* Corresponding author.
E-mail address: joseph.maldjian@utsouthwestern.edu

Primary injuries occur from tissue damage during the time of impact from mechanical forces that produce tissue strains and stresses.[6,7] Head impact generates both contact and inertial forces and can result in extra-axial and/or intra-axial intracranial tissue damage. Some head injuries may be acutely life threatening and require emergent neurosurgical interventions, while other sequelae of traumatic head injury are more subtle with little or no evidence of tissue damage on conventional anatomic imaging and only result in evidence of dysfunction of functional connectivity using advanced techniques, including resting state functional MR imaging (rs-fMR imaging) or magnetoencephalography (MEG).

Extra-axial tissue damage commonly results in epidural hematoma, subdural hematoma, subarachnoid hemorrhage, and/or subdural hygroma. Associated secondary complications of extra-axial injury often requiring emergent intervention include cerebral herniation, edema, hydrocephalus, or ischemia. Focal primary TBIs of intra-axial tissue also occur with closed head trauma and result from both direct impact of the brain with the cranial vault and transmitted linear and rotational forces on the brain. The rigid cranial vault and skull base provide a non-deformable internal surface of contact with the relatively soft, deformable, and mobile brain. Secondary effects of intra-axial hemorrhage include hypoxic-ischemic damage, oxidative stress from reactive oxygen species, neuroexcitatory response, cerebral edema, neuronal cell death, blood-brain barrier permeability, and autonomic dysfunction.[8–11] Cortical/subcortical contusions may also be associated with subarachnoid hemorrhage as a result of extension of parenchymal hemorrhage beyond the pia.

Diffuse traumatic axonal injury (DAI) typically involves a wide distribution with regional involvement of white matter axons, which are vulnerable to shearing strains owing to their long, highly structured architecture. Using the word diffuse is somewhat of a misnomer because the pattern is more multifocal with affected areas interposed with non-affected areas. White matter axons are particularly vulnerable to rapid shearing strains. Classically, a histologic grading scheme of diffuse axonal injury based on region of involvement is often used to describe the severity of DAI. Grade 1 involves the cerebral hemispheres, corpus callosum, brainstem, or cerebellum; grade 2 involves the corpus callosum, whereas grade 3 involves the brainstem.[12] These sites, particularly cortical/subcortical white matter, splenium of the corpus callosum, and brainstem, are also the areas frequently demonstrating abnormalities on conventional neuroimaging studies. Primary axotomy at the time of impact is considered rare. Instead, it is thought that mechanical forces produce axonal deformation and cytoskeletal disruption, which results in accumulation of transported materials appearing as multiple axonal swellings "axonal varicosities," or a single swelling referred to as "axonal bulb."[13] These findings correlate with axonal disconnection. Although contusional microhemorrhage, apoptosis, and necrotic cell death cascades likely occur with diffuse axonal injury, there has also been demonstration of neuronal plasmalemmal poration and disruption leading to either necrosis or reactive change without cell death.[14,15] The progression from disruption in axonal transport leading to axonal disconnection, apoptosis, and Wallerian degeneration has been traditionally thought to occur over the acute and subacute period following trauma; however, axonal degeneration may occur for years following injury. For these reasons, DAI is considered a disease of disconnection, which has made it an ideal candidate for study of functional connectivity using tools such as rs-fMR imaging.

This review covers rs-MR imaging and resting state magnetoencephalography (rs-MEG) acquisition, processing, and findings. A specific focus is given to machine learning and graph theory given the multiple applications of these methods in the literature and the potential for automated detection and diagnoses in the future.

NORMAL ANATOMY AND IMAGING TECHNIQUE

Conventional noncontrast head computed tomography (CT) and MR sequences remain the standard of care in clinical neuroimaging in the setting of TBI. Noncontrast head CT is rapid, accessible, and safe for all patients, plus it is very sensitive for detection of hemorrhage and other potentially life-threatening sequela of closed head injuries. These features make CT an ideal tool in the acute/hyperacute setting and for serial follow-up imaging when there are changes in clinical status. In the acute or early subacute setting, conventional MR imaging is typically reserved for patients with clinical/neurologic symptoms that are discordant with CT findings or when the injury extent may be better assessed by MR imaging. A conventional brain MR imaging protocol typically includes T1-weighted spin-echo or 3-dimensional (3D) T1, T2-weighted fast-spin-echo, T2 fluid attenuated inversion recovery (FLAIR), and echo planar diffusion-weighted imaging. Susceptibility-sensitive sequences, including T2 gradient recalled echo or 3D susceptibility weighted imaging (SWI), which are sensitive to blood products and can reveal microhemorrhages associated with DAI, are frequently included in the routine posttrauma MR imaging protocols. Examples of mild and severe DAI are shown in **Figs. 1** and **2**, respectively. Additional advanced MR techniques include evaluation with diffusion tensor imaging, arterial spin labeling perfusion, dynamic susceptibility contrast perfusion, and MR spectroscopy, but are beyond the scope of this article. Typical imaging findings of TBI on CT or conventional MR sequences range from frank intracranial hemorrhages to petechial foci of hemorrhage, as are often seen in diffuse axonal injury. However, these techniques may appear normal and often are insensitive to sequela of mTBIs.

RESTING STATE FUNCTIONAL MR IMAGING PROTOCOLS

fMR imaging relies on coupling of cerebral blood flow with neuronal activity (hemodynamic response) and most commonly uses an MR imaging technique sensitive to changes in blood hemoglobin oxygenation (BOLD, blood oxygenation-level–dependent signal). As neuronal activity increases in an area of the brain, hemodynamic responses cause an overcompensation of blood flow to the region, resulting in increased signal from a local change in the deoxy:oxyhemoglobin ratio. BOLD-sensitive sequences rely on susceptibility differences in oxyhemoglobin and deoxyhemoglobin. Even in optimal situations, signal change from active and inactive areas is relatively small, and this technique suffers from low signal-to-noise ratio. Understanding the physical mechanism of fMR imaging acquisition is important to consider in patients with TBI because there are unique features of these patients that may affect

analysis techniques and interpretation of fMR imaging results in these patients. Patients with TBI may have dysregulation in the coupling of hemodynamic response with neuronal activity, which may complicate whether abnormalities are due to actual decreased neuronal activity or alterations in hemodynamic response. Also, because fMR imaging relies on changes in susceptibility, intracranial blood products can cause artifacts that obscure true neuronal activation. fMR imaging can be acquired with a task (task-based fMR imaging), such as attending to a visual stimulus, or while the subject is at rest (rs-fMR imaging). rs-fMR imaging relies on low-frequency, spontaneous fluctuations in the BOLD signal that are present even in the absence of a stimulus or task.[16] No consensus exists on the optimal acquisition techniques for rs-fMR imaging. However, typically, acquisition entails an ultrafast single-shot, whole-head, gradient-echo echo planar imaging sequence with a TR ~2 to 3 seconds, over a period anywhere from 2 to 30 minutes.[17] Shorter acquisition times are less susceptible to patient motion, but fewer data points are available for analysis. Acquisition may occur with the patient's eyes open or closed.[18] Spatially discrete brain regions that exhibit strong interregional correlation, after excluding nonphysiologic sources of correlation, are assumed to be functionally connected. A suggested MR acquisition protocol for TBI patients is detailed in **Table 1** and should complement the existing clinical examination. A 3-T scanner would be preferred, and adjustments to the protocols optimized for particular scanners with techniques like parallel imaging can achieve data with better spatial or temporal resolution. Findings on fMR imaging in TBI patients reported in the literature are discussed later. Although this technique holds promise for further investigation in TBI patients,

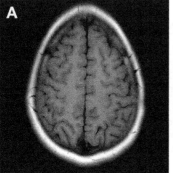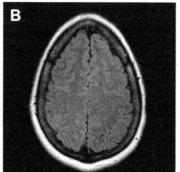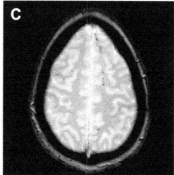

Fig. 1. Conventional MR findings of mild diffuse axonal injury. Axial T1 (*A*), axial T2 FLAIR (*B*), and axial SWI (*C*) demonstrate only petechial foci of susceptibility at the gray-white interfaces of bilateral frontal, and left parietal lobes. No other imaging findings are demonstrated on conventional sequences.

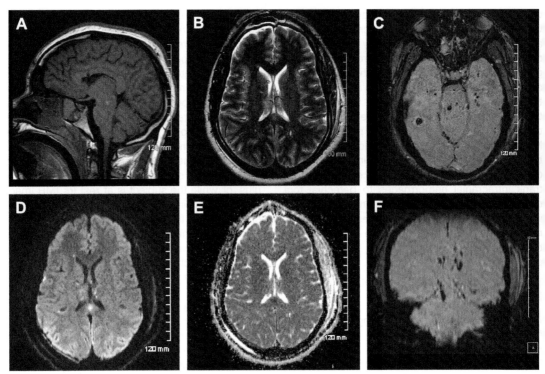

Fig. 2. Conventional MR findings of severe diffuse axonal injury. Sagittal T1 (*A*) demonstrates a petechial focus of T1 shortening compatible with subacute blood products in the midbrain. Axial T2 (*B*), axial diffusion-weighted images (*D*), and apparent diffusion coefficient map (*E*) demonstrate a focus of mild restricted diffusion in the splenium of the corpus callosum as well as foci of increased T2 signal in the periventricular white matter, right internal capsule, and right thalamus. Axial and coronal SWI (*C* and *F*) demonstrate numerous foci of susceptibility, consistent with foci of hemorrhage, in the brainstem, temporal lobes, periventricular white matter, and corpus callosum.

existing evidence is insufficient for routine clinical TBI diagnosis and/or prognostication at the individual patient level.[19] However, research is ongoing to determine the appropriate methods of application and interpretation in the clinical setting of TBI.

RESTING STATE FUNCTIONAL MR IMAGING FINDINGS

Subjects suffering from TBI tend to show impairment in high-level cognitive functions such as attention, memory, and executive function.[20,21]

Table 1
Suggested resting state functional MR imaging protocol for traumatic brain injury

Sequence	Sequence Parameters	Acquisition Parameters	Acquisition Time
Sagittal 3D T1 MPRAGE	TR 2500/TE 3	Isotropic, $1 \times 1 \times 1$ mm	~5–8 min
Axial thin T2/FLAIR or sagittal 3D T2/FLAIR	TR 8000/TE 80	$0.5 \times 0.5 \times 3$ mm or isotropic 3D ($1 \times 1 \times 1$ mm)	~4–5 min
Axial 3D SWI	TR 30/TE 20	$0.5 \times 0.5 \times 2$ mm	~3–4 min
BOLD rs-fMRI, axial GE-EPI	TR = 2000–3000 ms, TE = 30–40 ms, $\alpha = 80°–90°$	Near isotropic, $3 \times 3 \times 3$ mm to $4 \times 4 \times 4$ mm/matrix 64×64	~5–10 min
Diffusion tensor imaging, axial GE-EPI	TR = 4500/TE = 100, b = 0 and b = 1000 × 6–30 directions	$1.5 \times 1.5 \times 3$–5 mm/matrix 128×128	~10 min (with parallel imaging)

Because the integration of information across various regions of the brain is required for these high-level functions, researchers have often chosen to transform rs-fMR imaging data into a graph-based representation, also called a network representation. These graphs, or networks, consist of nodes connected by edges. The nodes can be brain regions, subnetworks, or individual voxels. Brain regions are determined by parcellating anatomic MR imaging and transferring these brain regions to the rs-fMR imaging through coregistration, whereas brain subnetworks are defined directly on the rs-fMR imaging data through a multivariate decomposition method, such as independent component analysis (ICA). For all of the parcellation schemes, the graph edges characterize a measure of connectivity between node pairs.

Graph Theoretic Measures

To make graphs amenable for quantitative analysis, graph theory is often used to convert the discrete graph into a set of descriptive numerical measures. Graph theoretic methods enable the study of functional integration through various metrics such as *small-worldness*, which measures the balance between network segregation and integration, and *network efficiency*, which is inversely proportional to the path length and thus strongest with the shortest path length. Functional segregation of the network can be studied through other metrics, such as the clustering coefficient, which quantifies how well connected the neighbors of a node are to one another. These network-based characterizations of the brain may provide insight into the dysfunction of interacting nodes in patients with TBI.[21] For example, it has recently been shown that network-based analyses offer the potential to understand subtle changes in cognitive function and the effects of rehabilitation.[22] It is important to bear in mind that these metrics provide sensitive but nonspecific markers of brain function.

Mounting Evidence for Connectivity Changes in Traumatic Brain Injury

In a graph analysis study by Pandit and colleagues,[23] TBI subjects exhibited a reduction in overall functional connectivity as evidenced by a reduction in the total number of connections present within the entire network. Longer average path lengths and reduced network efficiency in TBI patients particularly in a major network hub such as the posterior cingulate cortex were also found. However, the network segregation was not affected significantly. These findings suggest

patients suffering from TBI may show a significant deviation from the healthy brain's small world network. Overall, the patterns of network dysfunction caused by TBI are complex, but some unifying principles are emerging, such as the abnormal interactions between the sensory network and the default mode network (DMN) after TBI. Highly connected hub regions, such as the precuneus, are particularly susceptible to alterations in functional connectivity following TBI.[21]

Recently, Murugesan and colleagues[24] have developed a machine learning approach that can automatically distinguish between youth (9–13 years) athletes who have experienced varying levels of head impact exposure in the course of a single season of play. The levels include no or minimal exposure for control athletes and low- and high-impact exposure for football players. The method achieves high labeling accuracy using just features from the intrinsic networks extracted from rs-fMR imaging. The major components of their approach are shown in Fig. 3.

Evidence for Hypoconnectivity in Traumatic Brain Injury

Multiple studies have shown evidence of hypoconnectivity following TBI using seed-based analysis. Xiong and colleagues[25] found decreased functional connectivity in the thalamus, caudate nucleus, and right hippocampus in mTBI patients. Johnson and colleagues[26] found the DMN to have a reduced number of connections and a reduction in the detectable connection strengths. A decreased number of connections and decreased strength of connections were found in the posterior cingulate and lateral parietal cortices, and an increased number of connections were found in the medial prefrontal cortex even in less severe subconcussive head impacts, a milder injury which typically exhibits no clinical symptoms. Rigon and colleagues[27] investigated the differences in interhemispheric functional connectivity of resting state networks between chronic mild to severe TBI patients and normal controls by selecting components such as the DMN, frontoparietal, executive, and sensory motor areas. Their results suggest decreased interhemispheric connectivity for externally oriented networks, such as the frontoparietal and executive networks, but increased interhemispheric connectivity for the DMN following TBI.

Other studies using ICA also demonstrate hypoconnectivity following TBI. Stevens and colleagues[28] used ICA to extract 12 distinct resting

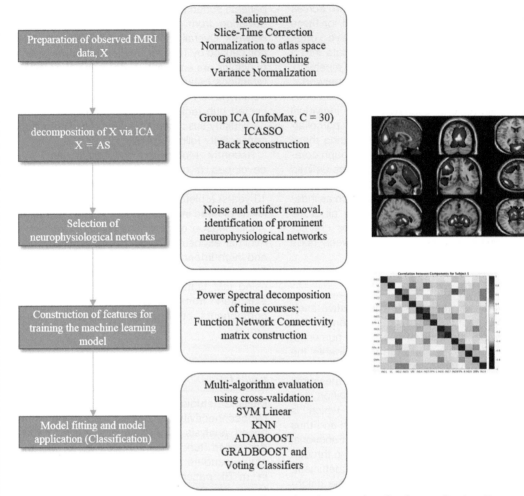

Fig. 3. Process flow for the training and application of a machine learning classifier that predicts head impact exposure using rs-fMR imaging. Left column highlights the main processing steps from preprocessing through classification. Right column provides details of each step presented by Murugesan and colleagues,[24] which automatically distinguishes athletes who, over the course of a single season of play, have experienced: no impact exposure, low-impact exposure, and high-impact exposure. ADABOOST, adaptive boosting; GRADBOOST, gradient boosting; ICASSO, software package for investigating ICA; KNN, k-nearest neighbors; SVM, support vector machine.

state networks from 30 mTBI patients and extended their study to all the extracted components. Diminished connectivity of the posterior cingulate cortex in the DMN was reported in mTBI. Iraji and colleagues[29] performed ICA analysis in 12 mTBI patients and reported reduced functional connectivity in the DMN and precuneus regions compared with controls. Palacios and colleagues[30] also used ICA on 75 mTBI patients, who also had CT within 2 to 3 hours of injury. The mTBI patients had significantly decreased connectivity in the frontal brain areas when conventional structural imaging (CT/MR) demonstrated evidence of TBI, and significantly decreased connectivity in the orbitofrontal network and the DMN when the conventional imaging was negative for evidence of TBI.

Evidence for Hyperconnectivity in Traumatic Brain Injury

There is also evidence for hyperconnectivity in TBI and it is considered to be a common response to TBI. Shumskaya and colleagues[20] studied the relationship between functional connectivity patterns and cognitive abnormalities using resting state networks extracted from group ICA of 43 moderate/severe TBI patients and found that attention abnormalities in TBI were associated with increased connectivity in the sensorimotor networks. In addition, longitudinal studies have shown that despite decreasing functional connectivity during recovery, connectivity remained higher in moderate to severe TBI relative to healthy controls.[31,32] This work suggests that hyperconnectivity in moderate and severe TBI patients may be present regardless of recovery phase (acute, subacute, or chronic phase) and does not represent a transient process as found in other mTBI studies. Thus, hyperconnectivity might become a useful prognostic tool to predict outcomes in moderate and severe TBI.[33] Differences in the results between studies may be attributed to differences in severity of TBI of the studied cohorts, region selection methods, time from injury, graph metrics used, the nature of connectivity studied, and extent of gray and white matter damage.

Automating Diagnosis with Machine Learning

Conventional neuroimaging techniques have limited ability to detect functional connectivity abnormalities, which underlie TBI-related neurocognitive deficits. Advanced neuroimaging, including rs-fMR imaging, can provide increased sensitivity to measure such deficits; however, these deficits can be subtle and diffuse and vary from patient to patient, which makes them hard to identify using standard statistical techniques. Therefore, it is important to develop tools that help automate clinical mTBI diagnostics using rs-fMR imaging. Promising machine learning methods have been developed for rs-fMR imaging interpretation that identify important diagnostic network features to predict mTBI severity, aim to automate mTBI diagnosis, and determine whether patients with TBI have similar functional network changes as patients with Alzheimer disease (AD).

Ravishankar and colleagues[34] used a machine learning framework to identify functional connectivity features associated with symptom severity in mTBI. In this study, 78 mTBI patients were imaged at 4 time points (3 days, 7 days, 21 days, and 3 months) after injury with 6-minute rs-fMR imaging. The investigators found that changes in the executive control and visual networks were most strongly associated with symptom scores. In particular, decreased connectivity between left executive control network and higher visual networks were found, which may correspond to some typical mTBI symptoms, including memory and visual deficits. This study suggests that rs-fMR imaging network features may be useful for predicting effects of mTBI and recovery trajectories.

Another machine learning approach developed by Iraji and colleagues[35] combines structural and functional network connectivity changes to predict whether a subject was a healthy control or an mTBI patient. In this study, 40 mTBI patients at the acute stage and 50 healthy controls were recruited. Sixty signatures were found that

distinguish patients from controls with 100% specificity and 93.75% sensitivity. Specifically, the emotion network demonstrated decreased intranetwork connectivity, whereas perception networks demonstrated increased interactions among action-emotion and action-cognition regions.

Machine learning is also being used to characterize a putative association between TBI and AD. Previously, Van Den Heuvel and colleagues[36] suggested TBI may be a risk factor for developing AD. More recently, Vanderweyen and colleagues[37] hypothesized that there is a common network abnormality between the functional connectome of TBI and AD, and a machine learning-based model was developed to test this association. The model, when trained on AD and healthy control subjects, achieved 82% accuracy in distinguishing AD from healthy controls. Notably, the same classifier also achieves an accuracy of 80% distinguishing TBI from healthy controls without any retraining on TBI, indicating that there are common network abnormality aspects in the connectomes of AD and TBI. Moreover, these results suggest that existing large, longitudinal Alzheimer datasets may be able to jump start the machine learning process, perhaps obviating gathering as much longitudinal TBI imaging data in order to develop a diagnostic tool for TBI.

Longitudinal Recovery Monitoring and Outcome Prediction

Complementary to the development of machine learning-based methods has been the concurrent development of statistical methods that predict TBI outcomes from subacute and longitudinal rs-fMR imaging functional connectivity measures. These methods may be able to predict the future recovery profile and determine which patients will require the most aggressive cognitive therapy and careful monitoring and which patients may do well with simply palliative care.

In a study of the DMN using rs-fMR imaging by Zhu and colleagues,[38] there is evidence that longitudinal changes in functional and structural connectivity of the default-mode network (DMN) can serve as a potential biomarker to monitor sports-related concussion recovery. This study tracked 11 control subjects and the recovery of 8 concussed collegiate football players over the course of 30 days after injury. Resting state and diffusion MR imaging (DTI) were acquired from each subject within 24 hours, 7 days, and 30 days after concussion. In both cohorts, DTI-based structural connectivity remained unchanged throughout the study; however, the cohorts differed significantly in the progression of overall DMN functional connectivity. Compared with the control group, the concussed group exhibited increased functional connectivity on day 1, significantly decreased functional connectivity on day 7, and partial recovery to that of the normal group by day 30. These results indicate rs-fMR imaging holds potential as a biomarker to monitor recovery in the concussed athlete.

Banks and colleagues[39] studied rs-fMR imaging differences between mTBI patients and healthy controls using a different set of functional connections, namely the functional connectivity of the thalamus with other regions and brain networks. This work examined longitudinal functional connectivity changes over a 4-month period in 13 mTBI subjects (mean age 39.3, 31% women) and 11 age- and gender-matched controls without mTBI (mean age 37.6, 36% women). Compared with controls, mTBI patients exhibited an increased functional connectivity between the thalamus and the DMN, whereas exhibiting a decreased functional connectivity between the thalamus and the dorsal attention network (DAN) and between thalamus and the frontoparietal control network. From 6 weeks to 4 months after injury, increased functional connectivity was identified between the thalamus and the DAN that was associated with decreased pain on the Brief Pain Inventory, and decreased postconcussive symptoms on the Rivermead Post-Concussion Symptoms Questionnaire. These findings suggest that thalamic connectivity may serve as a quantitative measure of recovery extent following mTBI.

MAGNETOENCEPHALOGRAPHY PROTOCOLS

MEG is a noninvasive form of brain imaging.[40] Clinically, MEG is used to identify seizure foci in patients with epilepsy.[41] Recent studies have shown MEG to be a useful tool in TBI research. One such study by Huang and colleagues[42] demonstrated changes in functional connectivity during rs-MEG in Veterans diagnosed with mTBI due to a blast. In this study, Veterans with blast-induced mTBI had increased functional connectivity in all frequency bands but the alpha band. Another study by Tarapore and colleagues[43] showed decreased functional connectivity in the alpha band in a group of civilian patients with mild, moderate, and severe TBI. A study by Alhourani and colleagues[44] found decreased local efficiency in different brain regions of patients with mTBI.

Acquisition

The high temporal resolution and wider dynamic range of MEG complements and extends standard rs-fMR imaging acquisition. Typical MEG scanners use between 250 and 300 sensors to measure the magnetic signals from the brain. These sensors are located within a dewar and do not come in direct contact with the subject's scalp. The acquisition is completely passive, and head position indicator coils are applied to track any head motion.[45] rs-MEG acquisition is similar to rs-fMR imaging from the subject's perspective. The subject is asked to keep their eyes open, closed, or look at a cross-hair displayed on a projector for 6 to 10 minutes. However, in MEG, the subject is often seated rather than in a supine position.

Reconstruction Techniques

The sources of these signals can be mapped from sensor space to source space (eg, brain space) using a variety of source localization algorithms. These algorithms are often simpler, yet more accurate, than those used in electroencephalography because the magnetic fields are relatively unaffected by the conductivity of the various tissues in and surrounding the brain, traveling seamlessly through the brain and skull. One source localization approach is beamforming, which builds a spatial filter and was originally developed for radar technology.[46] Beamforming methods used for MEG source reconstruction are often designated as source "scanning" methods because they search a grid for the best solution, usually by minimizing the noise in the output or source variance.[47] Compared with other methods, one benefit of the beamforming methods is that these methods do not limit the spatial solution to predetermined anatomic locations or regions of interest. Such data-driven solutions can minimize model bias for resting state analyses.

MAGNETOENCEPHALOGRAPHY FINDINGS
Frequency Domain

MEG data can also be analyzed in the frequency domain. The frequencies are primarily divided into functional categories, or spectral bands, of delta, theta, alpha, beta, and gamma. Changes in the magnitude and location of these frequencies during resting state scans may be informative of disease states. TBI literature often focuses on the delta band. Delta rhythms (0.5–4 Hz) are normally present during deep sleep but are also seen in pathologic states in adults. Pathologic delta waves originate in different locations depending on the disease. Predominantly, delta waves arise in areas of the cortex overlying white matter lesions.[48] Research on these rhythms and their causes is still ongoing.

Of particular interest to TBI is work by Huang and colleagues[49] showing increased delta waves after TBI. This work describes an automated algorithm for delta wave quantification applied to 45 mTBI patients and 10 moderate TBI patients with rs-MEG. Abnormalities were detected in the delta waves of 87% of the mTBI patients and 100% of the moderate TBI patients. In addition, the number of cortical regions with abnormal delta waves correlated significantly with the post–concussive symptom scores.[49–52] Preliminary data from another study also showed coup contrecoup injury patterns.

Automating Diagnosis with Machine Learning

Manual analysis of the MEG data is typically used as a cursory inspection to ensure that the data have been collected properly, whereas quantitative statistical analyses and automated machine learning interpretations are important to bringing rs-MEG into routine clinical use. Recently, several machine learning methods have been developed for rs-MEG interpretation that help identify important diagnostic network features to automate mTBI diagnosis and help predict mTBI severity. An approach that can automate individual diagnosis would overcome subjectivity in concussion diagnosis commonly based on clinical judgment from self-reported measures and behavioral assessments.

Vakorin and colleagues[53] investigated the type of alterations that occur in resting state oscillatory network phase synchrony in adults with mTBI and whether machine learning can accurately detect mTBI in individual subjects. rs-MEG was recorded and structural MR imaging was acquired from 20 patients with mTBI and 21 age-, gender-, and handedness-matched healthy controls. mTBI was associated with reduced network connectivity in the delta and gamma frequency range (>30 Hz) and increased connectivity in the slower alpha band (8–12 Hz). The most discriminatory features were found in the alpha band (8–12 Hz). Classification confidence was found to be correlated with clinical symptom severity scores. Overall, the results demonstrate that combining MEG network connectivity and machine learning is a promising approach to diagnose mTBI and may also help estimate mTBI severity.

Antonakakis and colleagues[54] investigated the utility of a different set of features extracted from rs-MEG for discriminating mTBI from healthy controls. This study analyzed cross-frequency coupling from rs-MEG in 30 mTBI patients and 50 controls. A classification accuracy of greater than 90% was achieved in distinguishing mTBI

patients from controls across many frequency band pairs. A maximum of 96% accuracy was achieved across the delta and low gamma bands, and this same coupling demonstrated 100% sensitivity and 93% specificity. Their findings showed that compared with mTBI patients, healthy controls formed a dense network of stronger local and global connections characteristic of higher functional integration. These results underscore the critical role development of machine learning tools for studying brain networks computed from rs-MEG serves and suggest that phase-to-amplitude coupling and tensorial representation of connectivity profiles may yield valuable biomarkers for the clinical diagnosis of mTBI.

PEARLS, PITFALLS, VARIANTS

There is significant heterogeneity in the current literature that may hinder direct translation to patient care. Imaging of patients with TBI faces many clinical challenges limiting its application. Timing of acquisition of rs-fMR imaging in patients with TBI, in relation to the patient's injury, provides several unique challenges.

First, it is difficult to image these patients in the hyperacute or acute setting because MR imaging is a relatively lengthy process that can preclude administration of critical resuscitative measures. Patients with TBI should only be sent to MR imaging if they are hemodynamically stable. Scanning patients under critical care who are intubated requires a team effort by technologists, nursing, respiratory therapists, and physicians to safely and effectively perform an MR imaging in the clinically critical patient. Frequently, a routine noncontrast head CT can be safely performed and will adequately answer the clinical question in the acute setting. Furthermore, when MR imaging is necessary, rs-fMR imaging acquisition is not typically included as part of an expedient brain MR imaging protocol, because it has not yet been proven clinically useful in these patients.

Second, in the acute setting, TBI patients have been demonstrated to have alterations in hemodynamic response that may confound rs-fMR imaging analysis and interpretation, if not properly accounted for in the analysis. Finally, hemorrhage and contusions may alter the BOLD signal or produce artifact that limits evaluation. Timing acquisition to minimize the effects of noninterest, while maximizing the effects of interest, is important; however, how to reliably establish this timing is yet to be defined because there is no clear consensus on the best time or times to perform rs-fMR imaging on TBI patients. Because the injury and subsequent healing process are dynamic, imaging only provides a single snapshot in time of that process. Longitudinal studies with consistent imaging and analysis techniques need to be performed to understand the most useful time or times for performing rs-fMR imaging before it will be accepted as a useful biomarker for diagnosis and prognosis in TBI.

Translation of research to individual clinical patients poses many difficulties. Translation of post-processing methods proposed in the literature may be difficult without the proper detailed documentation and computing resources. Application of group analyses to individual patients risks extrapolation from outside of the specific characteristics of the studied patient cohort and may lead to inaccurate interpretation of the results for an individual patient. Training machine learning methods to make individual diagnoses and prognoses is one step toward remedying this limitation. Given the complex biomechanics of closed head injuries and many additional variables involved in TBI, including patient characteristics, trauma mechanism, and post–trauma management, each individual injury is truly unique.

Pearls, Pitfalls, Variants

- Acquisition of rs-fMR imaging is difficult in the acute setting because of more pressing clinical needs.
- Hemorrhage and contusions may alter BOLD signal.
- Translation of research methods to individual clinical patients is difficult.
  - Postprocessing methods may not be reproducible.
  - Group analyses applied to an individual may be inaccurate.
    - Training machine learning methods may make individual diagnoses and prognoses possible.

DISCUSSION

Respecting the aforementioned limitations, rs-fMR imaging is a leading imaging candidate for translation to the clinic. Assignment of diagnosis and prognosis to patients carries serious ethical and medicolegal implications that must be considered; providing an inaccurate diagnosis or prognosis based on new techniques without adequate supportive evidence in the existing literature is unethical and may be negligent. In addition, because the topic of TBI has been recently in the news and social media, the interested public, including potential judges, jurors, and lawyers, may have preconceived ideas and biases. Furthermore, new and complex techniques, such as rs-fMR imaging, carry implicit risks of oversimplifying the pathophysiology, technique of acquisition, method of analysis, and interpretation for the lay public. In summary, care must be taken to ensure there is adequate evidence supporting the clinical utility of these techniques before incorporating them into routine clinical care.

In the future, the methods discussed in this review should be tested on large data sets to determine clinical relevance. Comorbidities such as depression and posttraumatic stress disorder should be included to determine their effects on the algorithms. In addition, the methods should be automated so that they can be easily reproducible in a clinical routine. One of the more promising avenues for rs-fMR imaging and rs-MEG may be the ability to predict recovery time and evaluate therapies. Both modalities allow us to study the healing process in a quantitative way that has not been available previously. In conclusion, there are many promising avenues for rs-fMR imaging and rs-MEG in TBI diagnosis and treatment. Moving these into the clinic should be approached with cautious optimism.

REFERENCES

1. Faul M, Xu L, Wald MM, et al. Traumatic Brain Injury in the United States: Emergency Department Visits, Hospitalizations and Deaths 2002–2006. Atlanta (GA): Centers for Disease Control and Prevention, National Center for Injury Prevention and Control; 2010.
2. Roof RL, Hall ED. Gender differences in acute CNS trauma and stroke: neuroprotective effects of estrogen and progesterone. J Neurotrauma 2000;17(5):367–88.
3. Roof RL, Hall ED. Estrogen-related gender difference in survival rate and cortical blood flow after impact-acceleration head injury in rats. J Neurotrauma 2000;17(12):1155–69.
4. Kleiven S, von Holst H. Consequences of head size following trauma to the human head. J Biomech 2002;35(2):153–60.
5. Champion HR. Abbreviated injury scale. In: Vincent JL, Hall JB, editors. Encyclopedia of intensive care medicine. Berlin, Heidelberg: Springer Berlin Heidelberg; 2012. p. 1–5.
6. McLean AJ, Anderson RWG. Biomechanics of closed head injury. In: Reilly P, Bullock R, editors. Head injury: pathophysiology and management of severe closed injury. London: Chapman & Hall Medical; 1997. p. 25–37.
7. El Sayed T, Mota A, Fraternali F, et al. Biomechanics of traumatic brain injury. Computer Methods Appl Mech Eng 2008;197(51–52):4692–701.
8. Stoica BA, Faden AI. Cell death mechanisms and modulation in traumatic brain injury. Neurotherapeutics 2010;7(1):3–12.

9. Toklu HZ, Tümer N. Oxidative stress, brain edema, blood–brain barrier permeability, and autonomic dysfunction from traumatic brain injury. In: Kobeissy FH, editor. Brain neurotrauma: molecular, neuropsychological, and rehabilitation aspects. Boca Raton (FL): CRC Press/Taylor & Francis; 2015. p. 43–8.

10. McGinn MJ, Povlishock JT. Pathophysiology of traumatic brain injury. Neurosurg Clin N Am 2016;27(4): 397–407.

11. Cornelius C, Crupi R, Calabrese V, et al. Traumatic brain injury: oxidative stress and neuroprotection. Antioxid Redox Signal 2013;19(8):836–53.

12. Adams JH, Doyle D, Ford I, et al. Diffuse axonal injury in head injury: definition, diagnosis and grading. Histopathology 1989;15(1):49–59.

13. Johnson VE, Stewart W, Smith DH. Axonal pathology in traumatic brain injury. Exp Neurol 2013;246:35–43.

14. Farkas O, Lifshitz J, Povlishock JT. Mechanoporation induced by diffuse traumatic brain injury: an irreversible or reversible response to injury? J Neurosci 2006;26(12):3130–40.

15. Farkas O, Povlishock JT. Cellular and subcellular change evoked by diffuse traumatic brain injury: a complex web of change extending far beyond focal damage. In: Maas JTW, Andrew IR, editors. Progress in brain research, vol. 161. Elsevier; 2007. p. 43–59.

16. Biswal B, Yetkin FZ, Haughton VM, et al. Functional connectivity in the motor cortex of resting human brain using echo-planar MRI. Magn Reson Med 1995;34(4):537–41.

17. Birn RM, Molloy EK, Patriat R, et al. The effect of scan length on the reliability of resting-state fMRI connectivity estimates. Neuroimage 2013;83:550–8.

18. Liu D, Dong Z, Zuo X, et al. Eyes-open/eyes-closed dataset sharing for reproducibility evaluation of resting state fMRI data analysis methods. Neuroinformatics 2013;11(4):469–76.

19. Wintermark M, Sanelli PC, Anzai Y, et al. Imaging evidence and recommendations for traumatic brain injury: advanced neuro- and neurovascular imaging techniques. AJNR Am J Neuroradiol 2015;36(2):E1–11.

20. Shumskaya E, van Gerven MAJ, Norris DG, et al. Abnormal connectivity in the sensorimotor network predicts attention deficits in traumatic brain injury. Exp Brain Res 2017;235(3):799–807.

21. Sharp DJ, Scott G, Leech R. Network dysfunction after traumatic brain injury. Nat Rev Neurol 2014;10(3): 156–66.

22. Hart MG, Ypma RJF, Romero-Garcia R, et al. Graph theory analysis of complex brain networks: new concepts in brain mapping applied to neurosurgery. J Neurosurg 2016;124(6):1665–78.

23. Pandit AS, Expert P, Lambiotte R, et al. Traumatic brain injury impairs small-world topology. Neurology 2013;80(20):1826–33.

24. Murugesan G, Famili A, Davenport E, et al. Changes in resting state MRI networks from a single season of football distinguishes controls, low, and high head impact exposure. IEEE 14th International Symposium on Biomedical Imaging (ISBI 2017). Melbourne, VIC; 2017. p. 464–7.

25. Xiong KL, Zhang JN, Zhang YL, et al. Brain functional connectivity and cognition in mild traumatic brain injury. Neuroradiology 2016;58(7):733–9.

26. Johnson B, Neuberger T, Gay M, et al. Effects of subconcussive head trauma on the default mode network of the brain. J Neurotrauma 2014;31(23): 1907–13.

27. Rigon A, Duff MC, McAuley E, et al. Is traumatic brain injury associated with reduced interhemispheric functional connectivity? A study of large-scale resting state networks following traumatic brain injury. J Neurotrauma 2016;33(11): 977–89.

28. Stevens MC, Lovejoy D, Kim J, et al. Multiple resting state network functional connectivity abnormalities in mild traumatic brain injury. Brain Imaging Behav 2012;6(2):293–318.

29. Iraji A, Benson RR, Welch RD, et al. Resting state functional connectivity in mild traumatic brain injury at the acute stage: independent component and seed-based analyses. J Neurotrauma 2015;32(14): 1031–45.

30. Palacios EM, Yuh EL, Chang YS, et al. Resting-state functional connectivity alterations associated with six-month outcomes in mild traumatic brain injury. J Neurotrauma 2017;34(8):1546–57.

31. Hillary FG, Rajtmajer SM, Roman CA, et al. The rich get richer: brain injury elicits hyperconnectivity in core subnetworks. PLoS One 2014;9(8):e104021.

32. Nakamura T, Hillary FG, Biswal BB. Resting network plasticity following brain injury. PLoS One 2009; 4(12):e8220.

33. Caeyenberghs K, Verhelst H, Clemente A, et al. Mapping the functional connectome in traumatic brain injury: what can graph metrics tell us? Neuroimage 2016. [Epub ahead of print].

34. Ravishankar H, Madhavan R, Mullick R, et al. Recursive feature elimination for biomarker discovery in resting-state functional connectivity. Conf Proc IEEE Eng Med Biol Soc 2016;2016:4071–4.

35. Iraji A, Chen H, Wiseman N, et al. Connectome-scale assessment of structural and functional connectivity in mild traumatic brain injury at the acute stage. Neuroimage Clin 2016;12:100–15.

36. Van Den Heuvel C, Thornton E, Vink R. Traumatic brain injury and Alzheimer's disease: a review. Prog Brain Res 2007;161:303–16.

37. Vanderweyen D, Munsell BC, Mintzer JE, et al. Identifying abnormal network alternations common to traumatic Brain injury and Alzheimer's disease patients using functional connectome data. In:

Zhou L, Wang L, Wang Q, et al, editors. Machine learning in medical imaging, vol. 9352. Cham (Germany): Springer; 2015. p. 229–37.

38. Zhu DC, Covassin T, Nogle S, et al. A potential biomarker in sports-related concussion: brain functional connectivity alteration of the default-mode network measured with longitudinal resting-state fMRI over thirty days. J Neurotrauma 2015;32(5):327–41.

39. Banks SD, Coronado RA, Clemons LR, et al. Thalamic functional connectivity in mild traumatic brain injury: longitudinal associations with patient-reported outcomes and neuropsychological tests. Arch Phys Med Rehabil 2016;97(8):1254–61.

40. Cohen D. Magnetoencephalography: detection of the brain's electrical activity with a superconducting magnetometer. Science 1972;175(4022):664–6.

41. Funke M, Constantino T, Van Orman C, et al. Magnetoencephalography and magnetic source imaging in epilepsy. Clin EEG Neurosci 2009;40(4):271–80.

42. Huang MX, Harrington DL, Robb Swan A, et al. Resting-state magnetoencephalography reveals different patterns of aberrant functional connectivity in combat-related mild traumatic brain injury. J Neurotrauma 2017;34(7):1412–26.

43. Tarapore PE, Findlay AM, Lahue SC, et al. Resting state magnetoencephalography functional connectivity in traumatic brain injury. J Neurosurg 2013;118(6):1306–16.

44. Alhourani A, Wozny TA, Krishnaswamy D, et al. Magnetoencephalography-based identification of functional connectivity network disruption following mild traumatic brain injury. J Neurophysiol 2016;116(4):1840–7.

45. Velmurugan J, Sinha S, Satishchandra P. Magnetoencephalography recording and analysis. Ann Indian Acad Neurol 2014;17:S113–9.

46. Van Veen BD, Buckley KM. Beamforming: a versatile approach to spatial filtering. IEEE ASSP Magazine 1988;5(2):4–24.

47. Hillebrand A, Barnes GR. Beamformer analysis of MEG data. Int Rev Neurobiol 2005;68:149–71.

48. Gloor P, Ball G, Schaul N. Brain lesions that produce delta waves in the EEG. Neurology 1977;27(4):326–33.

49. Huang MX, Nichols S, Robb A, et al. An automatic MEG low-frequency source imaging approach for detecting injuries in mild and moderate TBI patients with blast and non-blast causes. Neuroimage 2012;61(4):1067–82.

50. Nugent AC, Luber B, Carver FW, et al. Deriving frequency-dependent spatial patterns in MEG-derived resting state sensorimotor network: a novel multiband ICA technique. Hum Brain Mapp 2016;38(2):779–91.

51. Meng L, Xiang J. Frequency specific patterns of resting-state networks development from childhood to adolescence: a magnetoencephalography study. Brain Dev 2016;38(10):893–902.

52. Tewarie P, Hillebrand A, van Dijk BW, et al. Integrating cross-frequency and within band functional networks in resting-state MEG: a multi-layer network approach. Neuroimage 2016;142:324–36.

53. Vakorin VA, Doesburg SM, da Costa L, et al. Detecting mild traumatic brain injury using resting state magnetoencephalographic connectivity. PLoS Comput Biol 2016;12(12):e1004914.

54. Antonakakis M, Dimitriadis SI, Zervakis M, et al. Altered cross-frequency coupling in resting-state MEG after mild traumatic brain injury. Int J Psychophysiol 2016;102:1–11.

Applications of Resting-State Functional MR Imaging to Epilepsy

Alexander Barnett, MA[a,b], Samantha Audrain, MA[a,b],
Mary Pat McAndrews, PhD[a,b],*

KEYWORDS

- fMR imaging • Memory • Language • Functional connectivity • Medial temporal lobe

KEY POINTS

- Surgical resection of the anterior temporal lobe in epilepsy can result in impairments in language and memory; functional MR imaging (fMR imaging) biomarkers of risk would be valuable.
- Resting-state fMR imaging may be superior to task-related activation as an indicator of functional capacity.
- Resting-state functional connectivity between hippocampus and posterior cingulate cortex is predictive of memory change following temporal-lobe resection.
- Less work has been done to relating resting-state functional connectivity to language ability in people with temporal-lobe epilepsy, although some reports show promise.

WHAT CAN FUNCTIONAL MR IMAGING ADD TO EPILEPSY SURGICAL EVALUATIONS?

Most surgeries in adults with epilepsy involve patients with medial temporal-lobe epilepsy (mTLE) who experience recurrent seizures arising from one medial temporal lobe (MTL), including the hippocampus and surrounding entorhinal and parahippocampal cortices. In this situation, the concern is whether removal of anterior and medial temporal-lobe structures for seizure control will result in significant morbidity in the form of postsurgical cognitive decline. With respect to language, functional decline can result from excision of the anterior temporal neocortex of the dominant (typically left) hemisphere.[1–3] For memory, the functional adequacy of the epileptogenic MTL is critical, as better preoperative capacity is associated with greater decline,[4,5] typically with verbal memory associated with the left MTL and visuospatial memory with the right.[6–8] Functional MR imaging (fMR imaging) provides the means to assess adequacy of the epileptogenic tissue and risk of cognitive decline postoperatively, as well as characterize potential reorganization or compensation of neural networks that support language and memory.[9]

Clinical fMR imaging research has been directed largely at questions of task-related patterns of activation, focusing on specific regions of interest. The most robust findings concern reduced MTL activation during encoding in patients with mTLE[10–14] compared with healthy controls. Additionally, the strength (magnitude, spatial extent) of activation in the left temporal lobe predicts the degree of decline in verbal episodic memory and naming after left temporal lobectomy.[15–17] Recently, a panel of the American Academy of

Disclosure: The authors have no conflicts of interest to declare.
[a] Krembil Research Institute, University Health Network, 399 Bathurst Street, Toronto, ON M5T 2S8, Canada;
[b] Department of Psychology, University of Toronto, 100 St George Street, Toronto, ON M5S 3G3, Canada
* Corresponding author. Neuropsychology Clinic, Toronto Western Hospital, 4F-409, 399 Bathurst Street, Toronto, Ontario M5T 2S8, Canada.
E-mail address: Mary.McAndrews@uhn.ca

Neuroimag Clin N Am 27 (2017) 697–708
http://dx.doi.org/10.1016/j.nic.2017.06.002

Neurology evaluated the efficacy of fMR imaging in determining lateralization and predicting postsurgical memory and language outcome in patients with epilepsy, particularly focusing on comparison with the Wada procedure, which involves drug-induced inactivation of one hemisphere for assessing capacity of the contralateral hemisphere.[18] They reported evidence of material-specific asymmetry during verbal and nonverbal memory tasks (leftward and rightward, respectively), with fMR imaging as the superior predictor of verbal memory change postoperatively compared with the Wada procedure. In terms of language mapping, they argued that fMR imaging is as effective in lateralizing language functions as the Wada procedure, although data concerning language outcome were limited and relevant studies underpowered. The conclusion was that fMR imaging of language and verbal memory lateralization can be used as an alternative to the Wada procedure for predicting outcome in mTLE, although they cautioned that fMR imaging is not established as an alternative to the Wada procedure in terms of predicting global amnesia that can arise when functioning of the contralateral MTL is also impaired.

Although task-activation paradigms have shown considerable success in lateralizing language and predicting postoperative memory decline, there are important limitations. Relatively long scans with multiple runs are typically required for reliable data, and the capacity for full task engagement in patient populations is sometimes suspect. One must carefully consider task design and the sensitivity and specificity of various metrics of activation; for example, whether magnitude of activation in the epileptogenic MTL or asymmetry between hemispheres is a better indicator of capacity. Indeed, one study found that activation in a language task was superior to that from a memory task in predicting verbal memory decline following left anterior temporal lobectomy,[19] which may reflect relatively poor sensitivity or specificity to memory outcomes of the paradigms, the metrics, or both. Data analysis methods are also critical, including the selection method for regions of interest and how to determine appropriate thresholds. At this point, there is no consensus as to the best combination of methodologic features for clinical decisions, or the extent to which these variables affect the accuracy of predictions. Of importance, individual patients may use alternate strategies or activate different networks during a task, which can undermine a region of interest approach, and there is evidence that greater signal in the hippocampus does not correlate with better function.[20] Considerable effort has been aimed at

identifying ideal task-activation paradigms for clinical use,[19,21,22] but there is increasing interest in exploring whether resting-state networks may provide greater insight into the functional capacity of neural systems, rather than what is being activated by a particular task or situation, under the assumption that capacity is what is most important in the clinical context.

RESTING-STATE FUNCTIONAL MR IMAGING AND MEMORY IN MEDIAL TEMPORAL-LOBE EPILEPSY

Resting-state fMR imaging (rsfMR imaging) scans can be used to derive networks characterized by intrinsic functional connectivity among brain regions. Such resting connectivity measures could potentially be superior to task-based measures of activation or connectivity, as they eliminate variance or "noise" associated with atypical strategies or compensatory networks in patients in whom some degree of functional reorganization may have already taken place.[23] Examination of the Default Mode Network (DMN) may be particularly well-suited to address questions of functional adequacy of the MTL because the hippocampus and parahippocampal gyrus are constituent nodes, and the overall DMN shows considerable overlap with the constellation of brain regions commonly engaged during episodic recollection.[24,25] Studies have documented abnormal connectivity between the MTL and other DMN regions in patients with mTLE,[26–29] but only a few have examined the consequence of that disrupted connectivity to functional integrity as indexed by memory performance.

Our first study[30] focused on 2 nodes of the DMN: the hippocampus and posterior cingulate cortex (PCC), the latter of which is a hub within the network and is typically activated in recognition and recall tasks.[24] Patients with left or right mTLE showed reduced connectivity to the epileptogenic hippocampus and increased connectivity to the contralateral one compared with controls. Furthermore, stronger connectivity on the epileptogenic side was associated with better presurgical memory and greater postsurgical memory decline, whereas greater connectivity on the contralateral side was protective. We collected rsfMR imaging in a subset of patients following temporal-lobe resection and found an increase in contralateral connectivity, the magnitude of which was correlated with memory preservation, and therefore is suggestive of compensatory plasticity. A subsequent study examined the relationship between current memory performance and functional connectivity throughout 20 nodes of the

DMN.[31] Consideration of the full network resulted in correlations with memory that were even stronger than the simple 2-node solution. Better memory was associated with stronger posterior and interhemispheric connectivity (ie, between MTL structures and medial and lateral parietal cortices), whereas poorer memory was associated with stronger long-range posterior-to-anterior intrahemispheric connections. Of interest, the latter finding is quite similar to the long-range connectivity we have seen in patients with left mTLE when they are recalling personal autobiographical memories that are impoverished in detail compared with memories retrieved by control participants.[32] As this alternate pattern of connectivity (Fig. 1) has

been seen in different circumstances (resting state and directed memory retrieval), with distinct analytical techniques (multivariate correlations and structural equation modeling), and in association with different outcomes (reduced details in personal recollection and poorer performance on clinical measures of learning and recognition), it may signify a specific change in memory networks in mTLE.

Other studies, particularly a series by Voets and colleagues,[33] underscore the argument that networks beyond those considered "canonical" to memory processes in the healthy brain must be considered in patients with mTLE. They reported reduced resting-state functional connectivity

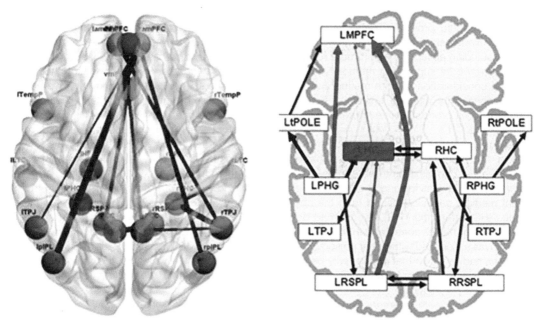

Fig. 1. Increased long-range intrahemispheric connectivity in patients with left mTLE. Figure on the left, in which blue lines indicate increased (relative to controls) long-range connectivity in rsfMR imaging from posterior medial and lateral parietal cortices to medial prefrontal regions in patients with left mTLE. Figure on the right indicates altered effective connectivity (relative to controls) during autobiographical memory retrieval, with increases in red and decreases in blue. Major differences are increased connectivity from retrosplenial to medial prefrontal cortex on the left and reduced connectivity involving left medial temporal regions. Red nodes in both figures indicate regions of reduced structural integrity of medial temporal cortex. dmPFC, dorsomedial prefrontal cortex; lamPFC, left anteromedial prefrontal cortex; LHC, left hippocampus; lHF, left hippocampal formation; lLTC, left lateral temporal cortex; LMPFC, left medial prefrontal cortex; lPCC, left posterior cingulate cortex; lPHC, left parahippocampal cortex; LPHG, left parahippocampal gyrus; lpIPL, left posterior inferior parietal lobule; lRSP, left retrosplenial cortex; LRSPL, left retrosplenial cortex; lTempP, left temporal pole; lTPJ, left temporoparietal junction; LTPJ, left temporoparietal junction; LtPOLE, left temporal pole; ramPFC, right anteromedial prefrontal cortex; RHC, right hippocampus; rHF, right hippocampal formation; rLTC, right lateral temporal cortex; rPCC, right posterior cingulate cortex; rPHC, right parahippocampal cortex; RPHG, right parahippocampal gyrus; rpIPL, right posterior inferior parietal lobule; rRSP, right retrosplenial; RRSPL, right retrosplenial cortex; rTempP, right temporal pole; rTPJ, right temporoparietal junction; RTPJ, right temporoparietal junction; RtPOLE, right temporal pole; vmPFC, ventromedial prefrontal cortex. (From [Left] McCormick C, Protzner AB, Barnett AJ, et al. Linking DMN connectivity to episodic memory capacity: what can we learn from patients with medial temporal lobe damage? Neuroimage Clin 2014;5:188–96; and [Right] Addis DR, Moscovitch M, McAndrews MP. Consequences of hippocampal damage across the autobiographical memory network in left temporal lobe epilepsy. Brain 2007;130:2327–42.)

(rsFC) between ipsilateral temporal neocortex and the DMN in patients with left mTLE, although unfortunately memory performance was not examined. A more recent study found that short-term memory was related to thalamic connectivity to specific regions in frontal and parietal cortices in the contralateral hemisphere, whereas long-term memory was associated with the strength of rsFC between ipsilateral thalamus and entorhinal cortex.[34] Of interest, when they assessed functional connectivity during memory encoding rather than rest, poorer subsequent memory performance was associated with reduced connectivity in a network that included bilateral MTL and extended to bilateral occipital and left orbitofrontal cortex.[28] There are too few studies comparing connectivity of networks during task activation versus rest to know whether "driving" the network could provide a better indicator of capacity. Nonetheless, these findings indicate that longstanding epilepsy may promote reorganization of networks supporting memory and indicate that consideration of both resting and task-based connectivity may be important in determining the most productive line to pursue for clinical purposes.

These are early days in the exploration of rsfMR imaging and memory in epilepsy, and of course there are many complexities to be addressed. For example, a few studies looking at connectivity and current memory capacity seeded from the hippocampus (HC) rather than PCC, as we had done. One found that higher contralateral HC-PCC connectivity was associated with better episodic memory, as we had, but also that connectivity between both hippocampi and other MTL structures (entorhinal cortex and parahippocampal gyrus) was negatively associated with memory performance.[35] Another group reported that connectivity between the ipsilateral left hippocampus and left PCC/precuneus and inferior parietal lobule (IPL) was negatively associated with memory, whereas stronger connectivity between the epileptogenic hippocampus and contralateral PCC/precuneus and IPL was associated with better memory.[36] A third pattern is represented by findings of poorer verbal memory in the context of strong ipsilateral hippocampus-to-PCC connectivity in patients with left mTLE, which aligns with the study by Holmes and colleagues[36] but contrasts with the study by McCormick and colleagues,[30] but stronger nonverbal memory in patients with right mTLE who demonstrated greater connectivity between the left hippocampus and medial prefrontal cortex.[37] Clearly, we need studies with larger cohorts and particularly those in which prediction of change after surgery is the primary outcome to discern the most

robust patterns of connectivity that are reliable indicators of functional capacity and risk.

The functional imaging literature to date typically refers to the hippocampus as a homogeneous structure, and yet there is evidence of considerable variability in the distribution of histopathology along the longitudinal axis in mTLE.[38–40] Furthermore, there is evidence that greater mesial temporal sclerosis in the anterior half of the hippocampus is associated with increased probability of seizure freedom after surgery.[41] Of interest, recent studies in normative populations have shown that anterior and posterior segments of the hippocampus have distinct multisynaptic patterns of rsFC connectivity with neocortical regions, which likely has important implications for the type of memory processes they support.[42–44] These anterior and posterior networks have been characterized in several ways. One model proposes that posterior regions support the fine-grained representations that enable retrieval characterized by recollection of details, rather than coarser "gist" information that anterior networks support.[45] Another model hypothesizes that coupling between the anterior hippocampus and the dorsal attention network is important for encoding new information, whereas retrieval depends more on posterior hippocampus–DMN connectivity.[46] Our own work indicates that posterior hippocampus–to-neocortex networks are especially involved with the type of relational memory processes that are particularly impaired in patients with mTLE.[47,48] Clearly, this is an important avenue for future investigations in individuals with mTLE, marrying rsfMR imaging to well-designed cognitive assays of clinically meaningful memory processes.

A key question regarding the added value of these functional connectivity measures in the clinical context is whether they complement or exceed structural integrity or task-evoked activation as indicators of memory capacity. In their study assessing thalamo-cortical connectivity and memory, Voets and colleagues[34] noted that hippocampal volume added unique information to thalamic-frontal rsFC in explaining short-term memory performance but volume did not add to the relationship between long-term memory and thalamic-medial temporal rsFC. We have found that rsFC is a stronger predictor of performance on clinically relevant memory tasks than is structural damage to the MTL or other DMN nodes.[30,31] These findings align with concepts articulated in the study of the Human Brain Connectome, that structure influences but does not fully determine the brain's dynamic and flexible functional repertoire.[49,50] Indeed, we found that the correlation between hippocampal volume and memory was in fact mediated by functional activation in the hippocampus during encoding,[10] indicating that anatomic constraints may be less important than how readily the affected tissue can be engaged.

RESTING-STATE FUNCTIONAL CONNECTIVITY AND LANGUAGE IN MEDIAL TEMPORAL-LOBE EPILEPSY

rsfMR imaging is also emerging as a potentially valuable tool for mapping the language network, a network composed of the inferior frontal gyrus, superior temporal gyrus, supramarginal gyrus, IPL, and pre–motor cortex. Although most fMR imaging research on this network has been done using task-based fMR imaging,[51] reliable network characterization has also been shown using rsFC.[52,53] Here, we review the literature on rsfMR imaging mapping of language network connectivity, discussing its reliability and stability in temporal-lobe epilepsy and healthy individuals. We also compare presurgical rsFC network characterization with traditional methods of presurgical language mapping, such as task-based language fMR imaging, the Wada procedure, and electrical stimulation mapping (ESM), highlighting the potential advantages of each. Finally, we review research examining the ability of rsFC to predict postsurgical language change.

As with memory, there are compelling reasons to develop a strong clinical grounding for rsFC in language processes. Any patient may be incapable of performing language tasks adequately or in the manner we designate, and thus our task-based patterns of activation may include regions that are engaged for the fMR imaging task but not truly indicative of language capacity. Language networks can be characterized from rsfMR imaging data using univariate, seed-based approaches[53] or multivariate approaches such as independent component analysis.[52] Using a very large database, Tomasi and Volkow[53] examined more than 900 healthy people collected from 22 research sites around the world and used a standard seed-to-voxel approach with 2 regions of interest (the Broca and Wernicke areas) to interrogate language network connectivity. Across each research site, both seeds demonstrated robust connectivity to language regions, including the inferior frontal gyrus (IFG; composed of pars orbitalis, triangularis, and opercularis), middle frontal gyrus, superior frontal cortex, inferior temporal cortex, superior temporal gyrus, inferior parietal cortex, caudate, putamen, and cerebellum, with the Broca area showing stronger connectivity to anterior language regions, and the Wernicke area communicating more with posterior regions.

Although the investigators found more bilateral connectivity than is typically captured by task-activation paradigms, they found leftward lateralization of connectivity, which supports lateralization of language to the left hemisphere, as is expected in the general population. These patterns were found to be highly reproducible within subjects across time intervals ranging from 45 minutes to 16 months,[54] providing evidence that rsFC reflects stable network measurements.

Although epilepsy specialists have noted the growing utility of rsfMR imaging in clinical decision making,[55] there are limited instances of this technique being applied in the presurgical mapping context. In one study involving patients with mTLE or tumor, language networks were extracted from rsfMR imaging scans using a machine-learning algorithm that was trained to classify voxels as being a part of canonical resting networks.[56] Before surgery, all patients also had ESM to identify eloquent cortex, and the investigators found strong agreement between ESM and rsFC language network classification. Because ESM is viewed as a gold standard for language mapping, this provides strong evidence that rsfMR imaging can identify eloquent cortex. In a comparison between language task–based fMR imaging and rsfMR imaging, greater leftward lateralization determined by task activation was associated with stronger resting-state connectivity between left IFG and other neocortical regions in the left hemisphere in controls and patients with mTLE.[57] In a subsequent study, this group showed that task-based patterns of activity and connectivity seem to be more left-lateralizing and selective, whereas resting language connectivity appears to reflect a broader, more bilateral set of "prepotent" language regions.[58] This suggests that task-based fMR imaging may be better suited for determining the language dominant hemisphere. However, Waites and colleagues[59] found that although task activation yielded similar language maps between patients and controls, resting-state connectivity produced striking differences between the 2 groups, with patients showing markedly less connectivity from seeded language regions at rest than controls. The investigators suggested that resting state was a more sensitive measure of difference in language networks between the 2 groups than task activation. Unfortunately, less has been done to compare resting-state connectivity with the Wada inactivation procedure in terms of predicting lateralization or functional capacity, although a recent study found that the 2 methods yielded highly concordant results of language lateralization.[60]

Although these findings are promising, if rsfMR imaging is to replace invasive procedures in surgical decision making, more work is needed to confirm that this measure is informative. Such work will need to compare rsfMR imaging with the current best practices of language activation tasks in a large sample, as well as investigate the ability of rsFC to predict postoperative language change. The few studies that have attempted to relate rsFC to presurgical and postsurgical language ability have used varying techniques with mixed success. For example, in one study, laterality indices produced from rsfMR imaging maps seeded from the IFG failed to predict preoperative language fluency in patients with left and right mTLE.[58] In another study, rsFC between language regions in the left hemisphere (posterior superior temporal gyrus, middle temporal gyrus, and pars triangularis of the IFG) was strongly correlated with verbal IQ in those with left mTLE.[61] Osipowicz and colleagues[62] used a multiscan approach to examine the ability of task-based fMR imaging, rsfMR imaging, and diffusion tensor imaging (DTI) to predict postoperative verbal fluency by examining the deviation of structure and function in patients from healthy controls at preoperative and postoperative time points. They found that a model including all 3 measures of postoperative deviation accounted for 52% of the variance in fluency outcome, with DTI explaining 32% of the variance, rsFC explaining 15%, and fMR imaging task-evoked activation explaining only 4%. No single modality significantly predicted outcome, nor did models using presurgical deviation from healthy controls, rendering this method ineffectual in the context of preoperative planning.

We previously reported that task-related connectivity between the left inferior frontal and left middle temporal gyri was a better indicator of current performance on clinical tests of naming and verbal fluency than magnitude of lateralized activation in individuals with mTLE.[21] For the present article, we probed a subset of these data (n = 10), which also included a resting-state scan, and here report that the correlation with naming (Boston Naming Test [BNT]) was stronger for task-based functional connectivity between those regions ($r = 0.50$), weaker for rsFC between those regions ($r = 0.25$), and weakest for the task-activation laterality index ($r = 0.16$). These preliminary findings appear to call into question the potential utility of rsFC to preoperative planning. However, we also found that when rsFC within a broader and more bilateral language network in individuals with left mTLE was compared with a healthy control template, greater similarity of patient connectivity to healthy control connectivity predicted better

BNT performance after surgery ($r = 0.74$, Fig. 2). Thus, more "normal" connectivity of resting-state language networks was associated with better language outcome. Furthermore, patients with greater degree (here, a resting-state graph theory measure of functional integration) in to-be-resected nodes in the anterior temporal lobes showed the greatest decline in naming after surgery ($r = -0.64$), indicating that greater integration of the anterior temporal lobe with the rest of the language network predicts worse language outcome after its removal. Note these results are from previously unpublished data (Audrain and colleagues, 2017) and we are currently analyzing a larger data set to assess how robust these preliminary findings may be.

Further success in using rsfMR imaging to predict postoperative change has been found using graph theory metrics.[63] This study selected 7 regions involved in expressive language to examine their relationship to neuropsychological outcome following anterior temporal-lobe resection. They found that integration of the left inferior frontal cortex (ie, the path length to all other brain regions) was the most significant predictor of outcome, with higher integration (shorter path length) predicting better verbal outcome in the left mTLE group. Interestingly, they also reported a somewhat complex relationship between graph theory properties and verbal episodic memory, in which increased integration and reduced centrality of the left inferior frontal cortex was associated with better verbal memory outcome for patients with left mTLE. Surprisingly, the graph theory measures of the hippocampus were not predictive of postsurgical memory change in either the left mTLE or right mTLE group. This finding is somewhat at odds with our study using simple correlation of DMN nodes to predict postsurgical memory change[30] and speaks to the impact that analysis choices can have on prediction. These findings indicate that in addition to the many ways one can characterize language networks, there are also many ways to relate resting-state measures to clinically meaningful cognitive performance. There is substantial work needed to determine the best methods for characterizing functionally relevant patterns of connectivity in a clinically useful way.

RESTING-STATE FUNCTIONAL MR IMAGING AND OTHER CLINICAL QUESTIONS IN EPILEPSY

A substantial development in the past decade of clinical epilepsy is that even "focal" epilepsies are considered as "network" disorders, and presurgical investigations are aimed at characterizing

Individual Patient rsFC

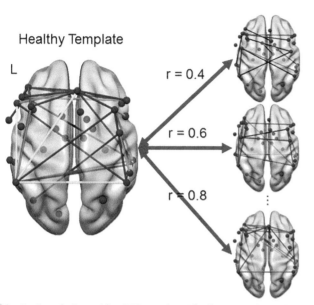

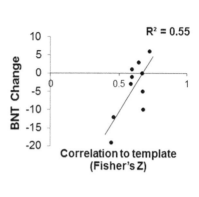

Fig. 2. Correlation with rsFC "template" for language in patients with mTLE. Each patient's language network rsFC was correlated with a healthy control template (created by taking the mean connectivity among language nodes in 19 healthy age-matched controls) to measure network similarity. The correlation coefficient was transformed into a z-score using a Fisher transformation and used to predict BNT performance, shown in the scatter plot on the right, which demonstrates that patients who had networks more similar to the template presurgically, had better language outcome. The brain maps are presented in neurologic convention with warmer-colored connectivity bars representing stronger connections between regions. Note: The brain maps displayed are for illustrative purposes only and are thresholded to demonstrate differences/similarities. The calculation of the correlation coefficients in this analysis included every pairwise connection among 33 bilateral brain regions involved in language.

that epileptic network to improve surgical outcomes.[64] Individuals with mTLE show a consistent pattern of disconnection of the MTL from the rest of the DMN in resting-state scans.[29,30,65,66] Simultaneous electroencephalogram (EEG)-fMR imaging data collection has allowed us to advance considerably on understanding the relationship between transient abnormalities associated with epileptiform discharges and intrinsic networks[67–69] and identifying patterns that may be predictive of postoperative seizure freedom.[70] Recently, there have been some important efforts to use resting-state connectivity, particularly coupled with measures of spatial clustering, to discern abnormalities associated with epileptic foci on an individual patient basis. One such study reported success in locating abnormal changes in connectivity that was closely related to EEG foci in 5 of 6 patients.[71] Although much work needs to be done, these early efforts are key steps in delivering on the promise of functional connectivity as a useful tool in the clinic, not dependent on capturing ictal events during a scanning session. To the extent that stable interictal defects that are clear biomarkers of epilepsy-associated damage can be identified, the need for more invasive

intracranial recording in patients in whom scalp EEG is insufficient to determine the likelihood of surgical success will be reduced.

POSSIBILITIES AND LIMITATIONS

A fundamental tenet of this enterprise is that resting-state networks provide a valid reflection of brain activity that underlies task performance, otherwise the objective of linking rsFC patterns to cognitive outcomes is unlikely to succeed. In addition to the specific studies reviewed previously, there are important examples in the literature of strong correspondence in the topology of networks active during particular cognitive states or tasks, including basic sensory and motor as well as more complex cognitive operations, including working memory and emotional processing, and intrinsic connectivity at rest.[72–74] Using large-scale connectivity across many brain regions and multiple cognitive tasks, Cole and colleagues[72] found a high degree of overlap between rest and task-evoked connectivity even at the local pairwise connectivity level, suggesting that the network supporting a given cognitive operation is shaped primarily by intrinsic architecture together with a limited set of task-evoked changes. Some strong cautions to this view have been offered, noting a modest amount of shared variance between rest and tasks that engage similar networks, arguments that scans during instruction to "do nothing in particular" merely reflect a poorly constrained and highly dynamic set of cognitive operations, and that rest may offer little insight into cognitive networks that are based on versatile process-specific alliances that form within and between intrinsic networks during the execution of particular cognitive operations.[75–78] Nonetheless, using machine-learning techniques, one group has demonstrated that it is possible to predict task-activation maps for a range of functions at an individual subject level from that person's resting-state connectivity[79] and, highly relevant to the concerns of this article, that algorithms trained on control resting connectivity can be used to predict activations associated with verbal fluency in patients being considered for neurosurgery.[80] These studies demonstrated remarkably good predictive accuracy, with poorer performance of the model associated with lower quality of the resting-state scans rather than individual differences in disease state, behavior, age, or other characteristics. Exporting this strategy and training data set on a broad scale, if feasible, would afford an excellent opportunity to discern the accuracy of predicting task-related topology in a variety of clinical populations.

There are operational concerns that need to be addressed to ensure this is a practical enterprise in clinical settings. First, there are many analytical approaches that can be taken, and it is important to decide which is most appropriate or best suited to specific questions. Approaches that use seed regions that are based on existing literature (eg, from the well-characterized DMN) may capture those networks in the healthy brain but become difficult to interpret if there has been substantial reorganization in the target clinical population. For example, the selection of a damaged hippocampus as seed may not lead to identifying the effective memory network in mTLE. Independent component analysis and related approaches are data-driven means to extract networks, but can sometimes split networks into a variable number of components across different subjects and still require one to select components of interest for interpretation. A semiautomated approach has been proposed for identification of these networks based on training templates,[52] and machine-learning techniques can enable identification of atypical networks given there is sufficient homogeneity within the patient population of interest. Finally, issues of thresholding for single-subject analyses are equally

important here as in activation paradigms; stringent yet arbitrary cutoffs may eliminate potentially meaningful connections, but without thresholds the signals can be noisy and uninterpretable.

In addition, there are concerns about reliability of resting-state connectivity metrics, particularly at the individual subject level. Test-retest reliability has been of concern in activation paradigms, particularly for complex tasks that can induce different strategies on subsequent scanning sessions.[81,82] There is some evidence that rsFC is more reliable than task-related activation magnitude or spatial extent,[83,84] and even sufficiently robust to identify individual subjects akin to a "fingerprint,"[85] but it is important to note that variables such as participant age, scan length, and other acquisition parameters can impact rsFC reliability.[86,87] Conversely, resting-state connectivity may be even more sensitive to nuisance variables, such as motion,[88,89] and to the extent that motion is confounded with the variable of interest (such as degree of cognitive impairment), it presents a genuine challenge for interpretation. In addition, investigations into the extent to which the pathology in mTLE and/or use of antiepileptic drugs in these conditions may influence (either globally or locally) the neurovascular coupling that is crucial for observing changes in local cerebral blood flow and blood oxygenation or other aspects of fMR imaging signals are just beginning.[90–93]

A final crucial step in advancing the clinical utility of rsfMR imaging, particularly for the individual patient with epilepsy considering surgery, is establishing sensitivity, specificity, and positive predictive value for these metrics. What is the degree of connectivity within the epileptogenic region that may signify a significant risk of cognitive morbidity should part of that network be excised? Our experience with postoperative memory change suggests that, even in the case of "lateralized" or material-specific memory functions, consideration of connectivity in the contralateral memory networks may be as important as characterizing adequacy of the to-be-resected MTL in devising clinical metrics. Fortunately, the barrier to conducting resting-state studies is considerably lower than with activation tasks in terms of amount of data required, the complexity of task influences, and the possibility of pooling data from multiple centers, making it more likely that the field will make rapid progress on some of these questions.

SUMMARY

Overall, there is very good evidence that rsfMR imaging is developing into a useful clinical tool for mapping language networks and characterizing functional integrity of memory networks in clinical populations and for providing predictions after surgical or other interventions. At present, however, much work still needs to be done in terms of comparisons to relevant "gold standards" in clinical practice, determining ideal analytical strategies and decision algorithms, and relating network properties to the behaviors we are most interested in measuring and predicting.

REFERENCES

1. Davies KG, Bell BD, Bush AJ, et al. Naming decline after left anterior temporal lobectomy correlates with pathological status of resected hippocampus. Epilepsia 1998;39:407–19.
2. Hermann BP, Wyler AR, Somes G, et al. Dysnomia after left anterior temporal lobectomy without functional mapping: frequency and correlates. Neurosurgery 1994;35:52–6 [discussion: 56–7].
3. Schwarz M, Pauli E, Stefan H. Model based prognosis of postoperative object naming in left temporal lobe epilepsy. Seizure 2005;14:562–8.
4. Chelune GJ. Hippocampal adequacy versus functional reserve: predicting memory functions following temporal lobectomy. Arch Clin Neuropsychol 1995;10:413–32.
5. Harvey DJ, Naugle RI, Magleby J, et al. Relationship between presurgical memory performance on the Wechsler Memory Scale-III and memory change following temporal resection for treatment of intractable epilepsy. Epilepsy Behav 2008;13:372–5.
6. Jones-Gotman M, Smith ML, Risse GL, et al. The contribution of neuropsychology to diagnostic assessment in epilepsy. Epilepsy Behav 2010;18:3–12.
7. McAndrews MP, Cohn M. Neuropsychology in temporal lobe epilepsy: influences from cognitive neuroscience and functional neuroimaging. Epilepsy Res Treat 2012;2012:925238.
8. Milner B. Disorders of learning and memory after temporal lobe lesions in man. Clin Neurosurg 1972;19:421–46.
9. Alessio A, Pereira FR, Sercheli MS, et al. Brain plasticity for verbal and visual memories in patients with mesial temporal lobe epilepsy and hippocampal sclerosis: an fMRI study. Hum Brain Mapp 2013; 34(1):186–99.
10. Barnett AJ, Park MT, Pipitone J, et al. Functional and structural correlates of memory in patients with mesial temporal lobe epilepsy. Front Neurol 2015; 6:103.
11. Detre JA, Maccotta L, King D, et al. Functional MRI lateralization of memory in temporal lobe epilepsy. Neurology 1998;50:926–32.
12. Powell HW, Richardson MP, Symms MR, et al. Preoperative fMRI predicts memory decline following anterior temporal lobe resection. J Neurol Neurosurg Psychiatry 2008;79:686–93.
13. Richardson MP, Strange BA, Thompson PJ, et al. Pre-operative verbal memory fMRI predicts post-operative memory decline after left temporal lobe resection. Brain 2004;127:2419–26.
14. Vannest J, Szaflarski JP, Privitera MD, et al. Medial temporal fMRI activation reflects memory lateralization and memory performance in patients with epilepsy. Epilepsy Behav 2008;12:410–8.
15. Binder JR. Functional MRI is a valid noninvasive alternative to Wada testing. Epilepsy Behav 2011; 20:214–22.
16. Bonelli SB, Thompson PJ, Yogarajah M, et al. Imaging language networks before and after anterior temporal lobe resection: results of a longitudinal fMRI study. Epilepsia 2012;53:639–50.
17. Sabsevitz DS, Swanson SJ, Hammeke TA, et al. Use of preoperative functional neuroimaging to predict language deficits from epilepsy surgery. Neurology 2003;60:1788–92.
18. Szaflarski JP, Gloss D, Binder JR, et al. Practice guideline summary: use of fMRI in the presurgical evaluation of patients with epilepsy: report of the Guideline Development, Dissemination, and Implementation Subcommittee of the American Academy of Neurology. Neurology 2017;88:395–402.
19. Binder JR, Swanson SJ, Sabsevitz DS, et al. A comparison of two fMRI methods for predicting verbal memory decline after left temporal lobectomy: language lateralization versus hippocampal activation asymmetry. Epilepsia 2010;51: 618–26.
20. Westmacott R, Silver FL, McAndrews MP. Understanding medial temporal activation in memory tasks: evidence from fMRI of encoding and recognition in a case of transient global amnesia. Hippocampus 2008;18:317–25.
21. Barnett AJ, Marty-Dugas J, McAndrews MP. Advantages of sentence-level fMRI language tasks in presurgical language mapping for temporal lobe epilepsy. Epilepsy Behav 2014;32:114–20.
22. Towgood K, Barker GJ, Caceres A, et al. Bringing memory fMRI to the clinic: comparison of seven memory fMRI protocols in temporal lobe epilepsy. Hum Brain Mapp 2015;36:1595–608.
23. McAndrews MP. Memory assessment in the clinical context using functional magnetic resonance imaging: a critical look at the state of the field. Neuroimaging Clin N Am 2014;24:585–97.
24. McDermott KB, Szpunar KK, Christ SE. Laboratory-based and autobiographical retrieval tasks differ substantially in their neural substrates. Neuropsychologia 2009;47:2290–8.
25. Rugg MD, Vilberg KL. Brain networks underlying episodic memory retrieval. Curr Opin Neurobiol 2013;23:255–60.

26. Frings L, Schulze-Bonhage A, Spreer J, et al. Reduced interhemispheric hippocampal BOLD signal coupling related to early epilepsy onset. Seizure 2009;18:153–7.

27. James GA, Tripathi SP, Ojemann JG, et al. Diminished default mode network recruitment of the hippocampus and parahippocampus in temporal lobe epilepsy. J Neurosurg 2013;119:288–300.

28. Voets NL, Adcock JE, Stacey R, et al. Functional and structural changes in the memory network associated with left temporal lobe epilepsy. Hum Brain Mapp 2009;30:4070–81.

29. Zhang Z, Lu G, Zhong Y, et al. Altered spontaneous neuronal activity of the default-mode network in mesial temporal lobe epilepsy. Brain Res 2010; 1323:152–60.

30. McCormick C, Quraan M, Cohn M, et al. Default mode network connectivity indicates episodic memory capacity in mesial temporal lobe epilepsy. Epilepsia 2013;54:809–18.

31. McCormick C, Protzner AB, Barnett AJ, et al. Linking DMN connectivity to episodic memory capacity: what can we learn from patients with medial temporal lobe damage? Neuroimage Clin 2014;5:188–96.

32. Addis DR, Moscovitch M, McAndrews MP. Consequences of hippocampal damage across the autobiographical memory network in left temporal lobe epilepsy. Brain 2007;130:2327–42.

33. Voets NL, Beckmann CF, Cole DM, et al. Structural substrates for resting network disruption in temporal lobe epilepsy. Brain 2012;135:2350–7.

34. Voets NL, Menke RA, Jbabdi S, et al. Thalamocortical disruption contributes to short-term memory deficits in patients with medial temporal lobe damage. Cereb Cortex 2015;25:4584–95.

35. Voets NL, Zamboni G, Stokes MG, et al. Aberrant functional connectivity in dissociable hippocampal networks is associated with deficits in memory. J Neurosci 2014;34:4920–8.

36. Holmes M, Folley BS, Sonmezturk HH, et al. Resting state functional connectivity of the hippocampus associated with neurocognitive function in left temporal lobe epilepsy. Hum Brain Mapp 2014;35:735–44.

37. Doucet G, Osipowicz K, Sharan A, et al. Extratemporal functional connectivity impairments at rest are related to memory performance in mesial temporal epilepsy. Hum Brain Mapp 2013;34:2202–16.

38. Babb TL, Lieb JP, Brown WJ, et al. Distribution of pyramidal cell density and hyperexcitability in the epileptic human hippocampal formation. Epilepsia 1984;25:721–8.

39. Thom M, Sisodiya SM, Beckett A, et al. Cytoarchitectural abnormalities in hippocampal sclerosis. J Neuropathol Exp Neurol 2002;61:510–9.

40. Woermann FG, Barker GJ, Birnie KD, et al. Regional changes in hippocampal T2 relaxation and volume: a quantitative magnetic resonance imaging study of hippocampal sclerosis. J Neurol Neurosurg Psychiatry 1998;65:656–64.

41. Babb TL, Brown WJ, Pretorius J, et al. Temporal lobe volumetric cell densities in temporal lobe epilepsy. Epilepsia 1984;25:729–40.

42. Kahn I, Andrews-Hanna JR, Vincent JL, et al. Distinct cortical anatomy linked to subregions of the medial temporal lobe revealed by intrinsic functional connectivity. J Neurophysiol 2008;100: 129–39.

43. Libby LA, Ekstrom AD, Ragland JD, et al. Differential connectivity of perirhinal and parahippocampal cortices within human hippocampal subregions revealed by high-resolution functional imaging. J Neurosci 2012;32:6550–60.

44. Ritchey M, Libby LA, Ranganath C. Cortico-hippocampal systems involved in memory and cognition: the PMAT framework. Prog Brain Res 2015; 219:45–64.

45. Poppenk J, Evensmoen HR, Moscovitch M, et al. Long-axis specialization of the human hippocampus. Trends Cogn Sci 2013;17:230–40.

46. Kim H. Encoding and retrieval along the long axis of the hippocampus and their relationships with dorsal attention and default mode networks: the HERNET model. Hippocampus 2015;25:500–10.

47. Adnan A, Barnett A, Moayedi M, et al. Distinct hippocampal functional networks revealed by tractography-based parcellation. Brain Struct Funct 2016;221:2999–3012.

48. McCormick C, St-Laurent M, Ty A, et al. Functional and effective hippocampal-neocortical connectivity during construction and elaboration of autobiographical memory retrieval. Cereb Cortex 2015;25: 1297–305.

49. Honey CJ, Kotter R, Breakspear M, et al. Network structure of cerebral cortex shapes functional connectivity on multiple time scales. Proc Natl Acad Sci U S A 2007;104:10240–5.

50. Sporns O. The human connectome: origins and challenges. Neuroimage 2013;80:53–61.

51. Price CJ. The anatomy of language: a review of 100 fMRI studies published in 2009. Ann N Y Acad Sci 2010;1191(1):62–88.

52. Tie Y, Rigolo L, Norton IH, et al. Defining language networks from resting-state fMRI for surgical planning—a feasibility study. Hum Brain Mapp 2014; 35(3):1018–30.

53. Tomasi D, Volkow ND. Resting functional connectivity of language networks: characterization and reproducibility. Mol Psychiatry 2012;17(8):841–54.

54. Zhu L, Fan Y, Zou Q, et al. Temporal reliability and lateralization of the resting-state language network. PLoS One 2014;9(1):e85880.

55. Tracy JI, Doucet GE. Resting-state functional connectivity in epilepsy: growing relevance for clinical decision making. Curr Opin Neurol 2015;28:158–65.

56. Mitchell RJ, Hacker CD, Breshears JD, et al. A novel data-driven approach to preoperative mapping of functional cortex using resting-state functional magnetic resonance imaging. Neurosurgery 2013;73(6): 969–83.

57. Doucet GE, Pustina D, Skidmore C, et al. Resting-state functional connectivity predicts the strength of hemispheric lateralization for language processing in temporal lobe epilepsy and normals. Hum Brain Mapp 2015;36:288–303.

58. Doucet GE, He X, Sperling MR, et al. From "rest" to language task: task activation selects and prunes from broader resting-state network. Hum Brain Mapp 2017;38(5):2540–52.

59. Waites AB, Briellmann RS, Saling MM, et al. Functional connectivity networks are disrupted in left temporal lobe epilepsy. Ann Neurol 2006;59: 335–43.

60. DeSalvo MN, Tanaka N, Douw L, et al. Resting-state functional MR imaging for determining language laterality in intractable epilepsy. Radiology 2016;281: 264–9.

61. Pravata E, Sestieri C, Mantini D, et al. Functional connectivity MR imaging of the language network in patients with drug-resistant epilepsy. AJNR Am J Neuroradiol 2011;32:532–40.

62. Osipowicz K, Sperling MR, Sharan AD, et al. Functional MRI, resting state fMRI, and DTI for predicting verbal fluency outcome following resective surgery for temporal lobe epilepsy. J Neurosurg 2016;124: 929–37.

63. Doucet GE, Rider R, Taylor N, et al. Presurgery resting-state local graph-theory measures predict neurocognitive outcomes after brain surgery in temporal lobe epilepsy. Epilepsia 2015;56:517–26.

64. Laufs H. Functional imaging of seizures and epilepsy: evolution from zones to networks. Curr Opin Neurol 2012;25:194–200.

65. Liao W, Zhang Z, Pan Z, et al. Default mode network abnormalities in mesial temporal lobe epilepsy: a study combining fMRI and DTI. Hum Brain Mapp 2011;32:883–95.

66. Pittau F, Grova C, Moeller F, et al. Patterns of altered functional connectivity in mesial temporal lobe epilepsy. Epilepsia 2012;53:1013–23.

67. Iannotti GR, Grouiller F, Centeno M, et al. Epileptic networks are strongly connected with and without the effects of interictal discharges. Epilepsia 2016; 57:1086–96.

68. Ridley B, Wirsich J, Bettus G, et al. Simultaneous intracranial EEG-fMRI shows inter-modality correlation in time-resolved connectivity within normal areas but not within epileptic regions. Brain Topogr 2017. [Epub ahead of print].

69. van Graan LA, Lemieux L, Chaudhary UJ. Methods and utility of EEG-fMRI in epilepsy. Quant Imaging Med Surg 2015;5:300–12.

70. Negishi M, Martuzzi R, Novotny EJ, et al. Functional MRI connectivity as a predictor of the surgical outcome of epilepsy. Epilepsia 2011;52:1733–40.

71. Dansereau CL, Bellec P, Lee K, et al. Detection of abnormal resting-state networks in individual patients suffering from focal epilepsy: an initial step toward individual connectivity assessment. Front Neurosci 2014;8:419.

72. Cole MW, Bassett DS, Power JD, et al. Intrinsic and task-evoked network architectures of the human brain. Neuron 2014;83:238–51.

73. Laird AR, Eickhoff SB, Rottschy C, et al. Networks of task co-activations. Neuroimage 2013;80:505–14.

74. Smith SM, Fox PT, Miller KL, et al. Correspondence of the brain's functional architecture during activation and rest. Proc Natl Acad Sci U S A 2009;106: 13040–5.

75. Buckner RL, Krienen FM, Yeo BT. Opportunities and limitations of intrinsic functional connectivity MRI. Nat Neurosci 2013;16:832–7.

76. Campbell KL, Schacter DL. Ageing and the resting state: is cognition obsolete? Lang Cogn Neurosci 2017;32(6):661–8.

77. Davis SW, Stanley ML, Moscovitch M, et al. Resting-state networks do not determine cognitive function networks: a commentary on Campbell and Schacter (2016). Lang Cogn Neurosci 2017;32(6): 669–73.

78. Morcom AM, Fletcher PC. Does the brain have a baseline? Why we should be resisting a rest. Neuroimage 2007;37:1073–82.

79. Tavor I, Parker Jones O, Mars RB, et al. Task-free MRI predicts individual differences in brain activity during task performance. Science 2016;352:216–20.

80. Parker Jones O, Voets NL, Adcock JE, et al. Resting connectivity predicts task activation in pre-surgical populations. Neuroimage Clin 2017;13:378–85.

81. Brandt DJ, Sommer J, Krach S, et al. Test-retest reliability of fMRI brain activity during memory encoding. Front Psychiatry 2013;4:163.

82. Clement F, Belleville S. Test-retest reliability of fMRI verbal episodic memory paradigms in healthy older adults and in persons with mild cognitive impairment. Hum Brain Mapp 2009;30:4033–47.

83. Shehzad Z, Kelly AM, Reiss PT, et al. The resting brain: unconstrained yet reliable. Cereb Cortex 2009;19:2209–29.

84. Zuo XN, Kelly C, Adelstein JS, et al. Reliable intrinsic connectivity networks: test-retest evaluation using ICA and dual regression approach. Neuroimage 2010;49:2163–77.

85. Finn ES, Shen X, Scheinost D, et al. Functional connectome fingerprinting: identifying individuals using patterns of brain connectivity. Nat Neurosci 2015;18: 1664–71.

86. Birn RM, Molloy EK, Patriat R, et al. The effect of scan length on the reliability of resting-state

fMRI connectivity estimates. Neuroimage 2013; 83:550–8.

87. Song J, Desphande AS, Meier TB, et al. Age-related differences in test-retest reliability in resting-state brain functional connectivity. PLoS One 2012;7: e49847.

88. Power JD, Barnes KA, Snyder AZ, et al. Spurious but systematic correlations in functional connectivity MRI networks arise from subject motion. Neuroimage 2012;59:2142–54.

89. Van Dijk KR, Sabuncu MR, Buckner RL. The influence of head motion on intrinsic functional connectivity MRI. Neuroimage 2012;59:431–8.

90. Gomez-Gonzalo M, Losi G, Brondi M, et al. Ictal but not interictal epileptic discharges activate astrocyte endfeet and elicit cerebral arteriole responses. Front Cell Neurosci 2011;5:8.

91. Marchi N, Lerner-Natoli M. Cerebrovascular remodeling and epilepsy. Neuroscientist 2013;19: 304–12.

92. Wandschneider B, Burdett J, Townsend L, et al. Effect of topiramate and zonisamide on fMRI cognitive networks. Neurology 2017;88(12):1165–71.

93. Yasuda CL, Centeno M, Vollmar C, et al. The effect of topiramate on cognitive fMRI. Epilepsy Res 2013;105:250–5.

Applications of Resting State Functional MR Imaging to Neuropsychiatric Diseases

Godfrey David Pearlson, MD[a,b,c,*]

KEYWORDS

- Neuropsychiatry • Resting state • Default mode • Functional MR imaging • Alzheimer
- Psychosis

KEY POINTS

- Numerous brain networks (eg, default mode network) normally communicate with each other constantly, and these functional communication patterns are often disrupted in association with numerous neuropsychiatric disorders.
- Resting state functional MR imaging is a quick, noninvasive, and convenient approach to explore these functional brain abnormalities in a quantitative manner.
- The resulting patterns of disruption are useful in a research context, but do not constitute unique "fingerprints" of diseases and are not yet practical for use in making diagnoses in individual patients.
- Care must be taken in gathering and analyzing resting state functional MR imaging data; there are numerous potential caveats and confounds, including head movement and other disease-associated but irrelevant sources of noise that can interfere with interpretation of results.

INTRODUCTION

The presence of spontaneous, slow, fluctuating, and temporally correlated activity in functional MR imaging (fMR imaging) time series, in addition to that observed during performance of specific tasks, was first mentioned in 1993 by Ogawa and colleagues.[1] It was realized subsequently that such resting activity, for example, occurring between the motor cortices of the 2 hemispheres, could yield informative connectivity data.[2] Later, similar resting activity was observed in visual and auditory cortices. More recently, functional connectivity (FC) was demonstrated within the brain's default mode network (DMN).[3] The DMN is a group of brain regions that manifests relatively higher levels of activity in the absence of goal-directed cognition.[4] Conversely, so-called task positive networks (TPNs) are active during task performance. TPNs' activities are anticorrelated with those of the DMN. Commonly identified TPNs include a cingulo-opercular network mediating cognitive set maintenance[5] and a fronto-parietal network involved in behavioral initiation and guidance. Additional "intrinsic connectivity networks" (ICNs)[6] subsume primary sensory and higher order association cortex; all are active to various degrees in states of both rest and cognitive

Disclosure Statement: The author has nothing to disclose.
a Department of Psychiatry, Yale University School of Medicine, New Haven, CT, USA; b Department of Neuroscience, Yale University School of Medicine, New Haven, CT, USA; c Olin Neuropsychiatry Research Center, Institute of Living, 200 Retreat Avenue, Hartford, CT 06106, USA
* Olin Neuropsychiatry Research Center, Institute of Living, 200 Retreat Avenue, Hartford, CT 06106.
E-mail address: godfrey.pearlson@yale.edu

neuroimaging.theclinics.com

engagement.[7] It is generally accepted that ICNs have functional relevance and are related to persisting individual differences such as temperament[8] and intelligence.[9]

Currently, resting state fMR imaging (RS fMR imaging) data are widely used by multiple researchers because they are relatively simple and easy to acquire, particularly in neuropsychiatrically (NP) impaired populations, because this approach requires minimal subject cooperation or alertness, is not effortful, and does not necessitate cognitive engagement with a task, as summarized in **Table 1**. Also, the DMN is examined most frequently in RS studies, because it is readily identifiable, but multiple intrinsic networks are also present at rest and may be relevant depending on context. Another advantage of RS data is that they are relatively straightforward to analyze, whether data driven or by seed-based analysis.

At rest, brain activity fluctuates slowly at frequencies less than 0.1 Hz, as straightforwardly demonstrable by analysis of RS fMR imaging. This activity is synchronized and coherent across brain regions in multiple reproducible circuits/networks termed variously as resting state networks (RSNs), ICNs, and so forth. These patterns of resting brain activity are conserved across the mammalian kingdom[10] with clear analogues being evident, for example, even in mice. From one perspective, the term "resting state" is a misnomer, because brain modules always remain active and functionally connected. RSNs manifest predictable age-related developmental and aging-related alterations,[11] and characteristic patterns with different levels of consciousness from coma to sleep and drowsiness to rest, and are modulated in the context of cognitive task-related behaviors.[12]

To expand on some of the above themes, spontaneously occurring, temporally synchronized spatially distributed, low-frequency signal fluctuations that reveal ICNs are measured in absence of an explicit or structured task. An entire "family" of ICNs exists, including the default mode, simple sensory-motor networks (visual, auditory, motor), and cognitively related (executive, salience, dorsal attention) networks that "lurk" in the background in absence of a task, but become prominent with task performance even as DMN activity is usually suppressed.[13] DMN has key nodes in medial prefrontal cortex, midline posterior cingulate cortex, precuneus and mesial temporal regions, including parahippocampal gyrus.[14] Some studies mention specifically inferior parietal lobule and anterior cingulate cortex (ACC).

It is useful to pose the question of why the DMN is so persistently present. In terms of its importance, DMN is conserved across the mammalian kingdom, for example, in awake and anesthetized rats[15] and monkeys,[10,16] is present in preterm infants,[11,17,18] and persists despite coma[19] and locked-in syndrome. Network activity can be altered by manipulating the level of consciousness with anesthesia.[20,21] It has been stated that the "…ability to efficiently integrate localized neuronal processing across widely distributed functionally-specialized brain regions in the service of complex cognition and behavioral control is characteristic of mature neural systems."[22] Functional RS activity is related to structural white matter connections, suggesting a generally linked structural functional underpinning to brain connectivity.[2] For example, direct comparisons between FC measured with RS temporal correlations and white matter anatomic connectivity quantified using diffusion tensor imaging (DTI) tractography show

Table 1
Utility of resting state functional MR imaging studies in neuropsychiatric illness

Advantage	Corresponding Disadvantage
Acquisition simple, quick, convenient	
Replicable brain BOLD patterns	Less replicable outside of core circuitry
Requires no cognitive effort on part of patient	Lack of cognitive referent: unable to "interrogate" brain, therefore unstandardized
Allows study of infants/children, drowsy/comatose, cognitively impaired hallucinated, and elderly individuals	
Analysis relatively straightforward	
Design simple enough to allow comparison across different studies	
Sensitive method	Equally sensitive to multiple confounds, as listed in Table 2

significant agreement, clearly so for the DMN.[23] This densely interconnected brain wiring plan is termed the "connectome,"[24] a concept that subsumes both underlying physical/structural connections and related functional interactions.[25] Logically, this arrangement is an efficient means to tie together diverse brain regions into circuits and to mesh them together into ordered, connected subsystems. These latter can call on a variety of similar, more distant modules in a flexible manner to serve the ever-changing needs of cognition.

On the one hand, the DMN activity that emerges from this brain organization seems to be a fundamental part of normal cerebral function. On the other hand, because it is evident in rats and during coma, it may be a conceptual overinterpretation to ascribe such higher-level functions to it as planning the future and self-reflection,[26] as is commonly done. One alternative "sentinel" hypothesis is that DMN mediates a general environmental monitoring for unexpected/salient events.[27] Buckner[28] and others[29] hypothesize alternatively that the major function of the DMN "is to support internal mental simulations that are used adaptively."[28] This latter idea is attractive because many NP disorders are characterized by disruptions to such internal simulations. Together with the straightforwardness of collecting RS data, this association has encouraged multiple investigators to examine DMN in multiple neurocognitive conditions.

As mentioned above, to some extent these functional patterns are dependent on hard-wired structural connections of the sort measured by DTI.[30] Where there are measurable differences in structural connectivity, one can examine to what extent these are accompanied by RS FC differences[30] and vice versa. The combination of measures may be more useful than either alone. Similarly, additional, potentially useful information is derived when RS data are used in conjunction with task-based fMR imaging assessments.

Useful RS fMR imaging data can be acquired quickly, typically in 5 to 7 minutes, especially when using multiband sequences.[31] Preprocessing approaches of the information gathered are generally similar to those used for conventional task-based fMR imaging. As noted in Table 1, RS data are quickly and straightforwardly gathered,[32] making this approach attractive in individuals with cognitive compromise, short attention spans, claustrophobia, compromised consciousness (coma, delirium), while being relatively stable within and across scan sessions.[33]

A useful recent general review of the RS field is that of Stevens,[22] who emphasizes that measurement of brain regional coactivation (ie, FC) is a statistical relationship showing that neural activation levels in spatially diverse brain regions are associated in the time dimension.[34] Following preprocessing, FC can be measured using multiple analytical techniques[32] (seed-based and independent component analysis are often used), and methods are generally convergent with regard to results.[35] Independent component analysis (ICA) has the attraction of identifying and potentially removing at least some head motion–induced artifacts. FC is generally assumed to represent neuronal communication across brain modules. "Effective connectivity" additionally allows claims about the causal effect that activity in one brain region has on a different region.[36]

RS FC is never an uncontaminated measure of brain connectivity; for example, MR imaging scanner acoustic noise, random cognition during the scan, bodily sensations, anxiety, eyes open versus closed,[37] and other factors all modulate the resulting FC data.

After region-to-region connectivity has been assessed from the above methods, graph-theoretical (GT) methods[38–40] provide additional information on network organization, essentially by considering all of the brain as one interconnected network. Typical indices are strength of linear correlation among nodes (defined as functionally similar brain regions) or distances between nodes. GT can also reveal how nodes are arranged topologically into subnetworks (modularity), the extent to which they belong to more local modular communities, whether they form hubs by connecting with numerous other modules as well as with other networks, and metrics of their path lengths.[38,41–43] GT also introduced terminology such as "small world architecture" that highlights efficiency of information transfer within/among networks.[44]

Despite the many advantages of information obtained from RS data, there need to be many cautions in collecting and interpreting this information. These cautions are summarized in Table 2, and some are discussed in detail later. A particular issue to pay attention to is that patients may show different DMN activity from control groups[28,45–50] in terms of coherence, spatial extent, relative magnitude of ICNs due to diverse factors that are epiphenomena of the illness under consideration related to treatment, lifestyle, demographic, and cognitive features.[51,52] Some of these specifics include medication, sleep[53,54] (one reason to acquire RS data with the subjects eyes open is to maximize the chance that subjects are awake during data-gathering acquisition, with consequently stronger temporal BOLD signal).[35] Physiologic variables such as breathing and cardiac rate[55,56] can

Table 2
Problems and pitfalls of resting state functional MR imaging studies in neuropsychiatric patients

Problem	Result	Suggested Solutions
NP patients more likely to move during image acquisition	Movement misinterpreted as actual activation	ICA to remove artifact image series, scrubbing
NP patients more likely to use substances, including recreational drugs, caffeine, nicotine	Confounding change in RS activity	Screen for substance control access to nicotine & caffeine
Disease-associated confounds: altered sleep, physical activity, BMI, breathing & cardiac rates medication treatment	Confounding change in RS activity	Pick analogous control group measure confound & covary
NP-associated elevated stress & corticosteroid levels	Confounding change in RS activity	Measure and covary
Severity of potentially confounding nonprimary disease symptoms, for example, dementia in PD, or nonprimary abused substances in addictions (eg, comorbid opioids in alcoholism)	Confounding changes in RS activity	Measure and covary; assess comparison study group with pure secondary issue, for example, pure opioid users
Unstandardized acquisition conditions, for example, eyes open vs closed, not checking if subject is asleep	Alters RS activity	Standardize acquisition conditions

Abbreviation: BMI, body mass index.

affect data, for example, a shared blood supply between different brain regions may falsely suggest shared variance in RS FC. A theoretic issue is the appropriate false positive rate control[57] to determine multiple comparison corrections. Dealing with global signal is another issue.[58]

A particularly insidious confound is that of head motion in the scanner, even small degrees of which produce signal artifacts that simultaneously exaggerate calculations of connectivity estimates for nearby voxels and decrease them for distant ones.[59–61] The bottom line is that RS connectivity estimates are typically both lower and inaccurate in neuropsychiatric populations and that a series of reports in these populations have had to be reconsidered.[59,62] Going forward, issues dealt with in Table 2 need to be carefully taken into account in study design and dealt with explicitly in the resulting reports.

Although clearly very important, the issue of study-related confounds may have been exaggerated by some. For example, it has been argued that because "it is unimaginable that… (patients with neuropsychiatric disorders) ….experience the MRI environment analogously to a paid healthy volunteer… will interfere with the so-called default pattern or with engagement of other so-called network profiles, producing a degree of 'abnormality'."[45] The author thinks this argument misses the

point however, because it is precisely because individuals with NP disorders do likely experience the scanner environment in different ways whether through paranoia, anxiety, aberrant sensory processing, and so forth, that these differences in and of themselves may produce characteristic illness-related patterns that differ from those of healthy volunteers, may be diagnostically useful, and thus constitute important signal rather than noise.

Thus, on the one hand, although it is extremely important to control for potential artifacts, especially head motion, it is equally important not to "throw out the baby with the bathwater." One useful validating approach with psychotic disorders, because these are heritable and familial, has been to treat neuroimaging differences from healthy controls as endophenotypes and to explore their occurrence in unaffected first-degree relatives.[63] On the other hand, a relative lack of specificity of DMN abnormalities among different NP disorders definitely interferes with the ability to use RS changes in the context of clinical diagnosis. To date, in fact, no RS pattern is yet practical for individual patient diagnostic use.

Although for simplicity's sake, the DMN is most frequently extracted and examined from RS data analysis of resting fMR imaging information, revealing multiple additional circuits, ICNs, some of which are involved in key aspects of cognitive processing, nevertheless are invariably present in the background at rest and therefore are amenable to analysis. Resting data have been demonstrated to correlate with both task-related behavioral performance and activation in task-associated brain regions.[64,65] Disease-related abnormalities often affect relationships within and among multiple ICNs, not just within the DMN. ICA is one convenient means of identifying ICNs. Using ICA-derived components, one can examine not only correlational relationships within distinct components (FC) but also such relationships pairwise across separate components (functional network connectivity; FNC). Some of the key questions that can be usefully posed for a particular disorder are shown in Box 1. Because this brief review is not meant to be exhaustive, and RS data have been used to examine literally dozens of NP disorders, in the later discussion, several disease states are focused on that have been most commonly considered in the literature.

ALZHEIMER DISEASE AND ITS PRECURSOR, AMNESTIC MILD COGNITIVE IMPAIRMENT

Typical, late life–onset Alzheimer disease (AD) is usually first identified and subsequently studied by cognitive symptoms, usually beginning with short-term memory deficits and gradually progressing to involve all cognitive functions and to interfere with activities of daily living. By the time that initial amnestic symptoms are apparent, the early clinical phase designated as amnestic mild cognitive impairment (MCI), the underlying pathologic process has likely existed for many years and has already crossed a critical threshold to allow symptomatic expression. In studying AD evolution, the ideal design is to have longitudinal studies of healthy individuals or those at increased risk. This arrangement allows for correlation of emerging early symptoms with associated brain changes. For the latter, MCI is useful but limited in that only a proportion of cases eventually evolve to the more severe state of AD. Furthermore, not all studies in the literature specify that they were studying the amnestic form of MCI that is the most relevant precursor of AD. Because the key underlying abnormality of AD is known, and its anatomic distribution affects key DMN hubs as detailed in later discussion, the disorder is especially suited for RS studies, and in some ways is the prototypical NP disorder to study with this approach. In addition, AD is relatively prevalent and can be identified clinically with reasonable accuracy, and much is known about the location and progression of the putative primary pathologic disease indicators, that is, specific regional beta-amyloid and tau deposition, that can now be quantified using PET in vivo.

Krajcovicova and colleagues[66] summarize several hundred studies of resting connectivity in patients with AD and MCI. Most focus on the DMN. Although there is now much useful evidence, the field still requires more information, especially on longitudinal relationships between RS DMN connectivity, PET amyloid measures of the presumed underlying primary abnormality, PET regional glucose metabolism, and clinical cognitive assessments as well as structural MR imaging brain biomarkers, such as age and sex normed percentile hippocampal volume. A useful review exploring the relationship with AD pathogenesis is

---

Box 1
A general format for considering resting state functional MR imaging changes associated with NP disorders

What are the disease-associated changes?

Sample size and effect sizes?

How reproducible are they, within and across subjects?

To what extent are the reported changes within (FC) and among (FNC) ICNs/RSNs associated or correlated with known structural differences on neuroimaging, neuropathology, or etiologic factors where these processes are well recognized?

To what extent are the changes cross-validated by functional abnormalities measured using different technologies, for example, magneto encephalography?

How specific are they to the disorder, for example, various psychotic disorders or dementias

Are the changes related to severity of typical symptoms or deficits characteristic of the disorder?

How confident can we be that reported changes are not an epiphenomenon of associated factors and behaviors that typically differ between NP and healthy control groups[16,26–31] in terms of spatial extent, relative prominence, and coherence of ICNs (see Table 2 for a list of such confounding associated factors)

included in the article by Simic and colleagues.[67] Some factors that need to be taken into account in studying this disorder are that the FC of the DMN diminishes with normal aging. Typically, there is a gradual decrease in task-induced deactivation in posterior cingulate cortex (PCC),[68] partially correlated with age-related cognitive changes, but occurring within substantially intact neural circuits. This relationship survives when corrected for gray matter volume loss.[69]

The most consistent finding in mild AD and MCI is decreased DMN FC, particularly evident in PCC and precuneus and in hippocampus/parahippocampal gyrus along with DMN connectivity to other brain circuits.[70,71] This result survives correction for gray matter reductions.[72] These changes correlate with the severity/progression of dementia.[73] Some reports document longitudinal alterations, for example, increases in frontal cortical connectivity that may be compensatory for the underlying abnormality, but that decline over time as the disease progresses.

One interesting set of relationships emerging from these investigations is that amyloid beta is deposited in DMN hub regions early in the pathogenesis of AD as documented by PET studies.[74] Higher PET amyloid plaque loads correlate with reduced FC measures of parietal cortex with all other brain voxels, as assessed by RS fMR imaging graph theory global centrality measures.[75] In the AD prodrome, amyloid plaque spatial distribution is also likely related to RS network FC.[76] As the disease progresses, RS abnormalities certainly extend beyond the DMN.[71]

Why key DMN areas seem especially affected by AD may be explained by the above, and various hypotheses have sought to unearth the pathologic basis for this. For example, dominant early-onset types of AD show very early DMN RS changes,[77] and DMN regions have very high aerobic glycolysis rates.[78] Also, default mode cortical hubs suffer high deposition of amyloid beta in AD, suggesting that DMN neurons may be affected by activity-dependent amyloid precursor protein processing that interacts with glutamate projection neurons.[67,79-81] Many core DMN regions are substantially involved in AD pathologic changes and manifest reduced glucose metabolism in early AD.

Pan and colleagues[82] performed a meta-analysis of 14 data sets from 12 studies that indicated that patients with amnestic MCI compared with healthy controls using a seed-based approach showed reduced amplitude of low-frequency fluctuations (ALFF) in bilateral precuneus/posterior cingulate, frontal-insular cortex, left occipital temporal cortex, and right supramarginal gyrus, and increased ALFF in right lingual gyrus, left middle occipital gyrus, left

hippocampus, and inferior temporal gyrus. Overall MCI was associated with widespread regional changes in resting brain activity, predominantly involving the DMN, salience, and visual networks. These data are generally supported by prior investigations, and by other meta-analyses of task-based studies.[83]

There is evidence for changes in the salience and central executive networks associated with MCI and AD in addition, for example, as summarized by Joo and colleagues.[84] Teipel and colleagues[85] summarize studies of cortical connectivity in AD across RS fMR imaging, electroencephalogram rhythms, and DTI-defined white matter bundles that explored interrelationships between different forms of brain connectivity. These studies can be revealing; for example Patel and colleagues[86] found no cognitive or white matter fractional anisotropy differences between 14 carriers and 22 noncarriers of ApoE4, but decreased FC in DMN regions previously implicated in AD on FC, suggesting that functional changes precede white matter structural abnormalities in these at-risk individuals.

Cortical connectivity in AD has sometimes been described as brain neural network abnormality.[81] For example, He and others[79,87,88] have adopted network analytical approaches to study AD and report that the disease is associated with disruption of normal global functional organization affecting not only local connectivity but also specialized hub nodes and important long-distance connections. Other graph theory–based investigations show altered overall network topology in AD consistent with increased randomness (greater path length and reduced clustering coefficient fitting a model of disrupted global information integration.[89] Wang and colleagues[90] reported reduced connectivity of the posterior DMN and executive control network in cognitively normal individuals carrying the ApoE4 allele. DMN connectivity is reported to be increased following treatment with cholinesterase inhibitor medications.[91-93]

A review of both cross-sectional and longitudinal papers in patients with MCI and mild AD compared with controls shows general agreement that these conditions manifest a reduced correlation of RS BOLD activity across several intrinsic brain circuits, including the DMN and attention-related networks. This finding contrasts with meta-analyses of task-based activation, where BOLD decreases occur mainly in frontoparietal and DMNs in MCI, whereas AD patients show reduced voxel activation in the visual network. Li and colleagues[83] and Sohn and colleagues[94] suggest that hippocampal over activation in amnestic MCI might represent compensatory processes, whereas other investigators have ascribed similar functions to DMN and various cognitive networks.

Key questions remaining in AD include elucidating the relationship between FC differences and symptoms cross-sectionally in amnestic MCI. Preliminary evidence suggests that FC in the DM and especially its posterior anatomy is disrupted in association with memory impairment in MCI and AD.[95] It is unclear to what extent RS fMR imaging patterns can be used to correctly diagnose MCI/AD, and what is the most useful adjunctive diagnostic information from other imaging modalities or other biomarkers such as cerebrospinal fluid measures. Clarification is also needed in terms of useful RS data in predicting future clinical course, from either MCI to AD or cognitive deterioration in the disorder at any stage. These questions are addressed in various reviews by Koch and colleagues,[96] Dai and colleagues,[97] and Zhang and colleagues.[73] DMN disconnection might predict conversion from amnestic MCI for example,[98] or show utility as an imaging marker to monitor progression.[99] The role of DMN changes in early AD/MCI needs to be further clarified in terms of how primary this is as a pathologic event.

The consistency between the known neuropathology of amnestic MCI/AD, regarding its distribution and evolution with disease progression, and corresponding resting brain activity changes provide some confidence for the use of RS activity in other conditions where the neuropathology or underlying disease neurobiology is less clear.

PARKINSON DISEASE

This disorder is characterized clinically by symptoms related to nigrostriatal motor system dysregulation, including motor slowing, difficulties in initiating movement, a characteristic tremor, and muscular rigidity. As in AD, much of the underlying abnormality of Parkinson disease (PD) is known, consisting here of dopamine neuronal loss in the substantia nigra pars compacta. Also, analogous to AD, by the time clinical symptoms are manifest, there has already been significant neuronal diminution.

Several studies have examined PD using RS fMR imaging[100]; plus, see reviews of Tahmasian and colleagues[101] and Muller-Oehring and colleagues.[102] In PD patients with significant tremor, movement artifact is an obvious problem.

Striatal neurons normally directly influence activity in DMN,[103] and FC decreases plus other abnormalities in that network have been documented in PD.[104,105] Because accessory symptoms, such as cognitive disturbances including dementia or visual hallucinations, can occur in some, but not all PD patients, it is important to note which studies have carefully classified PD patients by the presence or absence of such symptoms, because their presence may be associated with additional RS abnormalities. Several investigations specifically looked for RS alterations associated with symptoms, such as specific cognitive disturbance,[106] dementia,[107] and visual hallucinations.[108,109] One interesting observation is that FC between the DMN and the central executive network appears to be disrupted in PD,[104] perhaps in association with the above-mentioned cognitive symptoms. Under normal circumstances, activity in the substantia nigra and central executive network circuits is significantly positively correlated, perhaps to facilitate DMN suppression during executive circuit activation. This positive connectivity is significantly diminished in PD[104] in a manner that correlates with clinical severity. Other studies have looked carefully at treatment effects[101,110] using RS approaches. A small-scale longitudinal treatment study reported that DMN alterations were correlated with levodopa-induced clinical improvements, but that was during the course of a provocative task (face recognition).[111] A larger scale study with an RS design would be interesting to confirm and extend the original observation. The above studies highlight the importance of careful clinical descriptions of patients with a rather varied symptomatic profile and controlling for symptom status as well as for possible treatment confounds. Because both longitudinal evolution of symptoms in PD and treatment response vary considerably, the use of RS studies early in the course of disease, in terms of documenting utility as a biological marker, would be relevant to explore.

COMA

DMN activity diminishes as subjects are compared across normal consciousness, minimally conscious, vegetative state, with brain death.[112,113] DMN appears normal in cognitively normal individuals with locked-in-state.[19]

PSYCHOTIC ILLNESSES INCLUDING PSYCHOTIC BIPOLAR DISORDER

Compared with better-characterized pathologic conditions such as PD and AD, psychosis is clearly a collection of brain-based disorders, although the underlying pathophysiology remains unclear. However, a leading hypothesis is that psychosis is related to a disconnection of cortical circuits that becomes particularly prominent in late adolescence and early adult life.[114] Because of the widespread and numerous neurophysiologic abnormalities associated with schizophrenia and other psychotic disorders that likely involve apparent communication among numerous brain networks, independent component analysis-based approaches are often favored because they allow straightforward interrogation of data both within and between such networks. Although the first report of disrupted DMN activity in schizophrenia was derived from a task-based study,[115] reports of similar abnormalities derived from RS studies followed shortly thereafter, confirming the association with positive psychotic symptoms such as hallucinations.[116] Multiple publications have appeared subsequently, with some exploring the specificity of findings to schizophrenia as opposed to schizo-affective disorder and psychotic bipolar disorder from the Bipolar-Schizophrenia Network on Intermediate Phenotypes (BSNIP) consortium. As reviewed by Narr and Leaver,[117] connectomic studies of schizophrenia generally agree in showing distributed network alterations, particularly those using computational analyses separating the brain into functional nodes, and offering support for the disconnection hypothesis of psychosis.

Because psychotic illnesses typically begin during late adolescence and immediately thereafter, there is an intersection between RS FC MR imaging research and the study of normal adolescent development, with studies that track emerging psychosis in high-risk populations. A review of studies examining the onset of psychosis during the transition from the precursor prodromal state in schizophrenia is accompanied not only by progressive gray matter abnormalities but also by the emergence of anomalous FC patterns similar to those seen in more chronically ill individuals with the disorder.[118] The same investigators review abnormal FC in a prefrontal-thalamic network among clinical high risk for psychosis individuals in the North American Prodromal Longitudinal Study; subjects with the most pronounced abnormalities were most likely to show subsequent conversion to psychosis. The utility of such functional changes in predicting converting to psychosis for individuals has yet to be established.

Satterthwaite and Baker[114] make the important point that emergence of the typical late adolescent developmental trend toward segregation of large-scale brain association networks from the usual prior less organized state fails to occur in individuals developing psychotic illnesses, placing the disconnection hypothesis in a developmental context.

Novel Analyses

Some recent advances in analyzing RS activity in psychosis include dynamic connectivity approaches,[119,120] group information-guided independent component analysis,[121] and inclusion of low-frequency fluctuation measures such as ALFF/fractional ALFF.[122] Sometimes these are coupled with machine learning approaches.[121] To provide examples of the above, one recent refinement on RS analyses is the use of a "chronnectome" measure to better characterize activity variation in the time domain. Rather than averaging RS activity across the entire scan acquisition period, such dynamic connectivity approaches examine time-varying dynamic activity, using for example sliding time window methods. Such analyses can identify discrete FC states, the connectivity strength with-in each state, the amount of time (dwell time) spent within each state, and the transition times between them. Using such an approach, Du and colleagues[120] were able to demonstrate that schizophrenia patients spent more time in the states with nodes sparsely connected and exhibited weaker connectivity strength within each state, lower average values for node strength, clustering coefficient, global, and local efficiency than did healthy controls. These findings are consistent with impaired connectivity among DMN subsystems, with a reduction in the usual prominence for posterior cingulate and anterior medial PFC hubs. An earlier report from the same group[119] compared both schizophrenia and bipolar patients with healthy controls. Both static (average) and dynamic connectivity were examined. Patients made fewer transitions to some dynamic states compared with controls, and differences between the 2 clinical groups were more apparent using the dynamic approach, underlining its utility.

Use of RS measures is potentially problematic in that affected by concomitant prescribed medication as well as other factors that can impact RS measures that are disease-related confounds. Examples are that patients with psychotic disorders are more likely to have concomitant substance abuse problems, to have sleep disruption, or to be less likely to be able to stay still in a scanner, which can have artifactual effects on RS measures. On the other hand, DMN studies are useful in that they require little effort from subjects and do not encounter some of the problems of cognitive-based paradigms, as outlined elsewhere,[32] that are particularly applicable to this subject population.

One consistent result from the multisite BSNIP-1 study (Bipolar/Schizophrenia Network on Intermediate Phenotypes) is that, contrary to expectation, biological markers including RS fMR imaging data are much more similar across the presumed diagnostically distinct syndromes of schizophrenia, psychotic bipolar disorder, and schizoaffective disorder.[63] Many syndromes in psychiatry are diagnosed currently on the basis of cross-sectional symptoms and longitudinal outcome, but are not defined by biological criteria. It was hoped that biological measures such as RS FC would constitute "biomarkers" for these disorders, thus validating diagnostic distinctions as reflected for example in the American Psychiatric Association's Diagnostic and Statistical Manual. Somewhat unexpectedly, however, a series of such measures, including fMR imaging analyses, show many similarities across the 3 syndromes, in addition to several syndrome-specific alterations (for example, see Refs.[63,123]). Meda and colleagues[124] compared schizophrenia and psychotic bipolar probands and their unaffected relatives with healthy controls using ICA to probe spatial aspects of FNC in RSNs. They detected 3 different network pairs that were differentially connected in schizophrenia and psychotic bipolar illness: (a) frontal-occipital, (b) anterior DMN/prefrontal, (c) meso/paralimbic, (d) frontal-temporal/paralimbic, and (e) sensorimotor. The c-e pair was uniquely abnormal in schizophrenia; the c-d pair was uniquely abnormal in psychotic bipolar disorder, whereas the a-b combination was abnormal in both disorders. The paralimbic circuit found in networks c and d, and which uniquely distinguished bipolar probands, contains multiple regions previously identified in mood disorders of several types.

Analyzing the same data set using an ICA-based FC approach, Khadka and colleagues[125] documented abnormalities in 5 network components, 2 of which were unique to schizophrenia (posterior DMN and frontal-occipital), another 2 that were similarly abnormal in both schizophrenia and bipolar disorder (frontal-temporal/paralimbic, and midbrain/cerebellum), as well as 3 networks (frontal-occipital, frontal/thalamic/basal ganglia, and sensorimotor) that were shared by both probands and their relatives. In addition, several of these network abnormalities were related to current symptoms in the patient groups. Lui and colleagues[126] compared a similar diagnostic sample that measured ALFF with regional measures across groups. Schizophrenia and psychotic bipolar disorder probands had reduced activity in orbitofrontal cortex and cingulate gyrus compared with controls as well as with abnormal connectivity within striatal-thalamo-cortical networks. Such abnormalities were greater in schizophrenia, where probands showed more severe and widespread alterations particularly in thalamus

and bilateral parahippocampal gyri. The latter regional difference was related both to positive symptoms in cognitive deficits psychotic bipolar probands had uniquely increased FC between thalamus and bilateral insula.

A separate question that arises is whether psychotic and nonpsychotic bipolar patients differ from each other, and in comparison to patients with schizophrenia and healthy controls. This question was addressed in an analysis by Anticevic and colleagues[127] that examined connectivity in the ventral ACC, which has been linked to regulation of emotional behavior. This FC analysis used a ventral anterior cingulate seed to reveal altered connectivity along the dorsomedial prefrontal surface. Both schizophrenia and psychotic bipolar patients showed regional connectivity reductions, in contradistinction to those bipolar patients without a psychotic history who showed increased coupling compared with healthy controls. Schizophrenia patients and psychotic bipolar subjects were not significantly different from each other, again supporting the idea of commonalities among psychotic illnesses.

A useful review of by Sheffield and Barch[128] concluded that patients with schizophrenia show FC abnormalities in the RS within and between regions comprising the cortical-cerebellar-striatal-thalamic and task-positive and task-negative cortical networks. Furthermore, these FC abnormalities were shared across cognitive domains rather than being uniquely related to any particular type of cognitive impairment. A strong theme that emerged was that the normally strongly anticorrelated task-positive and task-negative functional networks were abnormally connected in schizophrenia, in association with the wide-ranging cognitive deficits frequently seen in schizophrenia patients.

Finally, an article by Meda and colleagues,[129] proceeding from the fact that DMN activity is highly heritable, used parallel independent component analysis to reveal underlying genetic associations of the RS DMN in psychotic bipolar disorder and schizophrenia. The analysis identified 5 subnetworks, each of which was significantly associated with 5 different SNP networks. Analysis of the implicated groups of genes uncovered several highly ranked SNPs that had been previously implicated in psychosis and mood disorder risk. Global enrichment analysis highlighted processes that included NMDA-related long-term potentiation, immune response signaling, axon guidance, and synaptogenesis that significantly influence DMN modulation in these psychotic illnesses.

Because white matter connectivity as revealed by DTI and RS FC is clearly related,[23] combining these 2 measures of brain connectivity provides a more comprehensive description of altered brain connections associated with psychosis. One such analysis revealed a complex picture in schizophrenia, where anatomic connectivity was uniformly decreased, and where FC was lower in the middle temporal gyrus but increased in cingulate and thalamus. Overall, the picture was one of decoupling between structural and FC localized to networks originating in PCC and the task-positive network and one DMN component.[30]

ACUTE DRUG INTOXICATION

Are there characteristic identifying patterns of different drugs or drug classes with regard to FC following acute drug challenges? This type of research is still at an early stage with regard to robust replication, but preliminary indications are that there may be differences in response patterns following acute challenge between drugs as diverse as tetrahydrocannabinol,[130] ketamine,[131] caffeine,[132,133] morphine and alcohol,[134] and nicotine.[135] The latter drug increases connectivity within limbic circuits.[136]

Acute drug challenge studies are particularly liable to artifacts of changes in regional cerebral blood flow (therefore arterial spin labeling is often a useful adjunct), to changes in restlessness, for example, with psychomotor stimulant drugs, cardiac rate (psychostimulants, cannabis), respiratory rate, for example, opioids, or somnolence, for example, benzodiazepines. The optimal design for such studies includes multiple sessions for each subject that are placebo-controlled and that use multiple drug doses together with biological drug-level monitoring.

CHRONIC DRUG AND ALCOHOL ABUSE

Fedota and Stein[136] note that conceptually addiction "is a disease of intercommunicating brain networks" subserving interactions between such domains as reward, learning, affect, and executive control, and thus, a suitable candidate for assessment of RS FC, although many of the above caveats associated with acute drug administration apply here. Heroin users are reported to show reduced RS connectivity in orbitofrontal cortex, thalamus, and cuneus,[137] and cocaine users have reduced bilateral prefrontal connectivity.[138] Ventral and dorsal striatal connectivity differences in cocaine users were reduced after methylphenidate administration.[139] Because nicotine is a widely used legal drug, it can be studied more straightforwardly than many other - substances. Chronic nicotine exposure diminishes network efficiency globally.[136] Nicotine

replacement in abstinent smokers improves patterns in RSN dynamics, along with cognitive withdrawal symptoms.[140] A very large-scale study of several hundred individual smokers showed reduced connectivity in executive and default networks.[141] Using a seed-based approach, Hong and colleagues[142] showed a correlational relationship between increasing severity of nicotine addiction and reduced dorsal ACC/ventral striatal connectivity. In contrast, the same set of experiments indicated that acute nicotine doses increased connectivity in cingulate-cortical circuits but had no effect on the above dorsal ACC/ventral striatal relationship. As pointed out by Fedota and Stein,[136] this may relate to low efficacy of nicotine replacement therapy in many smokers.

In conclusion, RS studies in NP disorders have already provided much useful information, but the field is regarded as being at a relatively preliminary stage and subject to several design issues that set limits on the overall utility.

REFERENCES

1. Ogawa S, Menon RS, Tank DW, et al. Functional brain mapping by blood oxygenation level dependent contrast magnetic resonance imaging. A comparison of signal characteristics with a biophysical model. Biophys J 1993;64(3):803–12.
2. Biswal B, Yetkin FZ, Haughton VM, et al. Functional connectivity in the motor cortex of resting human brain using echo-planar MRI. Magn Reson Med 1995;34(4):537–41.
3. Greicius MD, Krasnow B, Reiss AL, et al. Functional connectivity in the resting brain: a network analysis of the default mode hypothesis. Proc Natl Acad Sci U S A 2003;100(1):253–8.
4. Broyd SJ, Demanuele C, Debener S, et al. Default mode brain dysfunction in mental disorders: a systematic review. Neurosci Biobehav Rev 2009;33(3): 279–96.
5. Dosenbach NU, Fair DA, Miezin FM, et al. Distinct brain networks for adaptive and stable task control in humans. Proc Natl Acad Sci U S A 2007;104(26): 11073–8.
6. Greicius MD, Supekar K, Menon V, et al. Resting state functional connectivity reflects structural connectivity in the default mode network. Cereb Cortex 2009;19(1):72–8.
7. Laird AR, Eickhoff SB, Rottschy C, et al. Networks of task co-activations. Neuroimage 2013;80: 505–14.
8. Aghajani M, Veer IM, van Tol MJ, et al. Neuroticism and extraversion are associated with amygdala resting-state functional connectivity. Cogn Affect Behav Neurosci 2014;14(2):836–48.

9. Cole MW, Ito T, Braver TS. Lateral prefrontal cortex contributes to fluid intelligence through multinetwork connectivity. Brain Connect 2015;5(8):497–504.

10. Vincent JL, Patel GH, Fox MD, et al. Intrinsic functional architecture in the anaesthetized monkey brain. Nature 2007;447(7140):83–6.

11. Doria V, Beckmann CF, Arichi T, et al. Emergence of resting state networks in the preterm human brain. Proc Natl Acad Sci U S A 2010;107(46):20015–20.

12. Smith SM, Fox PT, Miller KL, et al. Correspondence of the brain's functional architecture during activation and rest. Proc Natl Acad Sci U S A 2009; 106(31):13040–5.

13. Raichle ME. The restless brain. Brain Connect 2011;1(1):3–12.

14. Raichle ME, MacLeod AM, Snyder AZ, et al. A default mode of brain function. Proc Natl Acad Sci U S A 2001;98(2):676–82.

15. Lu H, Zou Q, Gu H, et al. Rat brains also have a default mode network. Proc Natl Acad Sci U S A 2012;109(10):3979–84.

16. Belcher AM, Yen CC, Stepp H, et al. Large-scale brain networks in the awake, truly resting marmoset monkey. J Neurosci 2013;33(42):16796–804.

17. Fransson P, Skiold B, Horsch S, et al. Resting-state networks in the infant brain. Proc Natl Acad Sci U S A 2007;104(39):15531–6.

18. Fransson P, Aden U, Blennow M, et al. The functional architecture of the infant brain as revealed by resting-state fMRI. Cereb Cortex 2011;21(1): 145–54.

19. Noirhomme Q, Soddu A, Lehembre R, et al. Brain connectivity in pathological and pharmacological coma. Front Syst Neurosci 2010;4:160.

20. Boveroux P, Vanhaudenhuyse A, Bruno MA, et al. Breakdown of within- and between-network resting state functional magnetic resonance imaging connectivity during propofol-induced loss of consciousness. Anesthesiology 2010;113(5):1038–53.

21. Greicius MD, Kiviniemi V, Tervonen O, et al. Persistent default-mode network connectivity during light sedation. Hum Brain Mapp 2008;29(7):839–47.

22. Stevens MC. The contributions of resting state and task-based functional connectivity studies to our understanding of adolescent brain network maturation. Neurosci Biobehav Rev 2016;70:13–32.

23. Skudlarski P, Jagannathan K, Calhoun VD, et al. Measuring brain connectivity: diffusion tensor imaging validates resting state temporal correlations. Neuroimage 2008;43(3):554–61.

24. Sporns O, Tononi G, Kotter R. The human connectome: a structural description of the human brain. PLoS Comput Biol 2005;1(4):e42.

25. Craddock RC, Tungaraza RL, Milham MP. Connectomics and new approaches for analyzing human brain functional connectivity. Gigascience 2015;4:13.

26. Qin P, Northoff G. How is our self related to midline regions and the default-mode network? Neuroimage 2011;57(3):1221–33.

27. Mevel K, Chetelat G, Eustache F, et al. The default mode network in healthy aging and Alzheimer's disease. Int J Alzheimers Dis 2011;2011:535816.

28. Buckner RL. The brain's default network: origins and implications for the study of psychosis. Dialogues Clin Neurosci 2013;15(3):351–8.

29. Andrews-Hanna JR. The brain's default network and its adaptive role in internal mentation. Neuroscientist 2012;18(3):251–70.

30. Skudlarski P, Jagannathan K, Anderson K, et al. Brain connectivity is not only lower but different in schizophrenia: a combined anatomical and functional approach. Biol Psychiatry 2010;68(1):61–9.

31. Feinberg DA, Moeller S, Smith SM, et al. Multiplexed echo planar imaging for sub-second whole brain FMRI and fast diffusion imaging. PLoS One 2010;5(12):e15710.

32. Pearlson GD, Calhoun VD. Convergent approaches for defining functional imaging endophenotypes in schizophrenia. Front Hum Neurosci 2009;3:37.

33. Damoiseaux JS, Rombouts SA, Barkhof F, et al. Consistent resting-state networks across healthy subjects. Proc Natl Acad Sci U S A 2006;103(37): 13848–53.

34. Friston KJ. Functional and effective connectivity: a review. Brain Connect 2011;1(1):13–36.

35. Van Dijk KR, Hedden T, Venkataraman A, et al. Intrinsic functional connectivity as a tool for human connectomics: theory, properties, and optimization. J Neurophysiol 2010;103(1):297–321.

36. Friston KJ, Price CJ. Generative models, brain function and neuroimaging. Scand J Psychol 2001;42(3):167–77.

37. Yan C, Liu D, He Y, et al. Spontaneous brain activity in the default mode network is sensitive to different resting-state conditions with limited cognitive load. PLoS One 2009;4(5):e5743.

38. Bullmore E, Sporns O. Complex brain networks: graph theoretical analysis of structural and functional systems. Nat Rev Neurosci 2009;10(3): 186–98.

39. Smith SM, Miller KL, Salimi-Khorshidi G, et al. Network modelling methods for FMRI. Neuroimage 2011;54(2):875–91.

40. van den Heuvel MP, Hulshoff Pol HE. Exploring the brain network: a review on resting-state fMRI functional connectivity. Eur Neuropsychopharmacol 2010;20(8):519–34.

41. Sporns O. The human connectome: origins and challenges. Neuroimage 2013;80:53–61.

42. Rubinov M, Sporns O. Complex network measures of brain connectivity: uses and interpretations. Neuroimage 2010;52(3):1059–69.

43. Barkhof F, Haller S, Rombouts SA. Resting-state functional MR imaging: a new window to the brain. Radiology 2014;272(1):29–49.

44. Sporns O, Honey CJ. Small worlds inside big brains. Proc Natl Acad Sci U S A 2006;103(51): 19219–20.

45. Weinberger DR, Radulescu E. Finding the elusive psychiatric "lesion" with 21st-century neuro-anatomy: a note of caution. Am J Psychiatry 2016;173(1):27–33.

46. Morcom AM, Fletcher PC. Does the brain have a baseline? Why we should be resisting a rest. Neuroimage 2007;37(4):1073–82.

47. Rombouts SA, Stam CJ, Kuijer JP, et al. Identifying confounds to increase specificity during a "no task condition". Evidence for hippocampal connectivity using fMRI. Neuroimage 2003;20(2): 1236–45.

48. Khalili-Mahani N, Chang C, van Osch MJ, et al. The impact of "physiological correction" on functional connectivity analysis of pharmacological resting state fMRI. Neuroimage 2013;65:499–510.

49. Cole DM, Smith SM, Beckmann CF. Advances and pitfalls in the analysis and interpretation of resting-state FMRI data. Front Syst Neurosci 2010;4:8.

50. Murphy K, Birn RM, Bandettini PA. Resting-state fMRI confounds and cleanup. Neuroimage 2013; 80:349–59.

51. Smith SM, Nichols TE, Vidaurre D, et al. A positive-negative mode of population covariation links brain connectivity, demographics and behavior. Nat Neurosci 2015;18(11):1565–7.

52. Tavor I, Parker Jones O, Mars RB, et al. Task-free MRI predicts individual differences in brain activity during task performance. Science 2016;352(6282): 216–20.

53. Larson-Prior LJ, Zempel JM, Nolan TS, et al. Cortical network functional connectivity in the descent to sleep. Proc Natl Acad Sci U S A 2009; 106(11):4489–94.

54. Larson-Prior LJ, Power JD, Vincent JL, et al. Modulation of the brain's functional network architecture in the transition from wake to sleep. Prog Brain Res 2011;193:277–94.

55. Birn RM, Diamond JB, Smith MA, et al. Separating respiratory-variation-related fluctuations from neuronal-activity-related fluctuations in fMRI. Neuroimage 2006;31(4):1536–48.

56. Birn RM. The role of physiological noise in resting-state functional connectivity. Neuroimage 2012; 62(2):864–70.

57. Eklund A, Nichols TE, Knutsson H. Cluster failure: why fMRI inferences for spatial extent have inflated false-positive rates. Proc Natl Acad Sci U S A 2016; 113(28):7900–5.

58. Murphy K, Birn RM, Handwerker DA, et al. The impact of global signal regression on resting state correlations: are anti-correlated networks introduced? Neuroimage 2009;44(3):893–905.

59. Power JD, Barnes KA, Snyder AZ, et al. Spurious but systematic correlations in functional connectivity MRI networks arise from subject motion. Neuroimage 2012;59(3):2142–54.

60. Satterthwaite TD, Wolf DH, Loughead J, et al. Impact of in-scanner head motion on multiple measures of functional connectivity: relevance for studies of neurodevelopment in youth. Neuroimage 2012;60(1):623–32.

61. Power JD, Schlaggar BL, Petersen SE. Recent progress and outstanding issues in motion correction in resting state fMRI. Neuroimage 2015;105 536–51.

62. Satterthwaite TD, Wolf DH, Ruparel K, et al. Heterogeneous impact of motion on fundamental patterns of developmental changes in functional connectivity during youth. Neuroimage 2013;83:45–57.

63. Tamminga CA, Pearlson G, Keshavan M, et al. Bipolar and schizophrenia network for intermediate phenotypes: outcomes across the psychosis continuum. Schizophr Bull 2014;40(Suppl 2):S131–7.

64. Baldassarre A, Lewis CM, Committeri G, et al. Individual variability in functional connectivity predicts performance of a perceptual task. Proc Natl Acad Sci U S A 2012;109(9):3516–21.

65. Zou Q, Ross TJ, Gu H, et al. Intrinsic resting-state activity predicts working memory brain activation and behavioral performance. Hum Brain Mapp 2013;34(12):3204–15.

66. Krajcovicova L, Marecek R, Mikl M, et al. Disruption of resting functional connectivity in Alzheimer's patients and at-risk subjects. Curr Neurol Neurosc Rep 2014;14(10):491.

67. Simic G, Babic M, Borovecki F, et al. Early failure of the default-mode network and the pathogenesis of Alzheimer's disease. CNS Neurosci Ther 2014 20(7):692–8.

68. Hafkemeijer A, van der Grond J, Rombouts SA. Imaging the default mode network in aging and dementia. Biochim Biophys Acta 2012;1822(3): 431–41.

69. Damoiseaux JS, Beckmann CF, Arigita EJ, et al. Reduced resting-state brain activity in the "default network" in normal aging. Cereb Cortex 2008, 18(8):1856–64.

70. Jones DT, Machulda MM, Vemuri P, et al. Age-related changes in the default mode network are more advanced in Alzheimer disease. Neurology 2011;77(16):1524–31.

71. Agosta F, Pievani M, Geroldi C, et al. Resting state fMRI in Alzheimer's disease: beyond the default mode network. Neurobiol Aging 2012;33(8): 1564–78.

72. He Y, Wang L, Zang Y, et al. Regional coherence changes in the early stages of Alzheimer's disease

a combined structural and resting-state functional MRI study. Neuroimage 2007;35(2):488–500.

73. Zhang HY, Wang SJ, Liu B, et al. Resting brain connectivity: changes during the progress of Alzheimer disease. Radiology 2010;256(2):598–606.

74. Saint-Aubert L, Barbeau EJ, Peran P, et al. Cortical florbetapir-PET amyloid load in prodromal Alzheimer's disease patients. EJNMMI Res 2013; 3(1):43.

75. Drzezga A, Becker JA, Van Dijk KR, et al. Neuronal dysfunction and disconnection of cortical hubs in non-demented subjects with elevated amyloid burden. Brain 2011;134(Pt 6):1635–46.

76. Myers N, Pasquini L, Gottler J, et al. Within-patient correspondence of amyloid-beta and intrinsic network connectivity in Alzheimer's disease. Brain 2014;137(Pt 7):2052–64.

77. Reiman EM, Quiroz YT, Fleisher AS, et al. Brain imaging and fluid biomarker analysis in young adults at genetic risk for autosomal dominant Alzheimer's disease in the presenilin 1 E280A kindred: a case-control study. Lancet Neurol 2012;11(12):1048–56.

78. Sheline YI, Raichle ME. Resting state functional connectivity in preclinical Alzheimer's disease. Biol Psychiatry 2013;74(5):340–7.

79. Buckner RL, Sepulcre J, Talukdar T, et al. Cortical hubs revealed by intrinsic functional connectivity: mapping, assessment of stability, and relation to Alzheimer's disease. J Neurosci 2009;29(6): 1860–73.

80. Sheline YI, Raichle ME, Snyder AZ, et al. Amyloid plaques disrupt resting state default mode network connectivity in cognitively normal elderly. Biol Psychiatry 2010;67(6):584–7.

81. Mormino EC, Smiljic A, Hayenga AO, et al. Relationships between beta-amyloid and functional connectivity in different components of the default mode network in aging. Cereb Cortex 2011; 21(10):2399–407.

82. Pan P, Zhu L, Yu T, et al. Aberrant spontaneous low-frequency brain activity in amnestic mild cognitive impairment: a meta-analysis of resting-state fMRI studies. Ageing Res Rev 2016;35:12–21.

83. Li HJ, Hou XH, Liu HH, et al. Toward systems neuroscience in mild cognitive impairment and Alzheimer's disease: a meta-analysis of 75 fMRI studies. Hum Brain Mapp 2015;36(3):1217–32.

84. Joo SH, Lim HK, Lee CU. Three large-scale functional brain networks from resting-state functional MRI in subjects with different levels of cognitive impairment. Psychiatry Investig 2016;13(1):1–7.

85. Teipel S, Grothe MJ, Zhou J, et al. Measuring cortical connectivity in Alzheimer's disease as a brain neural network pathology: toward clinical applications. J Int Neuropsychol Soc 2016;22(2): 138–63.

86. Patel KT, Stevens MC, Pearlson GD, et al. Default mode network activity and white matter integrity in healthy middle-aged ApoE4 carriers. Brain Imaging Behav 2013;7(1):60–7.

87. He Y, Chen Z, Gong G, et al. Neuronal networks in Alzheimer's disease. Neuroscientist 2009;15(4): 333–50.

88. Supekar K, Menon V, Rubin D, et al. Network analysis of intrinsic functional brain connectivity in Alzheimer's disease. PLoS Comput Biol 2008;4(6): e1000100.

89. Wang K, Liang M, Wang L, et al. Altered functional connectivity in early Alzheimer's disease: a resting-state fMRI study. Hum Brain Mapp 2007;28(10): 967–78.

90. Wang J, Wang X, He Y, et al. Apolipoprotein E epsilon4 modulates functional brain connectome in Alzheimer's disease. Hum Brain Mapp 2015; 36(5):1828–46.

91. Dennis EL, Thompson PM. Functional brain connectivity using fMRI in aging and Alzheimer's disease. Neuropsychol Rev 2014;24(1):49–62.

92. Goveas JS, Xie C, Ward BD, et al. Recovery of hippocampal network connectivity correlates with cognitive improvement in mild Alzheimer's disease patients treated with donepezil assessed by resting-state fMRI. J Magn Reson Imaging 2011; 34(4):764–73.

93. Li W, Antuono PG, Xie C, et al. Changes in regional cerebral blood flow and functional connectivity in the cholinergic pathway associated with cognitive performance in subjects with mild Alzheimer's disease after 12-week donepezil treatment. Neuroimage 2012;60(2):1083–91.

94. Sohn WS, Yoo K, Na DL, et al. Progressive changes in hippocampal resting-state connectivity across cognitive impairment: a cross-sectional study from normal to Alzheimer disease. Alzheimer Dis Assoc Disord 2014;28(3):239–46.

95. Jacobs HI, Radua J, Luckmann HC, et al. Meta-analysis of functional network alterations in Alzheimer's disease: toward a network biomarker. Neurosci Biobehav Rev 2013;37(5):753–65.

96. Koch W, Teipel S, Mueller S, et al. Diagnostic power of default mode network resting state fMRI in the detection of Alzheimer's disease. Neurobiol Aging 2012;33(3):466–78.

97. Dai Z, Yan C, Wang Z, et al. Discriminative analysis of early Alzheimer's disease using multi-modal imaging and multi-level characterization with multi-classifier (M3). Neuroimage 2012;59(3):2187–95.

98. Serra L, Cercignani M, Mastropasqua C, et al. Longitudinal changes in functional brain connectivity predicts conversion to Alzheimer's disease. J Alzheimers Dis 2016;51(2):377–89.

99. Bai F, Watson DR, Shi Y, et al. Specifically progressive deficits of brain functional marker in amnestic

type mild cognitive impairment. PLoS One 2011; 6(9):e24271.

100. van Eimeren T, Monchi O, Ballanger B, et al. Dysfunction of the default mode network in Parkinson disease: a functional magnetic resonance imaging study. Arch Neurol 2009;66(7):877–83.

101. Tahmasian M, Bettray LM, van Eimeren T, et al. A systematic review on the applications of resting-state fMRI in Parkinson's disease: does dopamine replacement therapy play a role? Cortex 2015;73:80–105.

102. Muller-Oehring EM, Sullivan EV, Pfefferbaum A, et al. Task-rest modulation of basal ganglia connectivity in mild to moderate Parkinson's disease. Brain Imaging Behav 2015;9(3):619–38.

103. Kwak Y, Peltier S, Bohnen NI, et al. Altered resting state cortico-striatal connectivity in mild to moderate stage Parkinson's disease. Front Syst Neurosci 2010;4:143.

104. Putcha D, Ross RS, Cronin-Golomb A, et al. Altered intrinsic functional coupling between core neurocognitive networks in Parkinson's disease. Neuroimage Clin 2015;7:449–55.

105. Tessitore A, Esposito F, Vitale C, et al. Default-mode network connectivity in cognitively unimpaired patients with Parkinson disease. Neurology 2012;79(23):2226–32.

106. Disbrow EA, Carmichael O, He J, et al. Resting state functional connectivity is associated with cognitive dysfunction in non-demented people with Parkinson's disease. J Parkinsons Dis 2014; 4(3):453–65.

107. Rektorova I. Resting-state networks in Alzheimer's disease and Parkinson's disease. Neurodegener Dis 2014;13(2–3):186–8.

108. Franciotti R, Delli Pizzi S, Perfetti B, et al. Default mode network links to visual hallucinations: a comparison between Parkinson's disease and multiple system atrophy. Mov Disord 2015;30(9):1237–47.

109. Yao N, Shek-Kwan Chang R, Cheung C, et al. The default mode network is disrupted in Parkinson's disease with visual hallucinations. Hum Brain Mapp 2014;35(11):5658–66.

110. Krajcovicova L, Mikl M, Marecek R, et al. The default mode network integrity in patients with Parkinson's disease is levodopa equivalent dose-dependent. J Neural Transm (Vienna) 2012; 119(4):443–54.

111. Delaveau P, Salgado-Pineda P, Fossati P, et al. Dopaminergic modulation of the default mode network in Parkinson's disease. Eur Neuropsychopharmacol 2010;20(11):784–92.

112. Boly M, Tshibanda L, Vanhaudenhuyse A, et al. Functional connectivity in the default network during resting state is preserved in a vegetative but not in a brain dead patient. Hum Brain Mapp 2009;30(8):2393–400.

113. Vanhaudenhuyse A, Noirhomme Q, Tshibanda LJ et al. Default network connectivity reflects the level of consciousness in non-communicative brain-damaged patients. Brain 2010;133(Pt 1):161–71.

114. Satterthwaite TD, Baker JT. How can studies of resting-state functional connectivity help us understand psychosis as a disorder of brain development? Curr Opin Neurobiol 2015;30:85–91.

115. Garrity AG, Pearlson GD, McKiernan K, et al. Aberrant "default mode" functional connectivity in schizophrenia. Am J Psychiatry 2007;164(3) 450–7.

116. Whitfield-Gabrieli S, Thermenos HW, Milanovic S, et al. Hyperactivity and hyperconnectivity of the default network in schizophrenia and in first-degree relatives of persons with schizophrenia Proc Natl Acad Sci U S A 2009;106(4):1279–84.

117. Narr KL, Leaver AM. Connectome and schizophrenia. Curr Opin Psychiatry 2015;28(3):229–35.

118. Chung Y, Cannon TD. Brain imaging during the transition from psychosis prodrome to schizophrenia. J Nerv Ment Dis 2015;203(5):336–41.

119. Rashid B, Damaraju E, Pearlson GD, et al. Dynamic connectivity states estimated from resting fMR Identify differences among Schizophrenia, bipolar disorder, and healthy control subjects. Front Hum Neurosci 2014;8:897.

120. Du Y, Pearlson GD, Yu Q, et al. Interaction among subsystems within default mode network diminished in schizophrenia patients: a dynamic connectivity approach. Schizophr Res 2016;170(1) 55–65.

121. Du Y, Pearlson GD, Liu J, et al. A group ICA based framework for evaluating resting fMRI markers when disease categories are unclear: application to schizophrenia, bipolar, and schizoaffective disorders. Neuroimage 2015;122:272–80.

122. Meda SA, Wang Z, Ivleva EI, et al. Frequency-specific neural signatures of spontaneous low frequency resting state fluctuations in psychosis evidence from bipolar-schizophrenia network on intermediate phenotypes (B-SNIP) consortium Schizophr Bull 2015;41(6):1336–48.

123. Pearlson GD, Ford JM. Distinguishing between schizophrenia and other psychotic disorders Schizophr Bull 2014;40(3):501–3.

124. Meda SA, Gill A, Stevens MC, et al. Differences in resting-state functional magnetic resonance imaging functional network connectivity between schizophrenia and psychotic bipolar probands and their unaffected first-degree relatives. Biol Psychiatry 2012;71(10):881–9.

125. Khadka S, Meda SA, Stevens MC, et al. Is aberrant functional connectivity a psychosis endophenotype? A resting state functional magnetic resonance imaging study. Biol Psychiatry 2013;74(6) 458–66.

126. Lui S, Yao L, Xiao Y, et al. Resting-state brain function in schizophrenia and psychotic bipolar probands and their first-degree relatives. Psychol Med 2015;45(1):97–108.

127. Anticevic A, Savic A, Repovs G, et al. Ventral anterior cingulate connectivity distinguished nonpsychotic bipolar illness from psychotic bipolar disorder and schizophrenia. Schizophr Bull 2015; 41(1):133–43.

128. Sheffield JM, Barch DM. Cognition and resting-state functional connectivity in schizophrenia. Neurosci Biobehav Rev 2015;61:108–20.

129. Meda SA, Ruano G, Windemuth A, et al. Multivariate analysis reveals genetic associations of the resting default mode network in psychotic bipolar disorder and schizophrenia. Proc Natl Acad Sci U S A 2014;111(19):E2066–75.

130. Klumpers LE, Cole DM, Khalili-Mahani N, et al. Manipulating brain connectivity with delta(9)-tetrahydrocannabinol: a pharmacological resting state FMRI study. Neuroimage 2012;63(3):1701–11.

131. Niesters M, Khalili-Mahani N, Martini C, et al. Effect of subanesthetic ketamine on intrinsic functional brain connectivity: a placebo-controlled functional magnetic resonance imaging study in healthy male volunteers. Anesthesiology 2012; 117(4):868–77.

132. Rack-Gomer AL, Liu TT. Caffeine increases the temporal variability of resting-state BOLD connectivity in the motor cortex. Neuroimage 2012;59(3): 2994–3002.

133. Tal O, Diwakar M, Wong CW, et al. Caffeine-induced global reductions in resting-state BOLD connectivity reflect widespread decreases in MEG connectivity. Front Hum Neurosci 2013;7:63.

134. Khalili-Mahani N, Zoethout RM, Beckmann CF, et al. Effects of morphine and alcohol on functional brain connectivity during "resting state": a placebo-controlled crossover study in healthy young men. Hum Brain Mapp 2012;33(5):1003–18.

135. Tanabe J, Nyberg E, Martin LF, et al. Nicotine effects on default mode network during resting state. Psychopharmacology (Berl) 2011;216(2):287–95.

136. Fedota JR, Stein EA. Resting-state functional connectivity and nicotine addiction: prospects for biomarker development. Ann N Y Acad Sci 2015; 1349:64–82.

137. Qiu YW, Han LJ, Lv XF, et al. Regional homogeneity changes in heroin-dependent individuals: resting-state functional MR imaging study. Radiology 2011;261(2):551–9.

138. Kelly C, Zuo XN, Gotimer K, et al. Reduced interhemispheric resting state functional connectivity in cocaine addiction. Biol Psychiatry 2011;69(7): 684–92.

139. Konova AB, Moeller SJ, Tomasi D, et al. Effects of methylphenidate on resting-state functional connectivity of the mesocorticolimbic dopamine pathways in cocaine addiction. JAMA Psychiatry 2013;70(8):857–68.

140. Cole DM, Beckmann CF, Long CJ, et al. Nicotine replacement in abstinent smokers improves cognitive withdrawal symptoms with modulation of resting brain network dynamics. Neuroimage 2010;52(2):590–9.

141. Weiland BJ, Sabbineni A, Calhoun VD, et al. Reduced executive and default network functional connectivity in cigarette smokers. Hum Brain Mapp 2015;36(3):872–82.

142. Hong LE, Gu H, Yang Y, et al. Association of nicotine addiction and nicotine's actions with separate cingulate cortex functional circuits. Arch Gen Psychiatry 2009;66(4):431–41.

UNITED STATES POSTAL SERVICE ®

Statement of Ownership, Management, and Circulation
(All Periodicals Publications Except Requester Publications)

1 Publication Title	2 Publication Number		3 Filing Date
NEUROIMAGING CLINICS OF NORTH AMERICA	010 – 548		9/18/2017

4 Issue Frequency	5 Number of Issues Published Annually	6 Annual Subscription Price
FEB, MAY, AUG, NOV	4	$365.00

7 Complete Mailing Address of Known Office of Publication (Not printer) (Street, city, county, state, and ZIP+4®)

ELSEVIER INC.
230 Park Avenue, Suite 800
New York, NY 10169

Contact Person
STEPHEN R. BUSHING

Telephone (include area code)
215-239-3688

8 Complete Mailing Address of Headquarters or General Business Office of Publisher (Not printer)

ELSEVIER INC.
230 Park Avenue, Suite 800
New York, NY 10169

9 Full Names and Complete Mailing Addresses of Publisher, Editor, and Managing Editor (Do not leave blank)

Publisher (Name and complete mailing address)

ADRIANNE BRIGIDO, ELSEVIER INC.
1600 JOHN F KENNEDY BLVD. SUITE 1800
PHILADELPHIA, PA 19103-2899

Editor (Name and complete mailing address)

JOHN VASSALLO, ELSEVIER INC.
1600 JOHN F KENNEDY BLVD. SUITE 1800
PHILADELPHIA, PA 19103-2899

Managing Editor (Name and complete mailing address)

PATRICK MANLEY ELSEVIER INC.
1600 JOHN F KENNEDY BLVD. SUITE 1800
PHILADELPHIA, PA 19103-2899

10 Owner (Do not leave blank. If the publication is owned by a corporation, give the name and address of the corporation immediately followed by the names and addresses of all stockholders owning or holding 1 percent or more of the total amount of stock. If not owned by a corporation, give the names and addresses of the individual owners. If owned by a partnership or other unincorporated firm, give its name and address as well as those of each individual owner. If the publication is published by a nonprofit organization, give its name and address.)

Full Name	Complete Mailing Address
WHOLLY OWNED SUBSIDIARY OF REED/ELSEVIER, US HOLDINGS	1600 JOHN F KENNEDY BLVD. SUITE 1800 PHILADELPHIA, PA 19103-2899

11 Known Bondholders, Mortgagees, and Other Security Holders Owning or Holding 1 Percent or More of Total Amount of Bonds, Mortgages, or Other Securities. If none, check box. ☐ None

Full Name	Complete Mailing Address
N/A	

12 Tax Status (For completion by nonprofit organizations authorized to mail at nonprofit rates) (Check one)
The purpose, function, and nonprofit status of this organization and the exempt status for federal income tax purposes:
☒ Has Not Changed During Preceding 12 Months
☐ Has Changed During Preceding 12 Months (Publisher must submit explanation of change with this statement)

13 Publication Title	14 Issue Date for Circulation Data Below
NEUROIMAGING CLINICS OF NORTH AMERICA	MAY 2017

PS Form **3526**, July 2014 (Page 1 of 4 (see instructions page 4)) PSN: 7530-01-000-9931   PRIVACY NOTICE: See our privacy policy on www.usps.com

15 Extent and Nature of Circulation

			Average No. Copies Each Issue During Preceding 12 Months	No. Copies of Single Issue Published Nearest to Filing Date
a. Total Number of Copies (Net press run)			620	531
b. Paid Circulation (By Mail and Outside the Mail)	(1)	Mailed Outside-County Paid Subscriptions Stated on PS Form 3541 (include paid distribution above nominal rate, advertiser's proof copies, and exchange copies)	418	384
	(2)	Mailed In-County Paid Subscriptions Stated on PS Form 3541 (include paid distribution above nominal rate, advertiser's proof copies, and exchange copies)	0	0
	(3)	Paid Distribution Outside the Mails Including Sales Through Dealers and Carriers, Street Vendors, Counter Sales, and Other Paid Distribution Outside USPS®	94	87
	(4)	Paid Distribution by Other Classes of Mail Through the USPS (e.g. First-Class Mail®)	0	0
c. Total Paid Distribution (Sum of 15b (1), (2), (3), and (4))	▶		512	471
d. Free or Nominal Rate Distribution (By Mail and Outside the Mail)	(1)	Free or Nominal Rate Outside-County Copies included on PS Form 3541	36	60
	(2)	Free or Nominal Rate In-County Copies Included on PS Form 3541	0	0
	(3)	Free or Nominal Rate Copies Mailed at Other Classes Through the USPS (e.g. First-Class Mail)	0	0
	(4)	Free or Nominal Rate Distribution Outside the Mail (Carriers or other means)	0	0
e. Total Free or Nominal Rate Distribution (Sum of 15d (1), (2), (3) and (4))	▶		36	60
f. Total Distribution (Sum of 15c and 15e)	▶		548	531
g. Copies not Distributed (See instructions to Publishers #4 (page 3))	▶		72	0
h. Total (Sum of 15f and g)	▶		620	531
i. Percent Paid (15c divided by 15f times 100)	▶		93.43%	88.7%

* If you are claiming electronic copies, go to line 16 on page 3. If you are not claiming electronic copies, skip to line 17 on page 3.

16 Electronic Copy Circulation

		Average No. Copies Each Issue During Preceding 12 Months	No. Copies of Single Issue Published Nearest to Filing Date
a. Paid Electronic Copies	▶	0	0
b. Total Paid Print Copies (Line 15c) + Paid Electronic Copies (Line 16a)	▶	512	471
c. Total Print Distribution (Line 15f) + Paid Electronic Copies (Line 16a)	▶	548	531
d. Percent Paid (Both Print & Electronic Copies) (16b divided by 16c × 100)	▶	93.43%	88.7%

☒ I certify that 50% of all my distributed copies (electronic and print) are paid above a nominal price.

17 Publication of Statement of Ownership

☒ If the publication is a general publication, publication of this statement is required. Will be printed in the NOVEMBER 2017 issue of this publication.   ☐ Publication not required.

18 Signature and Title of Editor, Publisher, Business Manager, or Owner

STEPHEN R. BUSHING – INVENTORY DISTRIBUTION CONTROL MANAGER

Date 9/18/2017

I certify that all information furnished on this form is true and complete. I understand that anyone who furnishes false or misleading information on this form or who omits material or information requested on the form may be subject to criminal sanctions (including fines and imprisonment) and/or civil sanctions (including civil penalties).

PS Form **3526**, July 2014 (Page 3 of 4)   PRIVACY NOTICE: See our privacy policy on www.usps.com

Printed and bound by CPI Group (UK) Ltd, Croydon, CR0 4YY

03/10/2024

01040384-0012